PREDICTING HE
BEHAVIOUR
RESEARCH AND PRACTICE WITH
SOCIAL COGNITION MODELS

Edited by
**Mark Conner and
Paul Norman**

Open University Press
Buckingham · Philadelphia

Kinder Scout

Open University Press
Celtic Court
22 Ballmoor
Buckingham
MK18 1XW

and 1900 Frost Road, Suite 101
Bristol, PA 19007, USA

First published 1996

A catalogue record of this book is available from the British Library

ISBN 0 335 19320 X (pb)   0 335 19321 8 (hb)

Library of Congress Cataloging-in-Publication Data

Predicting health behaviour: research and practice with social
  cognition models / [edited] by Mark Conner & Paul Norman.
     p. cm.
  Includes bibliographical references and index.
  ISBN 0–335–19320–X (pb)   ISBN 0–335–19321–8 (hb)
  1. Health behavior. 2. Social perception. 3. Health attitudes.
I. Conner, Mark. 1962– .   II. Norman. Paul, 1962– .
RA776.9.P72 1995
613'.01'9—dc20   95–14732
                                                            CIP

Typeset by Graphicraft Typesetters Limited, Hong Kong
Printed in Great Britain by St Edmundsbury Press,
Bury St Edmunds, Suffolk

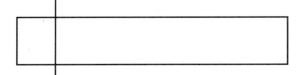

CONTENTS

LIST OF CONTRIBUTORS

Dr Charles Abraham is Senior Lecturer in Psychology at the School of Social Sciences, University of Sussex, England. His research interests involve the application of social cognition models to health behaviours, especially the prediction of young people's safer sexual practices. He has also written on the philosophical and psychological underpinnings of verbal reports in health and social psychological research.

Dr Paul Bennett is a Consultant Clinical Psychologist with Gwent Psychology Services and a Honorary Lecturer at the Department of Psychology, University of Wales, Swansea, Wales. His research interests include the impact of and coping with chronic illness, the social psychological determinants of health and health promotion.

Dr Henk Boer is Associate-Professor of Applied Social Psychology at the Department of Psychology, University of Twente, The Netherlands. His current research interests are in the field of communication and health-related behavioural change, with an emphasis on the psychosocial aspects of breast cancer and breast cancer screening.

Dr Mark Conner is Lecturer in Social Psychology at the Department of Psychology, University of Leeds, England. His research interests are in attitude theory and social cognitive determinants of health behaviours, with a particular interest in food choice.

Dr Reinhard Fuchs is Scientific Assistant and Lecturer at the Institut für Psychologie, Freie Universität Berlin, Germany. His major research interests concern the cognitive determinants of health behaviours (physical exercise, dietary behaviour and smoking) as well as the impact of these health behaviours on mental and physical health (in particular health-protective effects of physical exercise under stressful conditions).

Dr Paul Norman is Lecturer in Applied Social Psychology at the Department of Psychology, University of Wales, Swansea, Wales. His research interests are in social cognition and health behaviour, with particular interests in health promotion in general practice. From January 1996 he will be at the Department of Psychology, University of Sheffield, England.

Professor Ralf Schwarzer is Professor of Psychology at the Institut für Psychologie (WE 7), Freie Universität Berlin, Germany. He specializes in health psychology, including research on stress and social support. He is editor of *Anxiety, Stress, and Coping: an International Journal.* He is also Vice-President of the European Health Psychology Society (EHPS).

Professor Erwin R. Seydel is Professor of Applied Social Psychology at the Department of Psychology, University of Twente, The Netherlands. His current research interests are in the field of communication and health-related behavioural change, with an emphasis on psychosocial oncology and communication management.

Paschal Sheeran is Lecturer in Social Psychology at the Department of Psychology, University of Sheffield, England. His research interests are in the self-regulation of behaviour which has involved applying social cognitive theories to young people's HIV-preventive behaviour. He is also interested in the social psychology of identity and, in particular, the impact of social structural position upon self-conception.

Dr Paul Sparks is a Senior Research Scientist at the Department of Consumer Sciences, Institute of Food Research, Reading Laboratory, England. His research interests include attitude theory, the social and moral dimensions of food choice and the processes of social influence.

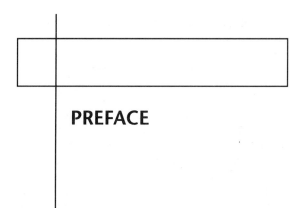

PREFACE

The study of behaviours that influence health and the factors determining which individuals will and will not perform such behaviours has become increasingly common in health psychology. The purpose of this book is to provide in a single source current research and practical details of how to apply five of the most widely used social cognition models to the prediction of the performance of health behaviours. Social cognition models start from the assumption that an individual's behaviour is best understood in terms of his or her perceptions of the social environment. Such an approach has been widely and successfully used by psychologists to understand a range of human behaviours and, in particular, health behaviours.

Much of the information in the book is not new. However, it is currently to be found in such a diverse range of publications, across a number of disciplines, as to make its access and application difficult. The bringing together of this information into a single volume is intended to make these approaches more accessible and, it is hoped, more widely and appropriately used. Moreover, by bringing together these models, similarities and differences between approaches can be examined and the whole approach critically evaluated. Both the relevant theoretical background and practical examples of how to apply each social cognition model are provided. As the five 'model' chapters focus on a number of different health behaviours, the book also contains considerable detail on a range of health behaviours and the particular problems of using the social cognition approach.

The introductory chapter was prepared by the editors, and examines the concept of health behaviour and briefly reviews epidemiological work looking at the variation in who performs such behaviours. It also outlines the general social cognitive approach taken to the understanding and prediction of health behaviour. This is followed by a review of the principal features of the social cognition models described in subsequent chapters. Finally, some advantages and disadvantages of this approach for the understanding of health behaviours are then outlined.

Following this introductory chapter are five individual chapters describing the most widely used social cognition models. Each chapter has been produced by prominent researchers in the area and follows a common structure. The first section of the 'model' chapters outlines the background to and the origins of the model. This is followed by a description of the model, including full details of each of its components, in the second section. The third section examines recent developments and expansions to the model. The fourth section contains a summary of research using this approach and examines a range of health behaviours. Sections 5 and 6 are intended to provide a clear demonstration of how the model might be applied. First, a detailed consideration of the procedures for developing appropriate measures for each of the components of the model is presented; and then an actual application of the model to a specific health behaviour is described and specific problems are considered. The final section looks at potential future directions for research with the model.

Chapter 2, by Sheeran and Abraham, looks at probably the most widely used of these models, the health belief model. Chapter 3, by Norman and Bennett, looks at the health locus of control concept. Protection motivation theory is described by Boer and Seydel in Chapter 4. These three models have all been developed specifically to predict the performance of health behaviours. Conner and Sparks describe a model derived from social psychology in Chapter 5, the theory of planned behaviour. In Chapter 6, Schwarzer and Fuchs look at models based around the concept of self-efficacy, a concept originating from Bandura's work on social learning.

In following a common structure, the chapters provide a clear introduction to the background, operationalization, current findings and developments within each model. Each chapter provides a general review of the research, applying that model to a variety of health behaviours and discussing the particular problems with applying the model. Each chapter also provides an extended example of the application of the model to a health behaviour and discusses the particular problems with applying the model.

In the final chapter of the book, the editors provide a critique of this general approach and outline a number of future directions for research in this area. In particular they focus on the need to develop models containing different stages in the adoption and maintenance of a new health behaviour. Each stage is seen to be qualitatively different in terms of which social cognitive variables are important in influencing behaviour. In addition, they highlight recent work that has examined non-deliberative, or automatic, influences on behaviour.

The book is not intended to be a 'cookbook' on how to apply social cognition models. Rather it is intended to introduce readers to the general social cognitive approach to the understanding of such behaviours, to describe the most commonly used social cognition models, their differences and similarities, and their advantages and disadvantages, and to enable researchers to apply each model appropriately to their own area of interest, and adequately to analyse and report the results. Potential directions for future research within this paradigm are described both in the model chapters and in the final chapter of the book.

The common format of the 'model' chapters is intended to help readers to access specific aspects of each approach and to aid comparisons. Such comparisons are also drawn out in the final chapter. This 'common' coverage will allow readers more easily to use the book as a 'user manual', while allowing the distinct features of each model to be clear and its applications to a specific set of health behaviours to be examined. The book should allow readers to see the advantages and disadvantages of each model and allow one to apply each model appropriately to the health behaviour of interest.

We should like to thank the authors of the chapters for all their hard work in producing such clear descriptions of these models and such extensive reviews of the relevant literature. We would also like to thank Open University Press for its help and encouragement during the preparation of this book.

Mark Conner and Paul Norman

LIST OF ABBREVIATIONS

A_B	attitude towards behaviour
AIDS	acquired immune deficiency syndrome
BI	behavioural intention
CID	Crevelling's identification
ELM	elaboration likelihood model
HAPA	health action process approach
HBM	health belief model
HIV	human immunodeficiency virus
HLC	health locus of control
HSM	heuristic-systematic model
IUD	intra-uterine device
MHLC	multidimensional health locus of control
PAP	precaution-adoption process
PBC	perceived behavioural control
PMT	protection motivation theory
SCM	social cognition model
SCT	social cognitive theory
SES	socioeconomic status
SET	self-efficacy theory
SEU	subjective expected utility
SN	subjective norm
SRT	self-regulation theory
TMC	transtheoretical model of change
TPB	theory of planned behaviour
TRA	theory of reasoned action

1   MARK CONNER AND
PAUL NORMAN

THE ROLE OF SOCIAL COGNITION IN HEALTH BEHAVIOURS

1 Introduction

The study of health behaviours is based upon two assumptions; that in industrialized countries a substantial proportion of the mortality from the leading causes of death is due to particular behaviour patterns, and that these behaviour patterns are modifiable (Stroebe and Stroebe 1995). It is increasingly recognized that individuals can make major contributions to their own health and well-being through the adoption of particular health-enhancing behaviours (e.g. exercise) and the avoidance of other health-compromising behaviours (e.g. smoking). The identification of the factors that underlie such 'health behaviours' has become the focus of a great deal of research in psychology and other health-related disciplines in recent years (e.g. Winett 1985; Rodin and Salovey 1989; Glanz et al. 1990; McQueen 1991; Hockbaum and Lorig 1992; McLeroy et al. 1993; Adler and Matthews 1994). This research has been motivated by two main factors: first, a desire to design interventions to change the prevalence of such behaviours and so produce improvements in individuals' and populations' health; second, a desire to gain a more general understanding of the reasons why individuals perform a variety of behaviours.

The health behaviours focused upon have been extremely varied, running from health-enhancing behaviours such as exercise participation and healthy eating, through health protective behaviours such as health screening clinic attendance, vaccination against disease and condom use in response to the threat of AIDS, to avoidance of health-harming behaviours such as smoking and excessive alcohol consumption, and sick-role behaviours such as compliance with medical regimens. A unifying theme across these behaviours has been that they have immediate or long-term effects upon the individual's health and are at least partially within the individual's control. Epidemiological studies have revealed considerable variation in who performs these behaviours. The approaches taken to understanding the factors underlying this variation have been many and varied. A broad distinction can be made between factors intrinsic to the individual (e.g. sociodemographic factors, personality, social support, cognitions) and factors extrinsic to the individual, which can be further divided into incentive structures (e.g. taxing tobacco and alcohol, subsidizing sporting facilities) and legal restrictions (e.g. banning dangerous substances, fining individuals for not wearing seat-belts). The first of these factors has received most attention from psychologists, and within these intrinsic factors, cognitive factors have been focused upon as the most important proximal determinants. Models of how such cognitive factors produce various 'social' behaviours are commonly referred to as social cognition models (SCMs) and have been widely used by psychologists. They are generally recognized to have provided a valuable contribution to the greater understanding of who performs health behaviours (Marteau 1989) and how extrinsic factors may produce behaviour change (e.g. Rutter *et al.* 1993). The justification for the focus on social cognitive determinants in SCMs is two-fold. First, these determinants are assumed to be important causes of behaviour which mediate the effects of many other determinants (e.g. social class). Second, these social cognitive factors are assumed to be more open to change than other factors (e.g. personality). Together these justifications imply that effective interventions should be based upon manipulations of those cognitive variables shown to be determinants of health behaviours. An outline of the importance of health behaviours in health outcomes and the role of SCMs in understanding the determinants of health behaviours provides the focus of this chapter.

2 Understanding health behaviours

Health behaviours have been defined as 'Any activity undertaken by a person believing himself to be healthy for the purpose of preventing disease or detecting it at an asymptomatic stage' (Kasl and Cobb 1966: 246). There are several limitations to this conception, including the omission of lay or self-defined health behaviours and the exclusion of activities carried out by people with recognized illnesses that are directed at self-management, delaying disease progression or improving general well-being. However, it demonstrates the limits to the range of behaviours considered to fall under this heading. The behaviours studied include a variety of behaviours such as medical service usage (e.g. physician visits, vaccination, screening), compliance with medical regimens (e.g. dietary, diabetic, anti-hypertensive regimens) and self-directed health behaviours (e.g. diet, exercise, breast or testicular self-examination, brushing and flossing teeth, smoking, alcohol consumption, contraceptive use). In this section we look briefly at the role of such behaviours in health outcomes, and the range of factors predictive of the performance of such behaviours.

2.1 The role of health behaviours in health outcomes

A number of studies have looked at the relationship between the perform-ance of a range of health behaviours and a variety of health outcomes (e.g. Doll and Peto 1976; Gottlieb and Green 1984; Cox *et al.* 1987; Black *et al.* 1988; Whitehead 1988; Blane *et al.* 1990; Blaxter 1990; Marmot *et al.* 1991; Cox *et al.* 1993). Such studies have demonstrated the importance of a variety of behaviours for both morbidity and mortality. For example, studies in Alameda County identified seven features of lifestyle – not smok-ing, moderate alcohol intake, sleeping seven to eight hours per night, exercising regularly, maintaining a desirable body weight, avoiding snacks and eating breakfast regularly – which together were associated with lower morbidity and higher subsequent long-term survival (Belloc and Breslow 1972; Belloc 1973; Breslow and Enstrom 1980). Such results have been replicated in a number of samples (e.g. Metzner *et al.* 1983; Brock *et al.* 1988).

In addition, research into the major causes of premature death in the Western world (e.g. cardiovascular diseases and cancer) has emphasized the importance for prevention of behaviours such as smoking, alcohol consumption, dietary choice, sexual behaviours and physical exercise (e.g. Goldman and Cook 1984; Smith and Jacobson 1988). Studies of prema-ture deaths attributable to lifestyle factors also confirm smoking, alcohol consumption, exercise and diet as major precursors together with gaps in primary prevention and screening uptake (Amler and Eddins 1987). Fin-ally, the impact of such health behaviours upon individuals' quality of life should be noted. As several authors have pointed out (e.g. Fries *et al.* 1989; Stroebe and Stroebe 1995), the above research evidence also generally supports the role of health behaviours in producing a positive impact on quality of life via delaying the onset of chronic disease and extending active lifespan.

2.2 Predicting the performance of health behaviours

Can we predict and understand who performs health behaviours? This would enable us to make a contribution to the understanding of the vari-ation in the distribution of health across society. It might also indicate targets for interventions designed to change health behaviours. As one might expect, a variety of factors account for individual differences in the propensity to undertake health behaviours, including demographic factors, social factors, emotional factors, perceived symptoms, factors relating to access to medical care, personality factors and cognitive factors (Rosenstock 1974; Taylor 1991; Adler and Matthews 1994).

Demographic variables show reliable associations with the perform-ance of health behaviours. For example, age appears to show a curvilinear relationship with many health behaviours, with high incidences of many health-risking behaviours such as smoking in young adults and much lower incidences in children and older adults (Blaxter 1990). Health behaviour also varies by gender, with females being generally less likely to smoke, consume large amounts of alcohol and engage in regular exercise, but more likely to monitor their diet, take vitamins and engage in dental care (Waldron 1988). Differences by socioeconomic status and ethnic status are also apparent for behaviours such as diet, exercise, alcohol consumption and smoking (e.g. Blaxter 1990). Generally, younger, wealthier, better educated individuals under low levels of stress with high levels of social support are more likely to practise health-enhancing behaviours. Higher levels of stress and/or fewer resources are associated with health-compromising behaviours such as smoking and alcohol abuse (Taylor 1991; Adler and Matthews 1994).

Social factors, such as parental models, seem to be important in instilling health behaviours early in life. Peer influences are also important, for example in the initiation of smoking (e.g. McNeil *et al.* 1988). Values of a culture also appear to be influential, for instance in determining the number of women exercising in a particular culture (e.g. Wardle and Steptoe 1991). Emotional factors play an important role in the practice of some health habits. For example, over-eating is linked to stress in some obese people. Self-esteem also appears to be an important influence in the practice of health behaviours by some. Perceived symptoms will control health habits when, for example, a smoker regulates his or her smoking on the basis of sensations in the throat. Accessibility of medical care services has been found to influence the use of such health services (e.g. Whitehead, 1988). Personality factors have been either positively (e.g. optimism) or negatively (e.g. negative affectivity) associated with the practice of health behaviours (Adler and Matthews 1994; Steptoe *et al.* 1994).

Finally, cognitive factors also determine whether or not an individual practises health behaviours. For example, knowledge about behaviour–health links (or risk awareness) is an essential factor in an informed choice concerning a healthy lifestyle. The reduction of smoking over the past 20 years in the Western world can be largely attributed to a growing awareness of the serious health risks posed by tobacco use brought about by widespread publicity. However, the fact that tobacco continues to be widely used among lower socioeconomic status groups, and the growing uptake of smoking among adolescent girls in some countries, illustrate the fact that knowledge of health risks is not a sufficient condition for avoidance of smoking. Similarly, few adults in the UK can be unaware that sweets promote dental caries, or that high fat consumption can increase the risk of heart disease; nevertheless, sugar and fat consumption in the UK over the past decade have scarcely shown any change (Department of Health 1992). A variety of other cognitive variables have been studied. These factors include perceptions of health risk, potential efficacy of behaviours in influencing this risk, perceived social pressures to perform the behaviour and control over performance of the behaviour. For instance, the belief that a particular health behaviour is beneficial and can help stave off a particular illness may contribute to the practice of the behaviour.

The relative importance of differing individual cognitive factors in the performance of various health behaviours has been the focus of numerous studies and the basis of a number of alternative models. Large numbers of different variables have been studied (for reviews see Cummings *et al.* 1980; Becker and Maiman 1983; Mullen *et al.* 1987; Weinstein 1993). For example, Cummings *et al.* (1980) had experts sort 109 variables derived from 14 different health behaviour models. On the basis of non-metric multidimensional scaling six distinct factors were derived:

1 Accessibility of health care services.
2 Attitudes to health care (beliefs about quality and benefits of treatment).
3 Perceptions of disease threat.
4 Knowledge about disease.
5 Social network characteristics.
6 Demographic factors.

Factors 2 to 5 represent social cognitive factors (beliefs, attitudes, knowledge). Such factors have been central to a number of models of the determinants of health behaviours for several reasons. These factors are enduring characteristics of the individual which shape behaviour and are acquired through socialization processes. They differentiate between individuals from the same background in terms of their propensity to perform health behaviours. They are also open to change and hence represent one route to influencing the performance of health behaviours. Cognitive factors have thus formed a particular area of study in the area of health promotion because they may mediate the effects of many of the other factors discussed earlier and because they are believed to be a good focus in attempting to change health behaviours. These cognitive factors constitute the focus of a small number of widely used models of health behaviours. Such models have been labelled social cognition models because of their use of a number of cognitive variables which are particularly important in one approach to understanding individual social behaviours (the social cognitive approach).

3 Social cognition approaches to health behaviours

Social cognition is concerned with how individuals make sense of social situations. The approach focuses on individual cognitions or thoughts as processes which intervene between observable stimuli and responses in specific real world situations (Fiske and Taylor 1991). Much social psychology over the past quarter century has started from this assumption that social behaviour is best understood as a function of people's perceptions of reality, rather than as a function of an objective description of the stimulus environment. The question of which cognitions are important in predicting behaviour has been the focus of a great deal of research. This 'social cognitive' approach to the person as a thinking organism has become dominant in much of social psychology in recent years (Schneider

1991). Much of the work in social cognition can be broadly split into how people make sense of others (person perception) and themselves (self-regulation) (Fiske and Taylor 1991: 14). The focus here is upon self-regulation processes and in particular how various social cognitive processes relate to behaviour.

Self-regulation processes can be defined as those 'mental and behavioral processes by which people enact their self-conceptions, revise their behavior, or alter the environment so as to bring about outcomes in it in line with their self-perceptions and personal goals' (Fiske and Taylor 1991: 181). As such, self-regulation can be seen as emerging from a clinical tradition in psychology which sees the individual as involved in behaviour change efforts designed to eliminate dysfunctional patterns of thinking or behaviour (Bandura 1982; Turk and Salovey 1986). Models of the cognitive determinants of health behaviour can be seen as part of this tradition. Self-regulation involves the setting of goals, cognitive preparations and the on-going monitoring and evaluation of goal-directed activities. Two phases are commonly distinguished: motivational and volitional (Gollwitzer 1990). The motivational phase involves the deliberation of incentives and expectations in order to choose between goals and implied actions. This stage ends with a decision concerning the goal to be pursued. The second, volitional, phase involves planning and action towards achieving the set goal. To date, most research has been concerned with developing models which explain the role of cognitive variables in the motivational phase. However, recent research has sought to redress this balance by developing models of the role of cognitive variables in volitional processes (e.g. Kuhl 1984; Kuhl and Beckmann 1985, 1994; Weinstein 1988; Heckhausen 1991; Bagozzi 1992, 1993; Gollwitzer 1993), with some applications to health behaviours (e.g. Schwarzer 1992; Norman and Conner, Chapter 7 in this volume).

Social cognition models (SCMs) describing what are the important cognitions and their interrelationships in the regulation of behaviour have been developed and extensively applied to the understanding of health behaviours. Two broad types of SCMs have been applied in health psychology, predominantly to explain health-related behaviours and response to treatment (Conner 1993). The first type can be labelled attribution models. These are concerned with individuals' causal explanations of health-related events (e.g. King 1982). However, most research within this tradition has focused on how people respond to a range of serious illnesses, including cancer (Taylor *et al.* 1984), coronary heart disease (Affleck *et al.* 1987), diabetes (Tennen *et al.* 1984) and end stage renal failure (Witenberg *et al.* 1983), rather than the health-enhancing and compromising behaviours of otherwise healthy individuals.

A second type of SCM examines various aspects of an individual's cognitions in order to predict future health-related behaviours and outcomes. The SCMs commonly used to predict health behaviours include the health belief model (HBM; e.g. Becker 1974; Janz and Becker 1984; Sheeran and Abraham, Chapter 2 in this volume), health locus of control (HLC; e.g. Wallston *et al.* 1978; Seeman and Seeman 1983; Norman and Bennett, Chapter 3 in this volume), protection motivation theory (PMT; e.g. Maddux and Rogers 1983; van der Velde and van der Pligt 1991; Boer and Seydel, Chapter 4 in this volume), theory of reasoned action/theory of planned behaviour (TRA/TPB; e.g. Ajzen and Fishbein 1980; Ajzen 1988, 1991; Conner and Sparks, Chapter 5 in this volume) and self-efficacy theory (SET; e.g. Bandura 1982, 1991; Schwarzer 1992; Schwarzer and Fuchs, Chapter 6 in this volume). Other models include self-regulation theory (SRT; Leventhal *et al.* 1984), the transtheoretical model of change (TMC; Prochaska and DiClemente 1984; Prochaska *et al.* 1992), the precaution-adoption process (PAP; Weinstein 1988) and the theory of trying (Bagozzi 1992). However, none of these latter models has been widely applied to the prediction of health behaviours at present.

These SCMs provide a basis for understanding the determinants of behaviour and behaviour change. They also provide a list of important targets which interventions designed to change behaviour might focus upon if they are to be successful. Each of these models emphasizes the rationality of human behaviour. The health behaviours to be predicted are considered to be the end result of a rational decision-making process based upon deliberative, systematic processing of the available information. Most assume that behaviour and decisions are based upon elaborate, but subjective, cost–benefit analysis of the likely outcomes of differing courses of action. As such they have roots going back to expectancy-value theory (Peak 1955) and subjective expected utility theory (SEU; Edwards 1954). It is assumed that individuals generally aim to maximize utility and so prefer behaviours which are associated with the highest expected utility.

The overall utility or desirability of a behaviour is assumed to be based upon the summed products of the probability (expectancy) and utility (value) of specific, salient outcomes or consequences. This can be represented as:

$$SEU_j = \sum_{i=1}^{i=m} P_{ij} \cdot U_{ij}$$

where SEU_j is the subjective expected utility of behaviour j, P_{ij} is the perceived probability of outcome i of action j, U_{ij} is the subjective utility or value of outcome i of action j, and m is the number of salient outcomes. Each behaviour may have differing subjective expected utilities because of the value of the different outcomes associated with each behaviour and the probability of each behaviour being associated with each outcome. While such a model allows for subjective assessments of both probability and utility, it is assumed that these assessments are combined in a rational, consistent way.

Such judgements underlie many of the widely used SCMs, including the health belief model, health locus of control, protection motivation theory,

theory of reasoned action/planned behaviour and self-efficacy theory (Weinstein 1993; van der Pligt 1994). While such considerations may well provide good predictions of which behaviours are selected, it has been noted by several authors that they do not provide an adequate description of the way in which individuals make decisions (e.g. Feather 1982; Edwards 1992; Jonas 1993; Frisch and Clemen 1994).

4 Overview of commonly used social cognition models

In this section we outline five of the most commonly used SCMs. We describe how each model conceptualizes the social cognitive variables important in determining behaviour and the way in which these variables are combined to predict behaviour. We also attempt to outline briefly what we see as the principal advantages and disadvantages of each model as currently conceptualized.

4.1 Health belief model

The health belief model (HBM) is perhaps the oldest and most widely used social cognition model in health psychology (Rosenstock 1966; Becker 1974; Sheeran and Abraham, Chapter 2 in this volume). The HBM has been considered more a loose association of variables that have been found to predict behaviour than a formal model (Conner 1993).

The HBM uses two aspects of individuals' representations of health behaviour in response to threat of illness: perceptions of illness threat and evaluation of behaviours to counteract this threat. Threat perceptions are seen to depend upon two beliefs, the perceived susceptibility to the illness and the perceived severity of the consequences of such illness. Together these two variables are believed to determine the likelihood of the individual following a health related action, although their effect is modified by individual differences in demographic variables, social pressure and personality. The particular action taken is believed to be determined by the evaluation of the available alternatives. The behavioural evaluation is considered to depend upon beliefs concerning the benefits or efficacy of the health behaviour and the perceived costs of or barriers to performing the behaviour. So individuals are likely to follow a particular health action if they believe themselves to be susceptible to a particular condition which they also consider to be serious, and believe that the benefits of the action taken to counteract the health threat outweigh the costs.

Two other variables commonly included in the model are cues to action and health motivation. Cues to action are assumed to include a diverse range of triggers to the individual taking action, which may be internal (e.g. physical symptom) or external (e.g. mass media campaign, advice from others) to the individual (Janz and Becker 1984). Furthermore, as Becker (1974) has argued, certain individuals may be predisposed to respond to such cues because of the value they place on their health.

The precise way in which these variables combine to produce behaviour has never been precisely specified (but see Becker and Rosenstock 1987). The HBM is thus frequently tested as six independent predictors of behaviour. There has been some variation in how these key variables are operationalized. Despite this lack of clear explication, the HBM has provided a useful framework for investigating health behaviours, has been widely used and has met with moderate success in predicting a range of health behaviours (for reviews see Janz and Becker 1984; Harrison *et al.* 1992; Sheeran and Abraham, Chapter 2 in this volume). Its strengths lie in the fact that it was developed by researchers directly working with health behaviours and so many of the concepts possess face-validity to those working in this area. The common sense operationalization of a number of cognitive variables relevant to the performance of health behaviour partly accounts for the model's popularity.

However, compared to other social cognitive models of health behaviours, the HBM suffers from a number of weaknesses. Several social cognitive variables found to be highly predictive of behaviour in other models are not incorporated in the HBM. For example, intentions to perform a behaviour and social pressure are key components of the theory of reasoned action/planned behaviour which do not appear in the HBM. Perceptions of control over the performance of the behaviour (self-efficacy ~~are~~ beliefs), which have been found to be such powerful predictors of beha- *now*. viour in models based upon self-efficacy theory (Bandura 1977), are not explicitly included in the HBM. In addition, in the lack of specification of a causal ordering among the variables in the HBM, as is done in other models, more powerful analysis of data and clearer indications of how interventions may have their effects are precluded. For example, several authors have noted that the threat variable is perhaps best seen as a more distal predictor of behaviour acting via influences upon outcome expectancies. Finally, the model is static; there is no distinction between a motivational stage dominated by cognitive variables and a volitional phase where action is planned, performed and maintained (Schwarzer 1992).

4.2 Health locus of control

The health locus of control (HLC) construct has also been widely applied in health psychology (Wallston 1992; Norman and Bennett, Chapter 3 in this volume). The HLC construct has its origins in Rotter's (1954) social learning theory. The main tenet of social learning theory is that the likelihood of a behaviour occurring in a given situation is a joint function of the individual's expectancy that the behaviour will lead to a particular reinforcement and the extent to which the reinforcement is valued. Rotter (1966) later developed the locus of control construct as a generalized expectancy, making the distinction between internal and external locus of control orientations: internals are seen to believe that events are a consequence of their own actions, whereas externals are seen to believe that events are unrelated to their actions and thereby determined by factors beyond their control. Wallston *et al.* (1978) built on Rotter's earlier work by developing the multidimensional health locus of control (MHLC) scale, which measures expectancy beliefs with respect to health along three dimensions; the extent to which individuals believe their health is under the influence of their own actions (i.e. internal HLC), powerful others and chance. The main prediction from HLC theory is that internals on the MHLC scale should be more likely to engage in health-promoting activities.

The HLC construct has been applied to a wide range of behaviours (for a review see Norman and Bennett, Chapter 3 in this volume). However, studies linking internal HLC control beliefs to the performance of preventive health behaviours have produced a mixed set of results, with some studies reporting a positive relationship (e.g. Duffy 1987) and others reporting a non-significant relationship (e.g. Brown *et al.* 1983). A number of researchers have commented that tests of the HLC construct have been inadequate because they have failed to consider the role of health value. It is argued that HLC beliefs should only predict health behaviour when people value their own health; no relationship is expected for individuals who place a low value on their health. Studies which have tested for the predicted interaction between internal HLC and health value have generally produced positive results (e.g. Weiss and Larsen 1990), although some studies have failed to find such an interaction (e.g. Wurtele *et al.* 1985).

Overall, the HLC construct has been found to be a relatively weak predictor of health behaviour, accounting for only small amounts of the variance in health behaviour, even when considered in conjunction with health value (Wallston 1992). However, a couple of developments in HLC work are worth noting. First, a number of researchers have attempted to construct more behaviour-specific locus of control scales. For example, Saltzer (1982) has developed a weight locus of control scale to predict weight reduction behaviour. In general, these scales have been found to be more predictive of behaviour than the more general MHLC scales (Lefcourt 1991). Second, Wallston (1989, 1992) has attempted to incorporate the HLC construct into a more general theory of health behaviour, which he has labelled as modified social learning theory. In this theory, health behaviour is seen to be a function of health value, health locus of control and self-efficacy, such that self-efficacy should only predict health behaviour when the individual values his or her health and has an internal HLC orientation. This modified model not only incorporates one of the most powerful predictors of health behaviour, self-efficacy, but also outlines a role for HLC as a more distal predictor of health behaviour.

4.3 Protection motivation theory

Protection motivation theory (PMT) was originally (Rogers 1975) proposed to provide conceptual clarity to the understanding of fear appeals. The theory has been revised on a number of occasions. As typically applied

(Maddux and Rogers 1983; Rogers 1983), PMT describes adaptive and maladaptive coping with a health threat as the result of two appraisal processes: threat appraisal and coping appraisal. Threat appraisal is based upon a consideration of perceptions of susceptibility to the illness and severity of the health threat. Coping appraisal involves the process of assessing the behavioural alternatives which might diminish the threat. This coping process is assumed to be based upon two components: the individual's expectancy that carrying out a behaviour can remove the threat (action-outcome efficacy) and a belief in one's capability to execute successfully the recommended courses of action (self-efficacy).

Together these two appraisal processes result in the intention to perform adaptive (protection motivation) or maladaptive responses. Adaptive responses are held to be more likely if the individual perceives him or herself to be facing a health threat to which he or she is susceptible and which is perceived to be severe. Fear arousal is assumed to operate via increasing perceptions of susceptibility and severity. Adaptive responses are also more likely if the individual perceives such responses to be effective in reducing the threat and believes that he or she can successfully perform the adaptive response. These two cognitive appraisals feed into protection motivation, which is an intervening variable that arouses, sustains and directs activity to protect the self from danger. Protection motivation is typically operationalized as intention to perform the health-protective behaviour or avoid the health-compromising behaviour. Actual behaviour is assumed to be a function of intentions.

PMT has been successfully applied to the prediction of a number of health behaviours (for a review see Boer and Seydel, Chapter 4 in this volume). The theory has also appeared in a number of different forms, originally being developed as a way to understand the response to fear appeals. In the 'revised theory' (Maddux and Rogers 1983), described here, it can be seen as a hybrid theory (Prentice-Dunn and Rogers 1986) with susceptibility, severity and response-efficacy components all originating from the HBM, and self-efficacy originating from Bandura's self-efficacy theory (Bandura 1977). As might be expected from our review of the HBM, the threat appraisal components have tended to be less predictive of intentions and actual behaviour than the response-efficacy and self-efficacy components (Boer and Seydel, Chapter 4 in this volume). This may be attributable to threat being better conceived of as a more distal determinant of intentions. This is not to dismiss threat appraisal but rather to assume that it is important earlier in the decision-making process (Weinstein 1988) and has its impact upon intentions and behaviour via influencing action-outcome expectancies. The response-efficacy component has been compared to action-outcome expectancy (Schwarzer 1992) and so threat may be best seen as impacting upon intentions via influencing this component.

Further revisions to the model (Rippetoe and Rogers 1987) have incorporated internal/external rewards from the current behaviour and perceived costs of the revised behaviour. However, few tests of this more complex version of the model have been reported. Overall, PMT appears to incorporate many of the important cognitive variables underlying the performance of health behaviours. However, variation in the way the theory has been conceived and operationalized has detracted from its explanatory power.

4.4 Theory of planned behaviour

The theory of planned behaviour (TPB) represents a model developed by social psychologists which has been quite widely applied to the understanding of a variety of behaviours (Ajzen 1988, 1991; Conner and Sparks, Chapter 5 in this volume). The TPB outlines how the influences upon an individual determine that individual's decision to follow a particular behaviour. This theory is itself an extension of the widely applied theory of reasoned action (Fishbein and Ajzen 1975; Ajzen and Fishbein 1980) which continues to attract a great deal of attention in social psychology (Sheppard *et al.* 1988; Tesser and Shaffer 1990; Olson and Zanna 1993).

The TPB suggests that the proximal determinants of behaviour are one's intention to engage in that behaviour and one's perceptions of control over that behaviour. Intentions represent a person's motivation in the sense of her or his conscious plan or decision to exert effort to perform the behaviour. Perceived behavioural control is a person's expectancy that performance of the behaviour is within his or her control. The concept is similar to Bandura's (1982) concept of self-efficacy (see Schwarzer and Fuchs, Chapter 6 in this volume). Control is seen as a continuum with easily executed behaviours at one end and behavioural goals demanding resources, opportunities and specialized skills at the other.

Intention is itself determined by three sets of factors. The first of these is attitudes, which are the overall evaluations of the behaviour by the individual. The second determinant of intentions is subjective norms. Subjective norms consist of a person's beliefs about whether significant others think he or she should engage in the behaviour. The third determinant of intentions is perceived behavioural control, which is the individual's perception of the extent to which performance of the behaviour is easy or difficult.

Each of the attitude, subjective norm and perceived behavioural control components is also held to have prior determinants. Attitudes are a function of beliefs about the perceived consequences of the behaviour based upon two perceptions: the likelihood of that outcome occurring as a result of performing the behaviour and the evaluation of that outcome. Subjective norm is a function of normative beliefs, which represent perceptions of specific significant others' preferences about whether one should or should not engage in a behaviour. This is quantified in the model as the subjective likelihood that specific salient groups or individuals (referents) think the person should perform the behaviour, multiplied by the person's motivation to comply with that referent's expectation. Motivation to comply is the extent to which the person wishes to comply with the specific wishes of the referent on this issue. Judgements of perceived behavioural control are influenced by beliefs concerning whether one has access to the necessary resources and opportunities to perform the behaviour successfully, weighted by the perceived power of each factor to facilitate or inhibit the execution of the behaviour. These factors include both internal control factors (information, personal deficiencies, skills, abilities, emotions) and external control factors (opportunities, dependence on others, barriers).

So, according to the TPB, individuals are likely to follow a particular health action if they believe that the behaviour will lead to outcomes which they value, if they believe that people whose views they value think they should carry out the behaviour and if they feel that they have the necessary resources and opportunities to perform the behaviour. The reliance upon combinations of each of the key variables according to expectancy-value theory should be noted.

The TPB (and more particularly the TRA) has been widely tested and successfully applied to the understanding of a variety of behaviours (for reviews see Sheppard *et al.* 1988; Ajzen 1991; Conner and Sparks, Chapter 5 in this volume). The theory incorporates a number of important cognitive variables which appear to determine health behaviours (intentions, outcome expectancies, perceived behavioural control). The role of social pressure from others is also incorporated in the model in the form of subjective norms. However, perhaps because the model was developed outside the health arena, it does not make an assessment of health threat as is included in models such as the HBM. Finally, the theory states a clear causal ordering among variables in how they relate to behaviour, allowing sophisticated analysis techniques to be applied to assessing the model.

4.5 Self-efficacy models

Self-efficacy theory (Bandura 1977) forms the basis of a further model of the determinants of health behaviour. In this approach human motivation and action are assumed to be based upon three types of expectancies: situation-outcome, action-outcome and perceived self-efficacy. Situation-outcome expectancies represent beliefs about what consequences will occur without interfering personal action. Susceptibility to a health threat represents one such situation-outcome expectancy. Action-outcome expectancy is the belief that a given behaviour will or will not lead to a given outcome. For example, the belief that quitting smoking will lead to a reduced risk of lung cancer would represent an action-outcome expectancy. Self-efficacy expectancy is the belief that a behaviour is or is not within your control. The belief that you are or are not capable of performing a particular behaviour, such as exercising regularly, would constitute such a self-efficacy expectancy.

There is also a clear causal ordering among these three types of expectancies (Schwarzer 1992). Situation-outcome expectancies are assumed to operate as distal determinants of behaviour and to influence behaviour principally via their impact on action-outcome expectancies. For example, perceptions of the threat from a health risk to which the individual perceives him or herself to be susceptible may motivate the individual to consider different actions to minimize this risk. Action-outcome expectancies in turn are assumed to impact upon behaviour via their influence upon intentions to engage in the behaviour and upon self-efficacy expectancies. Situation-outcome expectancies may in conjunction with consideration of action-outcome expectancies lead to the formation of intentions to take specific actions. Behaviours perceived to be efficacious in reducing a perceived risk are likely to lead to intentions to engage in such behaviours. Action-outcome expectancies impact upon self-efficacy expectancies because individuals believe they can produce the responses necessary to produce desired outcomes. Self-efficacy expectancies are assumed to have a direct impact upon behaviour and an indirect effect via their influence upon intentions. The first link is attributable to the fact that optimistic self-beliefs predict actual behavioural performance. The second link reflects the fact that individuals typically intend to perform behaviours they perceive to be within their control (Bandura 1992; Schwarzer 1992; Schwarzer and Fuchs, Chapter 6 in this volume).

Large numbers of applications of various aspects of self-efficacy theory have been attempted in health psychology, often with a high degree of success (see Schwarzer 1992). Self-efficacy and action-outcome expectancies along with intentions have been found to be important predictors of a range of health behaviours in a diverse range of studies (for reviews see Bandura 1992; Schwarzer 1992; Schwarzer and Fuchs, Chapter 6 in this volume). The model suggests a clear causal ordering among variables in their relationship to behaviour. Recent developments based upon self-efficacy theory have extended consideration of the role of these variables in determining motivations to perform a behaviour to consideration of the role of these variables in the volitional stage of behaviour (Schwarzer 1992; Schwarzer and Fuchs, Chapter 6 in this volume). The lack of explicit consideration of social influences on behaviour, such as are to be found in the TPB, may be seen as one drawback to these models. However, such considerations are frequently incorporated within the action-outcome expectancy component. Finally, a failure to incorporate measures of value associated with different outcomes in the action-outcome expectancy component may be seen as a deficiency given the large amount of evidence supporting an expectancy-value conceptualization of outcome beliefs.

5 Critique of the social cognition approach to understanding health behaviours

SCMs, such as those described in the previous section, represent one widely used approach to understanding health behaviours. Their application offers

us a number of distinct advantages. However, there are also distinct disadvantages to this whole approach and these models as currently applied.
In this section we provide a critique of the approach taken by these social
cognition models to understanding health behaviour.

The potential advantages of using social cognition models in health
psychology are simply rehearsed (Conner 1993). First, they provide a clear
theoretical background to research, guiding the selection of variables to
measure, the procedure for developing reliable and valid measures, and
how these variables are combined in order to predict health behaviours
and outcomes. As the previous section has demonstrated, there is considerable overlap in the variables these models identify as important in
predicting behaviour. This we take as convergent evidence that the key
cognitions have been identified. For example, intentions, self-efficacy and
expectancy-value considerations in one form or another play a role in
many of the most widely applied models (see Norman and Conner, Chapter 7 in this volume).

Second, to the extent that these models identify the variables important
in predicting health outcomes and behaviours they further our understanding of health. This understanding is useful in enabling us to develop effective
interventions designed to alter the cognitions underlying unhealthy behaviours. If these cognitions are causally related to behaviours then changes
in cognitions should lead to changes in behaviours and so promote positive
health outcomes. Third, the models provide us with a description of the
cognitive processes determining individuals' motivation to perform different behaviours.

There are also parallel potential disadvantages in too exclusive a focus
upon social cognition models as the only way to understand health behaviours. First, in providing such a clear theoretical framework to apply to the
understanding of health behaviour these models may lead us to neglect
variables (cognitive and non-cognitive) that are potentially important in
understanding a particular health behaviour or outcome. The most profit-
able application of these models uses variables specified both by the models
and by expert knowledge of the particular health behaviour. This is because
they only consider cognitive variables and many health behaviours and outcomes involve other types of variables. For example, the decision to use a
condom is likely to be a function of cognitions, emotional reactions and
also a complex interaction between the individuals involved. Social cognition models are unlikely to provide considerable predictive power in these
situations. In addition, even well established SCMs are open to extension
when empirically and theoretically justified (Fishbein 1993). For example,
such models may be improved by consideration of the biases in the processes by which individuals form the judgements of risk which feature so
prominently in many SCMs (van der Pligt 1994).

Second, while such models may provide us with likely targets for interventions designed to produce behaviour change, they do not specify how
such cognitions are best changed. Relatively few studies have attempted

to change these variables as the basis for changing health behaviours. Interventions designed to produce effective behaviour change need to consider not only the targets (e.g. cognitions) but also the persuasion process itself. This process of persuasion is described by other models of social cognitive processes (e.g. the elaboration likelihood model: Petty and Cacioppo 1986; the systematic-heuristic model: Chaiken *et al.* 1989; Eagly and Chaiken 1993). In addition, applications of such SCMs should not lead us to neglect alternatives to persuasion in producing behaviour change. Extrinsic changes to the rewards and costs of a given behaviour are frequently an effective way to produce the desired change. For example, increased taxation and legal restrictions can be effective means either in isolation or in tandem with persuasion in producing change in health behaviours.

Third, while SCMs have furthered our understanding of motivational processes and their influence upon behaviour, they have tended to neglect other aspects of behaviour change. For example, few of the models consider volitional processes beyond attempting to explain intentions (Gollwitzer 1990; Bagozzi 1993). However, many individuals who intend to change a health behaviour fail to do so. Hence, we need to consider in more depth the other important volitional processes associated with successful attempts to change and maintain behaviour change (see Norman and Conner, this volume; Schwarzer and Fuchs, Chapter 6 in this volume).

6 Conclusions: using social cognition models to understand and change health behaviours

We have attempted to justify the interest in understanding health behaviours as a basis for attempting to change their occurrence in order to increase both length and quality of life. SCMs provide one approach to understanding health behaviour in describing the important social cognitive variables underlying such behaviours. We believe that these models provide an important way of achieving the above aims by providing a means for identifying useful targets for persuasion. It would seem that there is already sufficient literature to support the contention that important determinants of health behaviours are identified in these models. Whether further refinement and development of these models leads to even better predictions of behaviour remains to be seen.

However, persuasive messages targeted at relevant cognitions may not be sufficient to produce the major behaviour change necessary for health benefits to accrue. It may be that strategies which employ multiple level interventions that take account not only of the psychosocial factors influencing performance of the behaviour (derived from SCMs), but also models of the process of persuasion, of how people change and the context in which changes are made, will be important (Winett 1985; Glanz *et al.* 1990; McQueen 1991; Hockbaum and Lorig 1992; McLeroy *et al.* 1993).

References

Adler, N. and Matthews, K. (1994) Health psychology: why do some people get sick and some stay well?, *Annual Review of Psychology*, 45, 229–9.

Affleck, G., Tennen, H., Croog, S. and Levine, S. (1987) Causal attribution, perceived control, and recovery from a heart attack, *Journal of Social and Clinical Psychology*, 5, 356–64.

Ajzen, I. (1988) *Attitudes, Personality and Behavior*. Milton Keynes: Open University Press.

Ajzen, I. (1991) The theory of planned behavior, *Organizational Behavior and Human Decision Processes*, 50, 179–211.

Ajzen, I. and Fishbein, M. (1980) *Understanding Attitudes and Predicting Social Behavior*. Englewood Cliffs, NJ: Prentice-Hall.

Amler, R.W. and Eddins, D.L. (1987) Cross-sectional analysis: precursors of premature death in the US. In R.W. Amler and H.B. Dull (eds) *Closing the Gap*. New York: Oxford University Press, 54–87.

Bagozzi, R.P. (1992) The self-regulation of attitudes, intentions and behavior, *Social Psychology Quarterly*, 55, 178–204.

Bagozzi, R.P. (1993) On the neglect of volition in consumer research: a critique and proposal, *Psychology and Marketing*, 10, 215–37.

Bandura, A. (1977) Self-efficacy: toward a unifying theory of behavioral change, *Psychological Review*, 84, 191–215.

Bandura, A. (1982) Self-efficacy mechanism in human agency, *American Psychologist*, 37, 122–47.

Bandura, A. (1991) Self-efficacy mechanism in physiological activation and health-promoting behavior. In J. Madden (ed.) *Neurobiology of Learning, Emotion and Affect*. New York: Raven Press, 229–70.

Bandura, A. (1992) Exercise of personal agency through the self-efficacy mechanism. In R. Schwarzer (ed.) *Self-efficacy: Thought Control of Action*. London: Hemisphere, 3–38.

Becker, M.H. (1974) The health belief model and sick role behavior, *Health Education Monographs*, 2, 409–19.

Becker, M.H. and Maiman, L.A. (1983) Models of health-related behavior. In D. Mechanic (ed.) *Handbook of Health, Health Care and the Health Professions*. New York: Free Press, 539–68.

Becker, M.H. and Rosenstock, I.M. (1987) Comparing social learning theory and the health belief model. In W.B. Ward (ed.) *Advances in Health Education and Promotion*, Vol. 2. Greenwich, CT: JAI Press, 245–9.

Belloc, N.B. (1973) Relationship of health practices to mortality, *Preventive Medicine*, 2, 67–81.

Belloc, N.B. and Breslow, L. (1972) Relationship of physical health status and health practices, *Preventive Medicine*, 9, 409–421.

Black, D., Morris, J.N., Smith, C. and Townsend, P. (1988) The Black report. In *Inequalities in Health: the Black Report and the Health Divide*. London: DHSS, 31–213.

Blane, D., Smith, G.D. and Bartley, M. (1990) Social class differences in years of potential life lost: size trends, and principal causes, *British Medical Journal*, 301, 429–32.

Blaxter, M. (1990) *Health and Lifestyles*. London: Tavistock.

Breslow, L. and Enstrom, J.E. (1980) Persistence of health habits and their relationship to mortality, *Preventive Medicine*, 9, 469–83.

Brock, B.M., Haefner D.P. and Noble, D.S. (1988) Alameda County Redux: replication in Michigan, *Preventive Medicine*, 17, 483–95.

Brown, N., Muhlenkamp, A., Fox, L. and Osborn, M. (1983) The relationship among health beliefs, health values, and health promotion activity, *Western Journal of Nursing Research*, 5, 155–63.

Chaiken, S., Liberman, A. and Eagly, A.H. (1989) Heuristic and systematic information processing within and beyond the persuasion context. In J.S. Uleman and J.A. Bargh (eds) *Unintended Thought*. New York: Guildford Press, 212–52.

Conner, M.T. (1993) Pros and cons of social cognition models in health behaviour, *Health Psychology Update*, 14, 24–31.

Cox, B.D., Blaxter, M., Buckle, A.L.J., Fenner, N.P. *et al.* (1987) *The Health and Lifestyles Survey: Preliminary Report*. London: Health Promotion Trust.

Cox, B.D., Huppert, F.A. and Whichelow, M.J. (1993) *The Health and Lifestyles Survey: Seven Years on*. Aldershot: Dartmouth.

Cummings, M.K., Becker, M.H. and Maile, M.C. (1980) Bringing models together: an empirical approach to combining variables used to explain health actions, *Journal of Behavioral Medicine*, 3, 123–45.

Department of Health (1992) *Health of the Nation*. London: HMSO.

Doll, R. and Peto, R. (1976) Mortality in relation to smoking: 20 years' observation of male British doctors, *British Medical Journal*, 2, 1525–36.

Duffy, M.E. (1987) Determinants of health promotion in midlife women, *Nursing Research*, 37, 358–62.

Eagly, A.H. and Chaiken, S. (1993) *The Psychology of Attitudes*. Fort Worth, TX: Harcourt Brace Jovanovich.

Edwards, W. (1954) The theory of decision making, *Psychological Bulletin*, 51, 380–417.

Edwards, W. (1992) *Utility Theories: Measurements and Applications*. Boston: Kluwer.

Feather, N.T. (1982) *Expectations and Actions: Expectancy-value Models in Psychology*. Hillsdale, NJ: Erlbaum.

Fishbein, M. (1993) Introduction. In D.J. Terry, C. Gallois and M. McCamish (eds) *The Theory of Reasoned Action: Its Application to AIDS-preventive Behaviour*. Oxford: Pergamon, xv–xxv.

Fishbein, M. and Ajzen, I. (1975) *Belief, Attitude, Intention, and Behavior*. New York: Wiley.

Fiske, S.T. and Taylor, S.E. (1991) *Social Cognition*, 2nd edn. New York: McGraw-Hill.

Fries, J.F., Green, L.W. and Levine, S. (1989) Health promotion and the compression of mortality, *Lancet*, i, 481–3.

Frisch, D. and Clemen, R.T. (1994) Beyond expected utility: rethinking behavioral decision making, *Psychological Bulletin*, 116, 46–54.

Glanz, K., Lewis, F.M. and Rimmer, B.K. (eds) (1990) *Health Behavior and Health Education: Theory, Research and Practice*. San Francisco, CA: Jossey-Bass.

Goldman, L. and Cook, E.F. (1984) The decline in ischaemic heart disease mortality rates: an analysis of the comparative efforts of medical interventions and changes in lifestyle, *Annals of Internal Medicine*, 101, 825–36.

Gollwitzer, P.M. (1990) Action phases and mind-sets. In E.T. Higgins and R.M.

Sorrentino (eds) *Handbook of Motivation and Cognition: Foundations of Social Behaviour*, Vol. 2. New York: Guilford Press, 53–92.

Gollwitzer, P.M. (1993) Goal achievement: the role of intentions, *European Review of Social Psychology*, 4, 142–85.

Gottlieb, N.H. and Green, L.W. (1984) Life events, social network, life-style and health: an analysis of the 1979 National survey of personal health practices and consequences, *Health Education Quarterly*, 11, 91–105.

Harrison, J.A., Mullen, P.D. and Green, L.W. (1992) A meta-analysis of studies of the Health Belief Model with adults, *Health Education Research*, 7, 107–16.

Heckhausen, H. (1991) *Motivation and Action*. Berlin: Springer-Verlag.

Hockbaum, G.M. and Lorig, K. (eds) (1992) Roles and uses of theory in health education practice, *Health Education Quarterly*, 19, 289–412.

Janz, N.K. and Becker, M.H. (1984) The health belief model: a decade later, *Health Education Quarterly*, 11, 1–47.

Jonas, K. (1993) Expectancy-value models of health behaviour: an analysis by conjoint measurement, *European Journal of Social Psychology*, 23, 167–83.

Kasl, S.V. and Cobb, S. (1966) Health behavior, illness behavior and sick role behavior, *Archives of Environmental Health*, 12, 246–66.

King, J. (1982) The impact of patients' perceptions of high blood pressure on attendance at screening, *Social Science and Medicine*, 16, 1079–91.

Kuhl, J. (1984) Volitional aspects of achievement motivation and learned helplessness: toward a comprehensive theory of action control, *Progress in Experimental Personality Research*, 13, 99–171.

Kuhl, J. and Beckmann, J. (eds) (1985) *Action Control: from Cognition to Behavior*. Berlin: Springer-Verlag.

Kuhl, J. and Beckmann, J. (eds) (1994) *Volition and Personality: Action versus State Orientation*. Gottingen: Springer-Verlag.

Lefcourt, H.M. (1991) Locus of control. In J.P. Robinson, P.R. Shaver, and L.S. Wrightsman (eds) *Measures of Personality and Social Psychological Attitude*. New York: Academic Press, 661–753.

Leventhal, H., Nerenz, D.R. and Steele, D.F. (1984) Illness representations and coping with health threats. In A. Baum and J. Singer (eds) *A Handbook of Psychology and Health*. Hillsdale, NJ: Erlbaum, 219–52.

McLeroy, K.R., Steckler, A.B., Simons-Morton, B., Goodman, R.M., Gottlieb, N. and Burdine, J.N. (1993) Social science theory in health education: time for a new model?, *Health Education Research*, 8, 305–12.

McNeil, A.D., Jarvis, M.J., Stapleton, J.A., Russell, M.A.H., Eiser, J.R., Gammage, P. and Gray, E.M. (1988) Prospective study of factors predicting uptake of smoking in adolescents, *Journal of Epidemiology and Community Health*, 43, 72–8.

McQueen, D. (ed.) (1991) Theme issue, *Health Education Research*, 6, 137–255.

Maddux, J.E. and Rogers, R.W. (1983) Protection motivation and self-efficacy: a revised theory of fear appeals and attitude change, *Journal of Experimental Social Psychology*, 19, 469–79.

Marmot, M.G., Davey Smith, G., Stansfeld, D., Patel, C., North, F., Head, J., White, I., Brunner, E. and Feeney, A. (1991) Health inequalities among British civil servants: the Whitehall II study, *Lancet*, 337, 1387–92.

Marteau, T.M. (1989) Health beliefs and attributions. In A.K. Broome (ed.) *Health Psychology: Processes and Applications*. London: Chapman Hall, 1–23.

Metzner, H.L., Carman W.J. and House, J. (1983) Health practices, risk factors and chronic disease in Tecumeseh, *Preventive Medicine*, 12, 491–507.

Mullen, P.D., Hersey, J.C. and Iverson, D.C. (1987) Health behaviour models compared, *Social Science and Medicine*, 24, 973–81.

Olson, J.M. and Zanna, M.P. (1993) Attitudes and attitude change, *Annual Review of Psychology*, 44, 117–54.

Peak, H. (1955) Attitude and motivation. In M.R. Jones (ed.) *Nebraska Symposium on Motivation*, Vol. 3. Lincoln: University of Nebraska Press, 149–88.

Petty, R.E. and Cacioppo, J.T. (1986) *Communication and Persuasion: Central and Peripheral Routes of Attitude Change*. New York: Springer Verlag.

Prentice-Dunn, S. and Rogers, R.W. (1986) Protection motivation theory and preventive health: beyond the health belief model, *Health Education Research*, 1, 153–61.

Prochaska, J.O. and DiClemente, C.C. (1984) *The Transtheoretical Approach: Crossing Traditional Boundaries of Therapy*. Homewood, IL: Dow Jones Irwin.

Prochaska, J.O., DiClemente, C.C. and Norcross, J.C. (1992) In search of how people change: applications to addictive behaviors, *American Psychologist*, 47, 1102–14.

Rippetoe, P.A. and Rogers, R.W. (1987) Effects of components of protection motivation theory on adaptive and maladaptive coping with a health threat, *Journal of Personality and Social Psychology*, 52, 596–604.

Rodin, J. and Salovey, P. (1989) Health psychology, *Annual Review of Psychology*, 40, 533–79.

Rogers, R.W. (1975) A protection motivation theory of fear appeals and attitude change, *Journal of Psychology*, 91, 93–114.

Rogers, R.W. (1983) Cognitive and physiological processes in fear appeals and attitude change: a revised theory of protection motivation. In J.T. Cacioppo and R.E. Petty (eds) *Social Psychophysiology: a Source Book*. New York: Guilford Press, 153–76.

Rosenstock, I.M. (1966) Why people use health services, *Millbank Memorial Fund Quarterly*, 44, 94–124.

Rosenstock, I.M. (1974) Historical origins of the health belief model, *Health Education Monographs*, 2, 1–8.

Rotter, J.B. (1954) *Social Learning and Clinical Psychology*. Englewood Cliffs, NJ: Prentice-Hall.

Rotter, R.B. (1966) Generalized expectancies for internal and external control of reinforcement. *Psychological Monographs: General and Applied*, 80 (whole no. 609), 1–28.

Rutter, D.R., Quine, L. and Chesham, D.J. (1993) *Social Psychological Approaches to Health*. London: Harvester-Wheatsheaf.

Saltzer, E.B. (1982) The weight loss of control (WLOC) scale: a specific measure for obesity research, *Journal of Personality Assessment*, 46, 620–8.

Schneider, D.J. (1991) Social cognition, *Annual Review of Psychology*, 42, 527–61.

Schwarzer, R. (1992) Self-efficacy in the adoption and maintenance of health behaviors: theoretical approaches and a new model. In R. Schwarzer (ed.) *Self-efficacy: Thought Control of Action*. London: Hemisphere, 217–43.

Seeman, M. and Seeman, T.E. (1983) Health behaviour and personal autonomy: a longitudinal study of the sense of control in illness, *Journal of Health and Social Behaviour*, 24, 144–60.

Sheppard, B.H., Hartwick, J. and Warshaw, P.R. (1988) The theory of reasoned action: a meta-analysis of past research with recommendations for modifications and future research, *Journal of Consumer Research*, 15, 325–39.

Smith, A. and Jacobson, B. (1988) *The Nation's Health: a Strategy for the 1990s.* London: Kings Fund.

Steptoe, A., Wardle, J., Vinck, J., Tuomisto, M., Holte, A. and Wichstrom, L. (1994) Personality and attitudinal correlates of healthy and unhealthy lifestyles in young adults, *Psychology and Health*, 9, 331–43.

Stroebe, W. and Stroebe, M.S. (1995) *Social Psychology and Health.* Buckingham: Open University Press.

Taylor, S. (1991) *Health Psychology.* New York: McGraw-Hill.

Taylor, S., Lichtman, R.R. and Wood, J.V. (1984) Attributions, beliefs about control and adjustment to breast cancer, *Journal of Personality and Social Psychology*, 46, 489–502.

Tennen, H., Affleck, G., Allen, D.A., McGrade, B.J. and Ratzan, S. (1984) Causal attributions and coping with insulin-dependent diabetes, *Basic and Applied Social Psychology*, 5, 131–42.

Tesser, A. and Shaffer, D.R. (1990) Attitudes and attitude change, *Annual Review of Psychology*, 41, 479–523.

Turk, D.C. and Salovey, P. (1986) Clinical information processing: bias inoculation. In R.E. Ingham (ed.) *Information Processing Approaches to Clinical Psychology.* New York: Academic Press, 305–23.

van der Pligt, J. (1994) Risk appraisal and health behaviour. In D.R. Rutter and L. Quine (eds) *Social Psychology and Health: European Perspectives.* Aldershot: Avebury Press, 131–52.

van der Velde, W. and van der Pligt, J. (1991) AIDS-related behavior: coping, protection motivation, and previous behavior, *Journal of Behavioral Medicine*, 14, 429–51.

Waldron, I. (1988) Why do women live longer than men?, *Journal of Human Stress*, 2, 2–13.

Wallston, K.A. (1989) Assessment of control in health care settings. In A. Steptoe and A. Appels (eds) *Stress, Personal Control and Health.* London: Wiley, 85–105.

Wallston, K.A. (1992) Hocus-pocus, the focus isn't strictly on locus: Rotter's social learning theory modified for health, *Cognitive Therapy and Research*, 16, 183–99.

Wallston, K.A., Wallston, B.S. and DeVellis, R. (1978) Development of multidimensional health locus of control (MHLC) scales, *Health Education Monographs*, 6, 160–70.

Wardle, J. and Steptoe, A. (1991) The European health and behaviour survey: rationale, methods and initial results from the United Kingdom, *Social Science and Medicine*, 33, 925–36.

Weinstein, W.D. (1988) The precaution adoption process, *Health Psychology*, 7, 355–86.

Weinstein, W.D. (1993) Testing four competing theories of health-protective behavior, *Health Psychology*, 12, 324–33.

Weiss, G.L. and Larson, D.L. (1990) Health value, health locus of control, and the prediction of health protective behaviors, *Social Behavior and Personality*, 18, 121–36.

Whitehead, M. (1988) The health divide. In *Inequalities in Health: the Black Report and the Health Divide.* Harmondsworth: Penguin, 217–356.

Winett, R.A. (1985) Ecobehavioral assessment in health life-styles: concepts and methods. In P. Karoly (ed.) *Measurement Strategies in Health Psychology.* Chichester: Wiley, 147–81.

Witenberg, S.H., Blanchard, E.B., Suls, J., Tennen, H., McCoy, G. and McGoldrick, M.D. (1983) Perceptions of control and causality as predictors of compliance with hemodialysis, *Basic and Applied Social Psychology*, **1**, 319–36.

Wurtele, S.K., Britcher, J.C. and Saslawsky, D.A. (1985) Relationships between locus of control, health value and preventive health behaviours among women, *Journal of Research in Personality*, **19**, 271–8.

| 2 | PASCHAL SHEERAN AND CHARLES ABRAHAM |

THE HEALTH BELIEF MODEL

1 General background

In the 1950s US public health researchers began developing models which would identify appropriate targets for health education programmes (Hochbaum 1958; Rosenstock 1966). There was clear evidence that demographic variables such as socioeconomic status, gender, ethnicity and age affected the extent to which people would adopt preventive health behaviours or use health services (Rosenstock 1974), but these could not be modified through health education and even when services were publicly financed the effects of socioeconomic status were not eliminated. It became clear that effective health education depended upon identifying how the different socialization histories indexed by demographic variables led to individual differences in the propensity to undertake preventive action and follow medical advice. This required measures of modifiable psychological characteristics which were correlated with health behaviour. Individual beliefs offered the ideal link between socialization and behaviour. Beliefs are enduring individual characteristics which shape behaviour and can be acquired through primary socialization. They are not, however, fixed and can differentiate between individuals from the same background. In fact they are the archetypal social cognitive construct.

The relationship between distinct health beliefs and between health beliefs and behaviours was conceptualized primarily in terms of Lewin's (1951) idea of valence, that is the rendering of a behaviour more or less attractive. This resulted in an expectancy-value model in which events believed to be more or less likely were seen to be positively or negatively evaluated by the individual. In particular the likelihood of experiencing a health problem, the severity of the consequences of that problem and the perceived benefits of a health behaviour in combination with its potential costs were seen as key beliefs guiding health behaviour.

Early research suggested that health beliefs were correlated with behaviour and could be used to differentiate between those who did and did not undertake these behaviours. The model was initially applied to preventive behaviours but later successfully extended to identify the correlates of health service usage and compliance with medical regimens (Becker *et al.* 1977b). Rosenstock (1974) attributes the first health belief model (HBM) research to Hochbaum's (1958) studies of the uptake of tuberculosis X-ray screening. Hochbaum found that perceived susceptibility to tuberculosis and the belief that people with the disease could be asymptomatic (so that screening would be beneficial) distinguished between those who had and had not attended for chest X-rays. Similarly, a prospective study by Kegeles (1963) showed that perceived susceptibility to the worst imaginable dental problems and awareness that visits to the dentist might prevent these problems were useful predictors of the frequency of dental visits three years later. Haefner and Kirscht (1970) took this one step further and demonstrated that a health education intervention designed to increase participants' perceived susceptibility, perceived severity and anticipated benefits resulted in a greater number of check-up visits to the doctor compared to controls over the following eight months. By the early 1970s, then, a series of studies had suggested that these key health beliefs provided a useful framework for understanding individual differences in health behaviour and for designing behaviour change interventions.

The model that emerged from this research had the advantage of specifying a discrete set of common sense cognitions that appeared to mediate the effects of demographic variables and were amenable to educational intervention. This model could be applied to a range of health behaviours and provided a basis for shaping public health behaviour and training health care professionals to work from their patients' subjective perceptions of illness and treatment. This was an important step forward for both public health research and social cognitive theory, and established social cognition modelling as central to health service research programmes.

The HBM was further consolidated when Becker *et al.* (1977b) published a consensus statement from the Carnegie Grant Subcommittee on Modification of Patient Behaviour for Health Maintenance and Disease Control. This paper considered a range of alternative approaches to understanding the social psychological determinants of health and illness behaviour and endorsed the HBM framework. The components of the model were defined and further research on the relationships between individual beliefs and health behaviours was called for.

2 Description of the model

The model that emerged focused on two aspects of individuals' representations of health and health behaviour: threat perception and behavioural evaluation. Threat perception was seen to depend upon two beliefs, perceived *susceptibility* to illness or health breakdown and anticipated *severity* of the consequences of such illness. Behavioural evaluation also consisted of two distinct sets of beliefs, those concerning the *benefits* or efficacy of a recommended health behaviour and those concerning the costs of or *barriers* to enacting the behaviour. In addition the model proposed that *cues to action* can trigger health behaviour when appropriate beliefs are held. These 'cues' included a diverse range of triggers including individual perceptions of symptoms, social influence and health education campaigns. Finally, an individual's general *health motivation* or 'readiness to be concerned about health matters' was included in later versions of the model (e.g. Becker *et al.* 1977b). There were therefore six distinct constructs specified by the HBM.

As Figure 2.1 indicates, no clear operationalization instructions linking perceived susceptibility and severity to threat and action were developed. Similarly, although it was suggested that perceived benefits were 'weighted against' perceived barriers (Becker *et al.* 1977b), no formula for creating an overall behavioural evaluation measure was developed. Therefore the model has usually been operationalized as a series of up to six separate independent variables which potentially account for variance in observed or reported health behaviours.

As we shall see below, even the definition of these six constructs was left open to debate. Rosenstock (1974) and Becker and Maiman (1975) illustrate how various researchers used somewhat different operationalizations of these constructs and a recent meta-analysis (Harrison *et al.* 1992) concluded that this lack of operational homogeneity continues to weaken the HBM's status as a coherent psychological model of the prerequisites of health behaviour. Nevertheless, a series of studies continued to show that these various operationalizations allowed identification of beliefs correlated with health behaviours (Janz and Becker 1984).

3 Summary of research

3.1 Overview of applications of the HBM and research strategies

The HBM has received greater research attention and has been applied to a broader range of health behaviours and subject populations than other social cognitive models. Table 2.1 illustrates the range of behaviours which have been examined. Three broad areas can be identified: (a) preventive health behaviours, which include health-promoting (e.g. diet, exercise) and health-risk (e.g. smoking) behaviours as well as vaccination and contraceptive practices; (b) sick role behaviours, which refer to compliance with recommended medical regimens, usually following professional diagnosis of illness; and (c) clinic use, which includes physician visits for a variety of reasons.

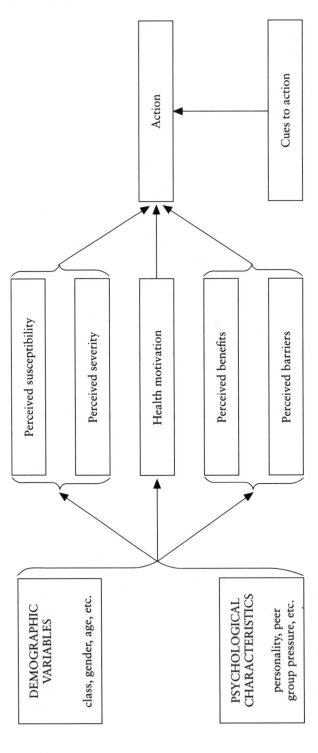

Figure 2.1 The health belief model.

Table 2.1 Examples of applications of the health belief model

Research area	Investigators
Preventive behaviours	
Screening	
• genetic	Becker *et al.* (1975) Tay–Sachs trait; Hoogewerf *et al.* (1990) faecal occult blood
• health	King (1984) Hypertension; Orbell *et al.* (1995) Cervical cancer; Simon and Das (1984) STD test
Risk behaviours	
• smoking	Gianetti *et al.* (1985), Mullen *et al.* (1987), Pederson *et al.* (1982), Stacy and Lloyd (1990)
• alcohol	Beck (1981), Gottlieb and Baker (1986), Portnoy (1980), Werch (1990)
Health behaviours	Aho (1979a), Langlie (1977) diet and exercise; Ogionwo (1973) cholera prevention
Influenza vaccination	Oliver and Berger (1979), Cummings *et al.* (1979), Larson *et al.* (1982), Rundall and Wheeler (1979)
Breast self-examination	Calnan (1985), Champion (1984), Owens *et al.* (1987), Ronis and Harel (1989)
Contraceptive use	Eisen *et al.* (1985), Hester and Macrina (1985), Lowe and Radius (1987)
Dental behaviours	Chen and Land (1986), Kegeles (1963) dental visits; Chen and Tatsuoka (1984) brushing/flossing
Sick role behaviours	
Anti-hypertensive regimen	Hershey *et al.* (1980), Kirsht and Rosenstock (1977), Nelson *et al.* (1978), Taylor (1979)
Diabetic regimen	Bradley *et al.* (1987), Brownlee-Duffeck *et al.* (1987), Harris and Lynn (1985)
Renal disease regimen	Cummings *et al.* (1982), Hartman and Becker (1978), Heinzelmann (1962)
Parental compliance with regimen for child's condition	Becker *et al.* (1977b) obesity regimen; Gordis *et al.* (1969) rheumatic fever regimen; Becker *et al.* (1972), Charney *et al.* (1967) *Otitis medea* regimen; Becker *et al.* (1978) asthma regimen
Clinic use	
Physician visits	
• preventive	Berkanovich *et al.* (1981), Leavitt (1979), Kirscht *et al.* (1976), Norman and Conner (1993)
• parent and child	Becker *et al.* (1972, 1977a), Kirscht *et al.* (1978)
• psychiatric	Connelly *et al.* (1982), Connelly (1984), Pan and Tantam (1989), Rees (1986)

Early HBM studies focused on preventive health behaviours. One of the first reviews of research (Becker *et al*. 1977a) examined 20 studies, 13 of which were investigations of preventive actions. These 13 studies examined seven distinct behaviours (X-ray screening for TB, polio and influenza vaccination, use of safety gloves, pap test, preventive dental visits and screening for Tay–Sachs trait). In contrast, six of the seven studies of sick role behaviours concerned compliance with penicillin prescriptions. When Janz and Becker reviewed the HBM literature in 1984, smoking, alcohol use, dieting, exercise and attendance at blood pressure screening had been added to the list of preventive behaviours which had been examined from a HBM perspective. Studies of sick role behaviours, however, greatly expanded in the interim period and included compliance with regimens for hypertension, insulin-dependent and non-insulin-dependent diabetes, end stage renal disease, obesity and asthma. Individual studies often examined a range of behaviours relevant to a particular regimen. For example, Cummings *et al*.'s (1982) study of end stage renal disease patients included measures of serum phosphorus and potassium levels, fluid intake, weight gain and patients' self-reports of diet and medication. Subsequent research has extended the range of behaviours examined to include contraceptive use, personal dental behaviours such as teeth brushing and flossing and screening for faecal occult blood and sexually transmitted disease. The range of behaviours addressed by HBM researchers, then, must be seen as impressive.

The diversity of content areas examined from this perspective is, to some extent, paralleled by the employment of a broad range of samples and data collection methods. While most HBM studies employ self-report measures of behaviour, several use physiological measures (e.g. Bradley *et al*. 1987), behavioural observation (e.g. Alagna and Reddy 1984) or medical records (e.g. Orbell *et al*. 1995) as outcomes. Many studies also employ longitudinal designs. Janz and Becker's (1984) review found that two-fifths (*n* = 18) were prospective. These studies are important since simultaneous measurements of both health beliefs and (especially self-reported) behaviour may be subject to memory and social desirability biases and do not permit causal inferences to be tested. While the majority of measures of health beliefs employ self-completion questionnaires, structured face-to-face (e.g. Cummings *et al*. 1982) and telephone (e.g. Grady *et al*. 1983) interviews have been employed. Use of random sampling techniques is commonplace and specific representation of low-income and minority groups is also evident in many studies (e.g. Becker *et al*. 1974; Mullen *et al*. 1987; Ronis and Harel 1989).

Findings from research studies employing the HBM are reviewed below. We first examine evidence for the predictive utility of the model's four major constructs: susceptibility, severity, benefits and barriers. Second, findings relating to cues to action and health motivation, which have received less empirical attention, are considered. Third, the issue of combining health beliefs and the potential importance of interactions among beliefs is examined. Finally, the extent to which health beliefs have been successful in mediating the effects of social structural variables or previous experience with a behaviour is investigated.

3.2 Utility of perceived susceptibility, severity, benefit and barrier constructs

Two quantitative reviews of research using the HBM with adults have been published (Janz and Becker, 1984; Harrison *et al.* 1992).[1] These reviews adopt different strategies in quantifying findings from research studies. Janz and Becker's (1984) review employs a vote count procedure (see Cooper 1986). A significance ratio was calculated 'wherein the number of positive and statistically significant findings for an HBM dimension are divided by the total number of studies which reported significance levels for that dimension' (p. 36). Janz and Becker's significance ratios tell us the percentage of times each HBM construct was statistically significant in the predicted direction across 46 studies. Across all studies, the significance ratios are very supportive of HBM predictions. Susceptibility was significant in 81 per cent of studies (30/37), severity in 65 per cent (24/37), benefits in 78 per cent (29/37) and barriers in 89 per cent (25/28). When prospective studies only (*n* = 18) are examined, findings appear to confirm a causal role for these health beliefs. The ratios were 82, 65, 81 and 100 per cent for susceptibility, severity, benefits and barriers based on 17, 17, 16 and 11 studies, respectively. Results show that barriers are the most reliable predictor of behaviour, followed by susceptibility and benefits, and finally severity.

Figure 2.2 presents significance ratios separately for preventive, sick role and clinic utilization behaviours based in each case on the number of studies examined by Janz and Becker.[2] Across 24 studies of preventive behaviours, barriers were significant predictors in 93 per cent of hypotheses, susceptibility in 86 per cent, benefits in 74 per cent and severity in 50 per cent. Barriers were also the most frequent predictor in 19 studies of sick role behaviours (92 per cent), with severity second (88 per cent) followed by benefits (80 per cent) and susceptibility (77 per cent). There were only three clinic use studies examined in the review. Benefits were significant in all studies, susceptibility was significant in two out of three and severity were significant in one out of three. Barriers were significant in one of the two studies of clinic use which examined this component. It is interesting to note that while severity has only a moderate effect upon preventive behaviour or clinic utilization, it is the second most powerful predictor of sick role behaviour. Janz and Becker suggest that these differences might be owing to respondents' difficulty in conceptualizing this component when they are asymptomatic or when the effects of the health threat are unfamiliar or only occur in the long term.

While findings from this vote count review seem to provide strong support for the HBM across a range of behaviours, difficulties with this

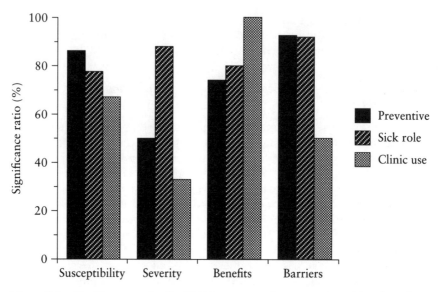

Figure 2.2   Significance ratios for HBM constructs for preventive, sick-role and clinic use behaviours (after Janz & Becker, 1984).

quantification strategy suggest caution in interpreting these results. In the first instance, significance ratios only tell us *how often* HBM components are significantly associated with behaviour. They do not tell us *how big an effect* these components have. Second, significance ratios give equal weighting to findings from studies with large numbers and to those from studies with small numbers and do not differentiate between bivariate relationships between a HBM component and behaviour and multivariate associations. In addition, Janz and Becker's analysis does not strictly take into account multiple measures of the same component or multiple behavioural outcomes.

Harrison *et al.*'s (1992) meta-analytic review of the HBM, however, takes cognizance of these considerations. These researchers originally identified 234 published empirical tests of the HBM. Of these, only 16 studies measured all four major components and included reliability checks. This figure clearly demonstrates the extent to which operationalizations of the HBM have failed to measure all components or provide psychometric tests of measures (see Conner 1993).

The meta-analysis involved converting results for HBM components for each study into a common effect size, namely Pearson's *r*. A weighted average of these effect sizes was then computed for each component (see Rosenthal 1984). Figure 2.3 presents findings from this analysis. Across all studies the average correlations between HBM components and behaviour were 0.15, 0.08, 0.13 and −0.21 for susceptibility, severity, benefits and barriers respectively. While these correlations are all statistically significant, they are small in substantive terms. Individual components account

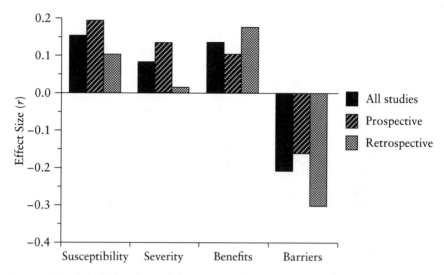

Figure 2.3 Effect sizes for HBM constructs for prospective and retrospective studies (after Harrison *et al.* 1992).

for between just one-half and 4 per cent of variance in behaviour across studies. Unlike Janz and Becker (1984), Harrison *et al.* found different associations for HBM components for cross-sectional versus longitudinal designs. Both benefits and barriers had significantly larger effect sizes in prospective than retrospective research, though in the case of severity the effect size was significantly larger in retrospective studies.

Overall, the results of quantitative reviews of the susceptibility, severity, benefits and barriers components suggest that these variables are very often significant predictors of behaviour but that their effects are small. A number of caveats are important here, however. The first is that the effects of individual health beliefs should be *combined* and the combined effect may be greater than the sum of individual effects. Second, Harrison *et al.* (1992) adopt extremely strict criteria for inclusion in their review and the effect sizes they obtained are based on findings from only 3515 respondents. Finally, Harrison *et al.* point out that their effect sizes also show considerable heterogeneity, which suggests that design or measurement differences across studies or different conceptualizations of the components are influencing their results. We can conclude that, while tests of these HBM components are supportive of their predictive utility, poor operationalizations of the model and failure to check both the reliability and the validity of constructs is a significant drawback with research to date.

3.3 Utility of cues to action and health motivation components

Cues to action and health motivation have been relatively neglected in empirical tests of the HBM. Neither Janz and Becker (1984) nor Harrison *et al.* (1992) include these components in their reviews because of the paucity of studies which employ these variables. One reason for researchers' failure to operationalize these components may be the lack of clear construct definitions. Grady *et al.* (1983), for example, found significant associations between the numbers of family members with breast and other cancers and participation in a breast self-examination teaching programme. These authors did not, however, refer to these measures as 'cues to action', while an almost identical variable in Keesling and Friedman's (1987) study of skin cancer prevention was conceptualized in this way.

Physicians' advice or recommendations have been found to be successful cues to action in the contexts of smoking cessation (Stacy and Lloyd 1990; Weinberger *et al.* 1981) and flu vaccination (Cummings *et al.* 1979). Postcard reminders have also been successful (e.g. Larson *et al.* 1982; Norman and Conner 1993), though the effect of other media cues to action is more doubtful. While Ogionwo (1973) found that a radio, film and poster campaign was successful in attempts to prevent cholera, Mullen *et al.* (1987) found no effect for memory of a mass media campaign upon smokers and Bardsley and Beckman (1988) reported a negative effect of an advert for alcoholism treatment. Knowing someone who is HIV positive or has AIDS has not been predictive of behavioural change among gay men (e.g. McCuskar *et al.* 1989a; Wolcott *et al.* 1990), though Aho (1979b) found that knowing someone who had experienced negative side-effects from influenza vaccination was negatively related to own inoculation behaviour. Measures of 'internal' cues to action, namely the presence or intensity of symptoms, have, not surprisingly perhaps, been generally predictive of behaviour (King 1984; Harris and Lynn 1985; Kelly *et al.* 1987).

Measurements of health motivation have generally comprised just a single item, usually expressing general 'concern' about health, though a small number of researchers have developed psychometric scales (e.g. Maiman *et al.* 1977; Champion 1984). Bivariate relationships between health motivation and health behaviour are generally small but statistically significant (e.g. Ogionwo 1973; Berkanovich *et al.* 1981; Champion 1984; Casey *et al.* 1985), with a small number of non-significant exceptions (e.g. Harris and Guten 1979; Rayant and Sheiham 1980). Findings from multivariate analyses are mixed, with some studies finding positive relationships (e.g. Portnoy 1980; Thompson *et al.* 1986) and others finding no association (e.g. King 1982; Wagner and Curran 1984). Very few studies have attempted to look at direct versus indirect effects of health motivation. One which did (Chen and Land 1986) found that health motivation was negatively related to perceived susceptibility and positively related to severity but did not directly affect behaviour. Chen and Land's (1986) measure of motivation, however, included items relating to control over health and perceived health status. This underlines problems with the discriminant validity of the health motivation construct. Further research is needed to clarify the relationship between this variable and related constructs, such as health locus of control (Wallston and Wallston 1982) and health value (Kristiansen 1985).

3.4 Combining HBM components

The general failure to operationalize the HBM in its entirety may be owing to the suggestion in early formulations that susceptibility and severity might be combined under a single construct, 'threat', and similarly, that benefits and barriers should be subtracted from one another rather than treated as separate components (Becker and Maiman 1975). There is evidence in the literature that some researchers use a threat index rather than measure susceptibility and severity separately (e.g. Kirscht *et al.* 1976) and combine benefits and barriers in a single index (e.g. Oliver and Berger 1979; Gianetti *et al.* 1985). Using a single measure of threat would seem to violate the expectancy-value structure of the HBM and therefore represent an incorrect operationalization of the model (see Feather 1982).

The issue of combining benefits and barriers would seem to be both a theoretical and an empirical issue. At a theoretical level, Weinstein (1988) suggests that there is a qualitative difference between benefits and barriers, at least in hazard situations, which means that they should be treated as distinct constructs. For example, while barriers relating to taking exercise or giving up salt are certain (e.g. time and effort, loss of pleasure), the benefits in terms of avoiding hypertension are more hypothetical. At an empirical level, the benefits component of the model may comprise distinct constructs, namely the efficacy of the behaviour in achieving an outcome (response efficacy) as well as possible psychosocial benefits such as social approval. Similarly, the barriers component may comprise both physical limitations on performing a behaviour (e.g. expense) and psychological costs associated with its performance (e.g. distress). It seems unlikely that a single index could adequately represent all these constructs. On the other hand, where researchers are unable to operationalize all these constructs, factor and reliability analyses might be used to determine whether benefits and barriers can legitimately be combined (e.g. Abraham *et al.* 1992).

A separate issue concerns whether susceptibility and severity scores should combine additively or multiplicatively as the HBM's expectancy value structure would suggest. This issue has been investigated experimentally from a protection motivation theory perspective by Rogers and Mewborn (1976). These researchers found no support for the predicted susceptibility by severity interaction (see also Weinstein 1982; Maddux and Rogers 1983; Rogers 1983; Ronis and Harel 1989). Lewis (1994), in the only HBM study which addresses this question, points out that the severity manipulation check in Rogers and Mewborn's study was not successful and their data do not represent a useful test of the interaction hypothesis. Lewis's data found no support for the interaction hypothesis using parametric and non-parametric statistical tests on retrospective data. In a prospective study, however, the susceptibility × severity interaction contributed a significant amount of unique variance ($sr^2 = 0.12$, $p < 0.05$). This finding comes from a small sample. However, as Lewis suggests, the equation

threat = susceptibility + (susceptibility × severity)

would seem to represent better the effects of the severity component, at least for some health behaviours, than a simple additive model. Kruglanski and Klar (1985) and Weinstein (1988) concur, suggesting that severity must reach a certain magnitude to figure in health decisions, but once that magnitude has been reached decisions are solely a function of perceived susceptibility. The relatively poor findings for the severity component in quantitative reviews appear to support these interpretations, though further research on this issue is clearly needed.

3.5 Utility of HBM components in mediating the impact of past experience or social structural position

In a useful review of literature on the impact of past experience with a behaviour upon its future performance, Sutton (1994) points out that almost all health behaviours are capable of being repeated. Janz and Becker (1984: 44) acknowledge that 'some behaviours (e.g. cigarette smoking; tooth-brushing) have a substantial habitual component obviating any ongoing psychosocial decision-making process', but do not address the question of whether health beliefs might have a role in breaking unhealthy habits. While the issue of whether cognitions mediate the effects of past experience has been a central concern of researchers using the theory of reasoned action (see Bentler and Speckart 1979), few HBM studies measure previous experience with a behaviour.

Only two studies were obtained that explicitly addressed the mediation hypothesis. In a prospective study, Cummings et al. (1979) found both direct and indirect effects for 'past experience with flu shots' upon subsequent inoculation behaviour. Perceived efficacy of vaccination (benefit) and the behavioural intention construct of the theory of reasoned action were both partial mediators of the effects of experience. Two studies by Otten and van der Pligt (1992) tested whether perceived susceptibility mediated the relationship between past and future preventive health behaviours. While past behaviour was predictive of both susceptibility assessments and a proxy measure of future behaviour (behavioural expectation; Warshaw and Davis 1985), susceptibility was negatively associated with expectation and did not mediate the effects of past behaviour. While Otten and van der Pligt's (1992) study is suggestive, these researchers underline the need for further longitudinal research on this issue.

Another important, but relatively neglected, issue concerns the ability of HBM components to mediate the effects of social structural position upon performance of health behaviours. Cummings et al. (1979) found that socioeconomic status (SES) was not related to health beliefs, though both SES and beliefs were significantly related to inoculation behaviour in bivariate analyses. Orbell *et al.* (1995), on the other hand, found that perceived susceptibility and barriers entirely mediated the effects of social class upon uptake of cervical screening. Direct effects were, however, obtained for both marital status and sexual experience. Salloway *et al.* (1978) obtained both direct and indirect effects for occupational status, sex and income and an indirect effect of education upon appointment-keeping at an inner-city hypertension clinic (see also Chen and Land 1990).

Salloway *et al.* (1978) are critical of Rosenstock's (1974) contention that the HBM may be more applicable to middle-class samples because of their 'orientation toward the future, toward deliberate planning, toward deferment of immediate gratification' and point out that working-class people 'are subject to real structural barriers and constrained by real differences in social network structure which are not present in middle class populations' (p. 113). Further research is clearly needed to determine the impact of SES upon health beliefs and behaviour and to discriminate between the effects of cognitions and the effects of non-psychological factors, such as financial constraints, culture of poverty/network effects and health system/provider behaviour barriers, upon the likelihood of health actions (Rundall and Wheeler 1979).

4 Developments

The theoretical and operationalization issues highlighted by the research reviewed above have not led to a reconceptualization of the model. However, two developments in the 1980s are worth consideration. In 1982 King 'extended' the model in a study of screening for hypertension. She included measures of individuals' causal understanding of high blood pressure derived from 'attribution theory' (Kelly 1967), which she theorized as determinants of health beliefs which in turn affected behaviour through intention-formation. The study is noteworthy because it sketches a process model that explores the cognitive foundations of health beliefs and the mechanism by which they might generate action. Using a prospective design King found that eight measures including intention could correctly classify 82 per cent of respondents as either attenders or non-attenders. She also reported that four measures, perceived severity, two measures of perceived benefits and the extent to which respondents identified one or many causes of high blood pressure, accounted for 18 per cent of the variance in behavioural intentions, which was in turn the best single predictor of actual attendance.

In 1974 Rosenstock suggested that a more comprehensive model could reveal how health beliefs are related to other psychological stages in decision-making. King's prospective study is an attempt to do precisely this and is a good early example of how pathways between cognition measures may be empirically examined to provide evidence relating to psychological processes rather than static belief strengths and valences. Unfortunately, the study appears to be unique in HBM-derived research. This failure to extend the model has distanced it from theoretical advances in social cognitive research and later attempts to situate health beliefs in a more comprehensive model of the cognitive prerequisites of action have abandoned the HBM in favour of new conceptual frameworks (see protection motivation theory; Prentice-Dunn and Rogers 1986; Boer and Seydel, Chapter 4 in this volume; Schwarzer and Fuchs, Chapter 6 in this volume).

By 1980 work on 'locus of control' by Rotter (1966) and Wallston *et al.* (1978) and on 'perceived self-efficacy' by Bandura (1977) had established perceived control as an important determinant of health behaviour. King therefore included a measure of perceived control derived from attribution theory, which was found to predict attendance. Later Janz and Becker (1984) also recognized the importance of perceived control but speculated that it might be thought of as a component of perceived barriers to a behaviour rather than an additional theoretical construct. The HBM therefore remained unmodified while Ajzen and Madden (1986) added perceived control to the theory of reasoned action to re-launch it as the theory of planned behaviour. Two years later, Rosenstock *et al.* (1988) acknowledged that Janz and Becker (1984) may have underestimated the importance of this construct and proposed that it be added to the HBM. Unlike King, however, Rosenstock *et al.* offered no new theoretical formulation specifying interactions between beliefs and self-efficacy. They suggested an addition to the HBM measures without an elaboration of its theoretical structure. This may have been short-sighted as recent reviews have suggested that key HBM components may have indirect effects on behaviour as a result of their effect on perceived control, which may be a more proximate determinant of action (Schwarzer 1992). Consequently, despite continued empirical investigation of the HBM framework in the late 1980s and early 1990s, no new conceptual reformulation emerged. The model has not evolved over three decades of research and continues to be a list of potentially useful cognitive predictors.

5 Operationalization of the model

In this section steps in developing a questionnaire based on the HBM are outlined. We briefly review available instruments and examine in detail a study by Champion (1984) which developed health belief scales for investigating frequency of breast self-examination. Determination of reliability and validity of scales is addressed in some depth. Finally, we identify some conceptual difficulties with HBM components and briefly address problems of response bias.

5.1 Developing an HBM questionnaire

Formulating clearly the research question, determining the sample, gaining access to that sample and deciding the mode of data collection (pencil and paper test or structured face-to-face or telephone interview) are generally prerequisites of instrument development. There are then two ways to determine the content of the items of the questionnaire. The first is to conduct a literature search for previous HBM studies in the area and determine whether previous instruments are published or available from the author(s). Scales should be checked to determine whether internal reliability is satisfactory (coefficients > 0.70) and whether the scale has face validity (respondents believe that the scale measures what it says it does). A scale obtained in this way might be used in its entirety or may require modification for use with the intended sample.

Perhaps the most widely used scales in studies of the HBM come from the Standardized Compliance Questionnaire (Sackett *et al.* 1974), which has been modified for use in a variety of settings (e.g. Cerkoney and Hart 1980; Bollin and Hart 1982; Connelly 1984). Unfortunately, this instrument may be quite difficult to obtain. Use of other previously developed scales is common, however, in the HBM literature. Both Calnan (1984) and Hallal (1982) employed measures derived from Stillman's (1977) research on breast cancer. Fincham and Wertheimer (1985) used items derived from Leavitt (1979) in their study of uptake of prescriptions, while Hoogewerf *et al.* (1990) examined compliance with genetic screening using items from Halper *et al.* (1980). There are also published HBM scales in the areas of compliance with hypertension regimens (Abraham and Williams 1991), children's obesity regimens (Maiman *et al.* 1977) and breast self-examination (Champion 1984).

If there is no previously developed HBM scale that might be used or modified for use, then the second route in determining the content of the questionnaire is for researchers to develop scales themselves. A useful example of this process of instrument development is provided by Champion's (1984) study of breast self-examination. The first step involves generating items which purport to measure HBM components (the item pool). Again, previous HBM studies can be used as a guide here. It is good practice, however, for researchers to conduct semi-structured interviews with 20 or 30 potential respondents in order to determine respondents' perceptions of the health threat and beliefs about the behaviour in an open-ended manner. This process will ensure that questionnaire items are salient to the population of interest and will provide guidance on how well medical terminology and other language use will be understood by respondents.

Alternatively, items might be generated in consultation with relevant experts on the behaviour of interest or items might be developed and, then, comments by experts invited. The latter procedure was adopted by Champion. She initially developed 20 to 24 items for each HBM component (excluding cues to action) but then retained only those items which at least six out of eight judges (faculty and doctoral students knowledgeable about the HBM) agreed represented the constructs in question. By this random presentation of items to judges, the *content validity* of each scale, the extent to which the items accurately and adequately reflect the content of that HBM component, is checked.

The next step in developing the instrument is the pilot study. While a small number of studies in the literature report pilots of the instruments employed in the main study (e.g. Eisen *et al.* 1985; Orbell *et al.* 1995), these, unfortunately, are exceptions rather than the rule and may explain some of the difficulties with previous research using the HBM. Champion's pilot questionnaires included the content valid items (10 to 12 items for each construct) and employed a five-point Likert scale for responses ('strongly agree' scored 5 and 'strongly disagree' scored 1). The questionnaires were posted to a convenience sample of women along with a prepaid return envelope. Three hundred and one women participated.

Reliability and validity analyses constitute the final step in determining the content of a questionnaire. Reliability analysis determines whether a scale accurately measures a construct, or, more formally, the amount of random error in measuring a construct. When a scale has high reliability the amount of random error is low. Error owing to sampling of the total content of a construct is measured by coefficients of internal reliability and can be determined by Cronbach's alpha coefficient or the Spearman–Brown formula (see Rust and Golombok 1990). Error over time can be determined by correlating scores on the same scale taken two weeks apart. Champion first determined alpha coefficients for each HBM component, dropping items which reduced the reliability of the scale. While coefficients for three constructs exceeded 0.70 (susceptibility = 0.78, severity = 0.78 and barriers = 0.76), the reliabilities for benefits and health motivation were just 0.62 and 0.61.

Two weeks after the original questionnaires were distributed these revised scales were sent to a subsample who had agreed to take part in a further study. Correlations were computed between scores on the scales at both time-points. These test–retest correlations were satisfactory (> 0.70) for four out of the five components (susceptibility = 0.86, severity = 0.76, benefits = 0.47, barriers = 0.76 and health motivation = 0.81). The *construct validity* of the scales (the extent to which scales measure what they are designed to measure) was next determined by factor analysing all of the scale scores. This statistical procedure sorts individual items into groupings or factors on the basis of correlations between items. Factor analysis showed that, with one exception, items all loaded on the factors (HBM components) they were supposed to, demonstrating satisfactory construct validity. *Criterion validity* was also determined by demonstrating that the HBM components were significantly related to previous practice of breast self-examination. Table 2.2 presents the items used to measure the susceptibility, severity, benefits and barriers components following the reliability and validity checks.

While there are some difficulties with Champion's (1984) analyses,[3] this paper is an important example of good practice in the design of a study using the HBM. Champion rightly contrasts her own study with previous research, pointing out that the validity and reliability of HBM measures has rarely been tested, that multiple-item measures are not

Table 2.2 Items representing susceptibility, severity, benefits and barriers components in a study of breast self-examination (Champion 1984)

Susceptibility
1 My chances of getting breast cancer are great.
2 My physical health makes it more likely that I will get breast cancer.
3 I feel that my chances of getting breast cancer in the future are good.
4 There is a good possibility that I will get breast cancer.
5 I worry a lot about getting breast cancer.
6 Within the next year I will get breast cancer.
  Cronbach's alpha = 0.78

Severity
 1 The thought of breast cancer scares me.
 2 When I think about breast cancer I feel nauseous.
 3 If I had breast cancer my career would be endangered.
 4 When I think about breast cancer my heart beats faster.
 5 Breast cancer would endanger my marriage (or a significant relationship).
 6 Breast cancer is a hopeless disease.
 7 My feelings about myself would change if I got breast cancer.
 8 I am afraid to even think about breast cancer.
 9 My financial security would be endangered if I got breast cancer.
10 Problems I would experience from breast cancer would last a long time.
11 If I got breast cancer, it would be more serious than other diseases.
12 If I had breast cancer, my whole life would change.
  Cronbach's alpha = 0.70

Benefits
1 Doing self breast exams prevents future problems for me.
2 I have a lot to gain by doing self breast exams.
3 Self-breast exams can help me find lumps in my breast.
4 If I do monthly breast exams I may find a lump before it is discovered by regular health exams.
5 I would not be so anxious about breast cancer if I did monthly exams.
  Cronbach's alpha = 0.61

Barriers
1 It is embarrassing for me to do monthly breast exams.
2 In order for me to do monthly breast exams I have to give up quite a bit.
3 Self-breast exams can be painful.
4 Self-breast exams are time consuming.
5 My family would make fun of me if I did self breast exams.
6 The practice of self breast exams interferes with my activities.
7 Doing self breast exams would require starting a new habit, which is difficult.
8 I am afraid I would not be able to do self breast exams.
  Cronbach's alpha = 0.76

routinely employed, that operational definitions vary across studies and that nominal-level operationalizations have limited statistical explorations of the relationships between measures.

5.2 Problems of operationalization: conceptual difficulties with HBM components

Champion's (1984) analysis of methodological problems in HBM research and the heterogeneity of effect sizes obtained by Harrison *et al.* (1992) highlight difficulties with the conceptual bases of HBM components. A variety of theorists have drawn attention to several problematic assumptions made by the HBM, namely that the relationships between HBM components and behaviour are both fixed and linear and that the components themselves are unidimensional. In this section we briefly review recent theorizing relevant to the conceptualization of each of the components of HBM.

Susceptibility
Becker and Maiman (1975: 20) acknowledge the wide variety of operationalizations of susceptibility:

> Hochbaum's questions apparently emphasized the concept of perceived *possibility* of contracting the disease; Kegeles' questions were directed at *probability* of becoming ill; Heinzelmann requested estimates of likelihood of *recurrence*, while Elling, Gordis, and Becker asked for similar *re-susceptibility* estimates from the mother concerning her child; and Rosenstock introduced '*self-reference*' versus '*reference to men (women) your age*' (as well as 'fixed-alternative' versus 'open-ended' items). (Italics in the original.)

Ostensibly, these different measurements are unproblematic. However, Tversky and Kahneman (1981) show that even quite small changes in the wording of risk choices have significant and predictable effects upon responses. Thus, considerable care needs be taken in the phrasing of items measuring perceived susceptibility, and multi-item measures are essential.

A variety of cognitive heuristics are also important in understanding people's susceptibility judgements. Slovic *et al.* (1977) point out that, in general, people seem to overestimate the frequency of rare causes of death and underestimate common causes of death. In particular, events that are dramatic or personally relevant, and therefore easy to imagine or recall, tend to be overestimated. There is also a tendency for people to underestimate the extent to which they are personally vulnerable to health and life-threatening problems. Weinstein (1980) has termed this phenomenon 'unrealistic optimism'. This sense of unique invulnerability has been demonstrated in the context of both relative risk comparisons of self to others (e.g. Weinstein 1984) and subjective versus objective risk appraisals (Gerrard and Warner 1991). Cognitive factors, including perceptions of control, egocentric bias, personal experience and stereotypical beliefs, have been posited as explanations for this tendency, as well as motivational factors, including self-esteem maintenance and defensive coping (see van der Pligt *et al.* 1993). These cognitive and motivational processes involved in risk estimation have clear implications for understanding the small effect sizes obtained between susceptibility estimates and health-protective behaviours (Harrison *et al.* 1992) and require further research.

Weinstein (1988) has recently drawn attention to a number of more fundamental difficulties with the HBM conceptualization of the susceptibility component. He points out that most studies request a risk estimate but often fail to provide respondents with the option of saying whether they have even heard of the threat in question. He is also critical of the static conceptualization of this component and suggests instead that beliefs about susceptibility should be characterized in terms of three stages. The first stage involves the awareness that the health threat exists. The second stage involves determining how dangerous the threat is and how many people are likely to be infected. This is inevitably an ambiguous question and many people will display unrealistic optimism at this stage. Only in the final stage, when the threat has been personalized, will personal susceptibility be acknowledged. While little research has, as yet, been conducted on Weinstein's processual account of risk perception, this approach does seem to offer insight into differential underestimates of susceptibility.

A final issue that should be addressed in the context of susceptibility concerns the interpretation of correlations between perceived susceptibility and health behaviour. One difficulty with cross-sectional HBM studies is that both positive and negative associations between risk and behaviour are easily interpreted. For example, suppose someone believes he is at risk of HIV infection and therefore decides that he will use a condom during sex. In this case high susceptibility leads to safer behaviour – the correlation is positive. The same person, having adopted safer sex, however, can now estimate his risk of infection as low. Here, safer behaviour leads to lowered susceptibility – the correlation is negative. Cross-sectional data, then, are problematic since we cannot determine whether beliefs give rise to behaviour or vice versa. In a review of this issue Weinstein and Nicolich (1993: 244) conclude that 'the correlation between perceived personal risk and simultaneous preventive behaviours should not be used to assess the effects of perceptions on behaviour. It is an indicator of risk perception accuracy.' They underline the need for longitudinal analyses and stress the importance of assessing cognitions immediately after risk information has been received by respondents, before they have had an opportunity to change their behaviour. Only under these circumstances can causal inferences about perceived susceptibility be confidently made.

Severity
Severity has been conceptualized as a multidimensional construct involving both the medical severity of a disease (pain, complications, etc.) and its

psychosocial severity (the extent to which the disease might interfere with valued social roles). Unfortunately, as Haefner (1974: 96) points out: 'In examining the literature, one becomes aware of the variation in the selection of particular dimensions of seriousness to be studied.' A number of recent studies have drawn attention to other important dimensions of the severity construct. Smith Klohn and Rogers (1991), in a study of osteoporosis prevention, used essays to manipulate three severity dimensions: visibility of disablement (high versus low), time of onset (near versus distant future) and rate of onset (gradual versus sudden). These researchers obtained a significant main effect for visibility and a significant interaction between visibility and time of onset on post-test intention measures. The more visibly disabling descriptions of the effects of osteoporosis were, the stronger were intentions to take preventive action. Moreover, low visibility consequences in the distant future were associated with less intention than high visibility effects with either time of onset. These findings underline the utility of presenting information about how quickly the consequences of a medical condition are likely to occur.

Ronis and Harel (1989) combined elements of the HBM and subjective expected utility (SEU) theory in a study of breast examination behaviours. Since breast examination leads to early detection and treatment, these researchers divided the severity component into severity given action (severity of breast cancer if treated promptly) and severity given inaction (severity of breast cancer if treated late). They found support for this distinction using confirmatory factor analysis. Path analysis showed that severity dimensions did not directly affect behaviour. Rather, the benefits component entirely mediated the effects of severity. This study is an interesting reconceptualization of the threat component of the HBM. Instead of directly influencing behaviour, threat appraisal is conceived as contributing to the subjective utility of taking action versus not taking action. Ronis and Harel also suggest that this reconceptualization could be extended to behaviours which reduce susceptibility to a health problem. In this instance, measures of susceptibility need to be made conditional upon behaviour. Clearly further research comparing the direct effects (Janz and Becker 1984), interactive (e.g. Lewis 1994) and mediational (Ronis and Harel 1989) models of severity should be a priority.

Benefits, barriers, cues to action and health motivation

A major conceptual difficulty shared by the remaining components of the HBM concerns acknowledgement of the multidimensionality of these constructs in operationalizations of the model. As was noted, the benefits component comprises both medical and psychosocial benefits of engaging in health-promoting behaviours. Similarly, the barriers component comprises practical barriers to performing the behaviour (e.g. time, expense, availability, transport, waiting time) as well as psychological costs associated with performing the behaviour (pain, embarrassment, threat to well-being or lifestyle and livelihood). More recent HBM formulations (Rosenstock *et al.* 1988) also include psychological barriers to performing the behaviour. While perceived confidence in one's ability to undertake correctly the recommended action – self-efficacy (Bandura 1986) – has received considerable attention, other psychological barriers might include poor understanding of complex recommendations (e.g. a learning disabled person with diabetes) or lack of social skills (e.g. successfully to negotiate condom use).

The cues to action component comprises a huge variety of possible social influences upon behaviour, ranging from awareness and memory of mass media campaigns, through leaflets and reminder letters, to descriptive and injunctive social norms from medical professionals and significant others. Weinstein (1988) argues that the cues to action component sits rather uneasily alongside the rational expectancy-value structure of the model's major components. Arguably, operationalizations of cues to action could ask respondents about the presence or absence of cues and also ask them to indicate the extent to which available cues influence their decisions (see Bagozzi 1986), thereby capturing an expectancy-value structure. What is crucial, however, is that the range of relevant cues is assessed. Similarly, operationalizations of the health motivation construct require theoretical specification in order to determine whether the related notions of health locus of control or health value need to be simultaneously assessed or more adequately represent the researcher's hypotheses. Finally, it is important also that measures of these components are relevant to intended samples. Identification of sample-relevant benefits, barriers and cues to action can be determined through open-ended pilot interviews and are likely to be better behavioural predictors than researcher-imposed conceptualizations of these components.

5.3 Problems of operationalization: response bias

A final issue concerns identifying and controlling for the effects of social desirability bias in studies of the HBM. It seems likely that respondents are generally aware of the purposes of interviews and questionnaires and may be motivated to exaggerate both the desirability of their beliefs and behaviours and the consistency between the two. Unfortunately, there is little evidence in the literature that this issue has received appropriate consideration. While longitudinal studies and objective outcome measures help to reduce bias, individual difference measures of social desirability should properly be used in all HBM studies. Sheeran and Orbell (1995) have shown that responses to HBM components may also be subject to bias when questionnaire items are not randomized and can easily be 'read' by respondents. One very effective means of controlling for this type of bias is to ask respondents to complete both actual and ideal questionnaire responses. Where this is not feasible, then ratings by judges or a subgroup of the main sample might be covaried with respondents' answers.

6 Applications of the model to HIV-preventive behaviour

The spread of human immunodeficiency virus (HIV) has prompted research into modifiable determinants of HIV-preventive behaviours such as condom use and restriction of sexual partners. This work began with homosexual men but was extended to sexually active adolescents when they were identified as potentially at risk. The HBM had been employed to explore contraceptive behaviour (e.g. Herold 1983; Hester and Macrina 1985) and was presented as a potentially useful theoretical framework for HIV-preventive education.

6.1 Utility of the model in identifying the cognitive determinants of HIV-preventive sexual behaviour among homosexual men

In an early cross-sectional study of the determinants of HIV risk behaviour among homosexual men in Chicago, Emmons *et al.* (1986) found effects for both perceived susceptibility and perceived efficacy/benefits of behaviour change. Perceived susceptibility was found to be significantly but weakly associated with reported efforts to reduce numbers of sexual partners and strongly but negatively associated with avoidance of anonymous partners. Although perceived efficacy was generally very high, variance on this measure was associated with reported behaviour change, including attempts to reduce partner numbers, avoidance of anal intercourse and safer intercourse practice. These results suggested that HBM-specified beliefs could contribute to the promotion of HIV-preventive behaviour among homosexual men. However, the negative association between susceptibility and anonymous partner contact suggested that respondents' awareness of their past behaviour could be shaping reported beliefs, thereby highlighting the need for longitudinal research.

A follow-up longitudinal study of this cohort (Joseph *et al.* 1987) revealed that health beliefs had little impact on reported behaviour over the subsequent six months. The perceived efficacy effect disappeared and perceived susceptibility was only associated with avoidance of anonymous partners. This relationship remained negative, clarifying that increased susceptibility may render certain groups less likely to take preventive behaviour. The only cognitive variable which was consistently related to a range of time 2 behaviour measures was descriptive norms, that is perceptions that peers were changing their behaviour. Discussing these findings, Joseph *et al.* (1987) noted that HIV-relevant cognitions may change over time and that only beliefs held immediately before a behaviour influence it (see also Boldero *et al.* 1992).

Similar results were reported by McCusker and colleagues, using HBM measures to study the behaviour of homosexual men in Boston. A cross-sectional study (McCuskar *et al.* 1989b) showed that only age and lifetime partners were associated with number of partners and that only reported effort to change behaviour significantly distinguished between condom users and non-users. Although health belief measures were not significantly related to behaviour, perceived susceptibility and severity were associated with reported effort, suggesting that they may affect behaviour indirectly through more proximal cognitions. A 12-month longitudinal follow-up (McCuskar *et al.* 1989a) found that only previous number of partners predicted subsequent partner numbers and that susceptibility was significantly related to adoption of condom use during receptive, but not insertive, intercourse. In all cases past behaviour was found to be the most powerful predictor of subsequent behaviours.

The importance of past behaviour was confirmed by Siegel *et al.* (1989), who found that the number of years for which homosexual men had engaged in regular intercourse with men was significantly associated with reported safer sexual behaviour six months later. In this study drug use during sex, perceived emotional support and perceived difficulty of behaviour change/self-efficacy also predicted safer sexual behaviour. Aspinwall *et al.* (1991) found that previous numbers of partners accounted for 51 per cent of the variance in reported partner number six months later, with health beliefs accounting for 5 per cent of the variance and health belief interactions, and with HIV status, partner HIV status and age adding a further 10 per cent. Only prior behaviour and perceived barriers to behaviour change were significantly associated with subsequent safer sexual behaviour, accounting for 12 per cent of the variance.

Collectively, these studies suggested that HIV risk behaviour is self-perpetuating, that increased levels of perceived susceptibility could prompt denial in those already aware of their HIV risk and that other measures, including descriptive norms, perceived self-efficacy and contextual factors such as drug use, are more important predictors of HIV-preventive behaviour than HBM-specified variables.

6.2 Utility of the model in identifying the cognitive determinants of HIV-preventive sexual behaviour among young heterosexuals

There have been fewer studies of the antecedents of adolescent HIV-preventive behaviour (Boyer and Kegeles 1991). An early cross-sectional survey showed that adolescents who believed that condoms were effective in preventing HIV transmission and who felt susceptible to HIV infection were significantly more likely to report always using condoms during intercourse (Hingson *et al.* 1990). However, HBM-specified beliefs accounted for less than 15 per cent of the variance in behaviour measures. Rosenthal *et al.* (1992) were critical of the measures employed by Hingson *et al.* and reported another cross-sectional study showing that HBM measures were not associated with young men's HIV risk behaviour or young women's behaviour with regular partners. Perceived susceptibility, however, accounted for 13 per cent of the variance in young women's reported HIV risk behaviour with *casual* partners.

Longitudinal studies are required to test the relevance of findings from studies of homosexual men to adolescent sexual behaviour. In one such study the present authors employed a HBM framework to model the psychological antecedents of adolescent condom use on the east coast of Scotland (Abraham *et al.* 1995). This study attempted to assess the degree to which health beliefs would predict consistency of condom use over the subsequent year.

School lists of pupils below the minimum school leaving age were used to select random quota samples of teenagers from two cohorts (16- and 18-year-olds). A postal questionnaire containing HBM-based items was constructed after piloting and a response rate of 64 per cent yielded 690 questionnaires. These respondents were sent a second questionnaire one year later, including items concerning their sexual behaviour and condom use over the previous year. A 52 per cent response rate resulted in a longitudinal sample of 333. Of these, 122 who reported new sexual partners over the study year were retained for analysis. These respondents were of particular interest because they had been in a situation in which condom use should have been an issue according to available HIV-relevant health education campaigns. This sample consisted of 81 women (66.4 per cent) and 41 men (33.6 per cent).

As well as HBM measures, the initial questionnaire included an intention item because previous work had suggested that the effects of health beliefs may be partially or wholly mediated by intentions (e.g. Cummings *et al.* 1979). A measure of perceived condom-use norms was also included because supportive risk-reduction norms had been found to be associated with preventive behaviours among homosexual men (Joseph *et al.* 1987). Intention to use condoms was operationalized using a five-point Likert item: 'In future I intend to use a condom if I have sex with someone new' (strongly agree to strongly disagree) and perceived condom-use norm was measured by two seven-point items (Cronbach's alpha = 0.75): 'How many heterosexual men/women of your age would agree with the statement "I will use a condom if I have sex with someone new"').

Eight HBM measures were included. Perceived susceptibility was measured using four items (Cronbach's alpha = 0.76): 'How likely do you think it is that you will get the AIDS virus in the next five years?' (seven response options from 'extremely unlikely' to 'extremely likely'); and three items concerning HIV spread, 'Thinking of heterosexual people in Scotland of your age, how many do you think will have been infected by the AIDS virus in (one year/five years/ten years) time?' (seven response options, 'none' through 'about half' to 'all'). Perceived severity was measured using two seven-point items (Cronbach's alpha = 0.63): 'How many people who get the AIDS virus develop AIDS?' and 'How many people who get AIDS actually die of it?' ('none' to 'all').

Eight five-point Likert items were used to measure perceived benefits of and barriers to condom use. Principal components analysis with varimax rotation yielded three factors for the time 1 sample (Abraham *et al.* 1992). However, one of the resulting measures fell below acceptable reliability for respondents with new partners at time 2 and was divided into two single-item measures; perceived condom offensiveness ('I would be offended if someone who wanted to have sex with me suggested protecting themselves against the AIDS virus') and perceived condom casualness ('People would think I wanted casual sex if I carried condoms'). Three items were employed to measure perceived condom effectiveness (Cronbach's alpha = 0.76): 'Using a condom is effective in preventing a man from passing the AIDS virus to a woman', 'Using a condom is effective in preventing a woman from passing the AIDS virus to a man' and 'Using condoms is a good way to avoid unwanted pregnancy'. A measure of perceived condom attractiveness also consisted of three items (Cronbach's alpha = 0.55): 'Most people find condoms awkward to use', 'Condoms would not spoil the pleasure of having sex' and 'A person thinking of having sex with me would probably be pleased if I suggested using a condom'.

Cues to action were measured by asking whether respondents remembered eight specified United Kingdom AIDS-education campaigns (score range 0–8). Finally, a single Likert item ('Health is less important than enjoyment') was used to measure relative health value.

In addition, three measures of previous sexual behaviour, lifetime partners, prior condom use and intercourse frequency, were included. Respondents were asked to record the number of people they had ever had sexual intercourse with, whether or not they had ever used a condom during sex (yes/no) and how often they had had sexual intercourse in the previous year (never, once, more than once). Finally, three demographic measures were included, gender, age and socioeconomic status. Socioeconomic status was indexed using the Registrar General's classification of father's occupation.

The follow-up questionnaire included four items assessing respondents' consistency of condom use ('How often do you use condoms during sex?'; five response options, 'never/almost never' through 'sometimes' to 'almost always/always') and three consecutive items asking how often in the past year they had: 'had sexual intercourse', 'used a condom during intercourse' and 'not used a condom during intercourse' (five response options, 'never', 'once', 'most months', 'most weeks' and 'most days'). A ratio score was calculated by dividing the reported frequency of condom use during intercourse in the previous year by the reported frequency of intercourse over the year. This was significantly correlated with responses to the other two items (rs = 0.61, 0.71) and the three response distributions formed a reliable measure (Cronbach's alpha = 0.83).

A four-step hierarchical multiple regression was conducted to assess the extent to which the time 1 variables were able to predict reported condom use consistency. In order to assess what predictive power HBM measures and the perceived norm measure would add to the effect of intention, intention was entered in step 1 followed by the other cognitive variables in step 2. Previous behaviour measures were entered in step 3 followed by demographic variables in step 4. As can be seen from Table 2.3, the

Table 2.3 Predictors of consistent condom use among adolescents with new partners in the previous year

Step	Independent variable	Beta	p
1	Intention	0.15	0.13
	$F = 3.20$, d.f. $= 1$, 120, $p = 0.08$		
2	Susceptibility	0.00	0.97
	Severity	0.02	0.78
	Condom offensiveness	−0.05	0.54
	Condom casualness	−0.08	0.38
	Condom attractiveness	0.10	0.27
	Condom effectiveness	−0.08	0.40
	Campaign memory	0.01	0.94
	Relative health value	0.05	0.55
	Condom use	−0.09	0.40
	$F = 1.26$, d.f. $= 10$, 111, $p = 0.26$		
3	Lifetime partners	−0.22	0.05
	Intercourse frequency	−0.27	0.06
	Previous condom use	0.19	0.07
	$F = 1.98$, d.f. $= 13$, 108, $p = 0.03$, $R^2 = 0.19$, adj. $R^2 = 0.10$		
4	Age	−0.21	0.02
	Gender	0.31	0.00
	Socioeconomic status	−0.13	0.13
	$F = 2.94$, d.f. $= 16$, 105, $p = 0.00$, $R^2 = 0.31$, adj. $R^2 = 0.24$		

regression equation failed to reach significance until the previous behaviour measures were entered in step 3.

These results suggest that the HBM measures are not useful predictors of adolescent condom use and confirm the findings of studies of homosexual men by emphasizing the importance of previous behaviour as a correlate of safer sexual behaviour. Of course, health beliefs specified by the HBM may be prerequisite to adolescent HIV-preventive behaviour. In a well-informed population prerequisite beliefs may be so widely accepted that they no longer effectively distinguish between people who do and do not take precautions. In this study, for example, perceived severity and perceived condom effectiveness were uniformly high and were therefore unlikely to discriminate between degrees of condom use. In such populations, further cognition measures, which distinguish between those who do and do not adopt recommended behaviours, are required.

The failure of our intention measure significantly to predict condom use consistency may be more complex. This finding is less convincing because the intention measure employed only a single item. In addition, the observed intention–behaviour relationship is likely to have been weakened by a failure to measure the two variables at the same level of specificity; that is, the intention item referred to new partners while the behaviour items referred to condom use in general. Finally, an interesting gender difference appears to have affected the intention–behaviour relationship. Zero order correlations show that the intention and behaviour measures are significantly correlated for men ($r = 0.33$, $p < 0.05$) but not for women ($r = 0.15$). Similar gender effects on adolescents' HIV-preventive intentions were reported by Petosa and Kirby (1991) and these findings lend support to the results of qualitative studies suggesting that young women may be disempowered in sexual negotiation so that their good intentions are not translated into action (Holland *et al.* 1990). Although these are plausible reasons for the failure of this intention measure to account for significant proportions of the variance in reported consistency of condom use, it should be noted that intentions also failed to predict behaviour in one of the few previous prospective studies of the cognitive antecedents of adolescent condom use (Breakwell *et al.* 1994).

The effects of previous behaviour suggest that condom use may be self-perpetuating (see Abraham and Sheeran 1993) and that those reporting greatest previous sexual activity are least likely to report consistent condom use. This suggests that those most at risk from HIV may be the least likely to take precautions. Finally, women, older teenagers and those from higher class backgrounds reported less consistent condom use. The effects of age and class are likely to be mediated by higher numbers of sexual partners. However, the age effect mirrors Schaalma *et al.*'s (1993) observation that older Dutch teenagers had more negative perceptions of condoms, thereby emphasizing the importance of condom promotion interventions with this group.

Overall, available evidence recommends that young men and women's HIV-preventive behaviour should be considered separately and suggests that cognitions other than those specified by the HBM will be required to promote safer sexual behaviour effectively among adolescents (Brown *et al.* 1991).

6.3 Implications of HBM-based studies of HIV-preventive behaviour

Research in this area has highlighted the complexity of HIV-preventive behaviour and the limitations of the HBM. HIV is not highly infectious and the consequences of infection are delayed but fatal. The salience of a fatal outcome may lead to a rapid consensus regarding severity while limited transmission routes and delayed effects produce a general failure to acknowledge personal susceptibility. Such ceiling and floor effects may limit the extent to which these measures can distinguish between those who do and those who do not take precautions (Abraham *et al.* 1992). Moreover, as we have noted above, increasing perceptions of threat among individuals who already acknowledge personal susceptibility may prompt maladaptive coping in the form of denial and thereby increase the likelihood of risk behaviour (see also van der Pligt *et al.* 1993).

It has been suggested that the theory of reasoned action may offer a better account of HIV-preventive behaviour than the HBM (Montgomery *et al.* 1989; Brown *et al.* 1991), both because it acknowledges the importance of others' approval in the subjective norm construct and because intention formation provides a mechanism through which beliefs might influence behaviour. Studies employing measures derived from the theory of reasoned action offer some support for this suggestion, showing that social norms are important determinants of HIV-preventive behaviour (Joseph *et al.* 1987: Fisher *et al.* 1992) and that the effect of health beliefs can be accounted for by intentions. Warwick *et al.* (1993), for example, demonstrated that the effects of health beliefs on a subsequent measure of condom use at last intercourse were entirely mediated by an intention measure. However, intentions themselves may be unreliable antecedents of HIV-preventive behaviour (Boldero *et al.* 1992; Warwick *et al.* 1993; Breakwell *et al.* 1994; Abraham *et al.* 1995) and more detailed measures of commitment and planning may be required to distinguish accurately between those who do and do not take precautions (Schwarzer 1992; Gollwitzer 1993; Abraham and Sheeran 1994).

The social nature of sexual behaviour goes beyond an awareness of others' approval. Sexual behaviour is fundamentally interactive and has high emotional and arousal content. Consequently, the social skills involved in interpersonal negotiation and individual differences in emotional responses to sexual stimuli may be better predictors of safer sexual behaviour than the socially learnt beliefs specified by the HBM (Abraham and Sheeran 1993). There is evidence suggesting that perceived self-efficacy, which may be an important cognitive component of skill (Bandura 1992), is a useful predictor of safer sexual behaviour (Rosenthal *et al.* 1991; Schaalma *et al.* 1993) and that representations of anticipated affective states such as anticipated regret may also guide HIV-preventive behaviour (Richard and van der Pligt 1991; Richard *et al.* 1995). Further exploration of the cognitive components of skills required to overcome situational barriers to safer sex practice, such as drug and alcohol use, would be especially useful to health educators.

Studies have revealed different psychological antecedents of HIV-preventive behaviour among HIV-seropositive gay men and other gay men, teenage men and women, those of different ages, those in monogamous and non-monogamous relationships and those with more or less sexual experience (Aspinwall *et al.* 1991; Richard and van der Pligt 1991; Abraham *et al.* 1992; Schaalma *et al.* 1993). Campaigns which target specific beliefs may therefore have different effects on specified sub-groups. In other words, the relationships between health beliefs and behaviour may vary across groups with very different sexual histories. This also suggests that different groups may require different skills. Young women's difficulties in implementing their good intentions (Abraham *et al.* 1994) highlight the issue of gendered power relations in heterosexual encounters (Holland *et al.* 1990) and imply that young women may need to develop powerful negotiating strategies before their individual beliefs and values can affect safer sex practice. More detailed consideration of sexual scripts may be necessary before this can be achieved (Miller *et al.* 1993).

Finally, the term 'HIV-preventive behaviour' obscures the behavioural complexity of safer sex practice. Condom use, for example, involves a series of behaviours including getting condoms, carrying them, negotiating their use and handling and using them correctly. In practice, then, research in this area is attempting to identify the psychological prerequisites of a series of behaviours among a range of different groups. Moreover, it concerns the maintenance of these behavioural sequences over time rather than a single performance (Montgomery *et al.* 1989). Overall, it appears that the HBM is too distant from the cognitive processes involved in the regulation of such complex behaviours to offer a productive theoretical framework for this work.

7 Future directions

The HBM has provided a useful theoretical framework for investigators of the cognitive determinants of a wide range of behaviours for more than 30 years. Its common sense constructs are easy for non-psychologists to assimilate and apply and it can be readily and inexpensively operationalized. It has focused researchers' and health care professionals' attention on modifiable psychological prerequisites of behaviour and provided a basis for practical interventions across a range of behaviours (e.g. Jones *et al.* 1987). Research to date has, however, been predominantly cross-sectional in design and further prospective studies are required to clarify the causal direction of observed belief–behaviour relationships. The proposed mediation of socioeconomic influences on health also remains unclear. Research identifying which beliefs or cognitions mediate the effects of socioeconomic status in relation to particular health behaviours (e.g. Orbell *et al.* 1995) would be especially valuable.

Despite the impressive record of HBM-inspired research, numerous limitations have been identified which detract from the contribution this framework can make to future modelling of the cognitive determinants of behaviour. Its common sense, expectancy-value framework simplifies health-related representational processes, and qualitative distinctions between beliefs encompassed by each construct may be important to understanding why an individual does or does not undertake a specified behaviour. Such broadly defined theoretical components mean that different operationalizations may not be strictly comparable. Further elaboration of HBM constructs, as seen in Weinstein's (1988) 'precaution adoption process', may therefore be necessary. The model also excludes cognitions which have been shown to be powerful predictors of behaviour. In contrast to the theory of reasoned action, it fails to address the importance of intention formation or the influence that others' approval may have upon our behaviour. It portrays individuals as asocial economic decision-makers and consequently fails to account for behaviour under social and affective control. This is especially evident in its application to sexual behaviour, where, despite initial optimism, it has failed to distinguish between 'safer' and 'unsafe' behaviour patterns.

The model is also limited because it does not articulate anticipated relationships between cognitions. Despite King's (1982, 1984) innovative extension the model has not distinguished between proximal and distal antecedents of behaviour. More recent models, such as the theory of planned behaviour (Ajzen and Madden 1986; Conner and Sparks, Chapter 5 in this volume) and protection motivation theory (Prentice-Dunn and Rogers 1986; Boer and Seydel, Chapter 4 in this volume) propose direct and indirect cognitive influences on behaviour. This facilitates a more powerful analysis of data and a clearer indication of how interventions might have their effects. For example, if a certain level of perceived severity is a threshold condition for the operation of perceived susceptibility on behaviour this would explain its generally weak associations with behaviour but would suggest that it be retained as a more distal cognitive antecedent (Schwarzer 1992). Intentions and perceived self-efficacy may mediate the effects of beliefs on behaviour (Cummings *et al.* 1979; Warwick *et al.* 1993), confirming Rosenstock's (1974: 371) suggestion that HBM constructs could be seen as 'the setting for . . . subsequent responses at other stages in the decision process' leading to action. More recent work has focused upon specifying cognitions which distinguish between those who intend and do undertake a behaviour and those who intend and do not (Schwarzer 1992; Gollwitzer 1993). Health beliefs may, therefore, be seen as increasingly distant from action facilitation and regulation processes.

Notes

1 There is also a substantial literature using children as participants which will not be considered here (see Gochman and Parcel 1982, for review).
2 The number of hypotheses examined for each HBM component varies across behaviour types. The relevant numbers for vulnerability, severity, benefits and barriers in the case of preventive behaviours are 21, 18, 19 and 14, respectively. In the case of sick role behaviours the number of hypotheses are 13, 16, 15 and 12, respectively.
3 Champion's (1984) paper mistakenly refers to the regression of breast self-examination practice upon HBM components as evidence for *construct* rather than *criterion* validity. There is also some difficulty with interpretation of the factor analysis in that a three-factor solution for the perceived severity component was not pursued. An item relating to having 'relative and friends with breast cancer' (p. 83) was not interpreted as a cue to action – a component of the HBM which was ignored in Champion's analysis. Finally, further item development on the benefits component should properly have been conducted in order to improve its poor reliability.

References

Abraham, I.L. and Williams, B.M. (1991) Hypertensive elders perception and management of their disease: health beliefs or health decisions?, *Journal of Applied Gerontology*, 10, 444–54.

Abraham, S.C.S. and Sheeran, P. (1993) In search of a psychology of safer-sex promotion; beyond beliefs and texts, *Health Education Research: Theory and Practice*, 8, 245–54.

Abraham, S.C.S. and Sheeran, P. (1994) Modelling and modifying young heterosexuals' HIV-preventive behaviour; a review of theories, findings and educational implications, *Patient Education and Counselling*, 23, 173–86.

Abraham, S.C.S., Sheeran, P., Abrams, D. and Spears, R. (1995) Health beliefs and teenage condom use: a prospective study, manuscript submitted for publication.

Abraham, S.C.S., Sheeran, P., Spears, R. and Abrams, D. (1992) Health beliefs and the promotion of HIV-preventive intentions amongst teenagers: a Scottish perspective, *Health Psychology*, 11, 363–70.

Aho, W.R. (1979a) Smoking, dieting and exercise: age differences in attitudes and behaviour relevant to selected health belief model variables, *Rhode Island Medical Journal*, 62, 95–102.

Aho, W.R. (1979b) Participation of senior citizens in the Swine Flu inoculation programme: an analysis of health belief model variables in preventive health behaviour, *Journal of Gerontology*, 34, 201–8.

Ajzen, I. and Madden, T.J. (1986) Prediction of goal-directed behaviour: attitudes, intentions and perceived behavioral control, *Journal of Experimental Social Psychology*, 22, 453–74.

Alagna, S.W. and Reddy D.M. (1987) Predictors of proficient technique and successful lesion detention in breast self-examination, *Health Psychology*, 3, 113–27.

Aspinwall, L.G., Kemeny, M.E., Taylor, S.E., Schneider, S.G. and Dudley, J.P. (1991) Psychosocial predictors of gay men's AIDS risk-reduction behaviour, *Health Psychology*, 10, 432–44.

Bagozzi, R.P. (1986) Attitude formation under the theory of reasoned action and a purposeful behaviour reformulation, *British Journal of Social Psychology*, 25, 95–107.

Bandura, A. (1977) Self-efficacy: towards a unifying theory of behavioural change, *Psychological Review*, 84, 191–215.

Bandura, A. (1986) *Social Foundations of Thought and Action*. Englewood-Cliffs, NJ: Erlbaum.

Bandura, A. (1992) Exercise of personal agency through the self-efficacy mechanism. In R. Schwarzer (ed.) *Self-efficacy: Thought Control of Action*. Washington, DC: Hemisphere, 3–38.

Bardsley, P.E. and Beckman, L.J. (1988) The health belief model and entry into alcoholism treatment, *International Journal of the Addictions*, 23, 19–28.

Beck, K.H. (1981) Driving while under the influence of alcohol: relationship to attitudes and beliefs in a college sample, *American Journal of Drug and Alcohol Abuse*, 8, 377–88.

Becker, M.H., Drachman, R.H. and Kirscht, P. (1972) Predicting mothers' compliance with pediatric medical regimens, *Journal of Pediatrics*, 81, 843.

Becker, M.H., Drachman, R.H. and Kirscht, P. (1974) A new approach to explaining sick-role behaviour in low income populations, *American Journal of Public Health*, 64, 205–16.

Becker, M.H., Haefner D.P., Kasl, S.V., Kirscht, J.P., Maiman, L.A. and Rosenstock, I.M. (1977a) Selected psychosocial models and correlates of individual health-related behaviors, *Medical Care*, **15**, 27–46.

Becker, M.H., Haefner D.P. and Maiman L.A. (1977b) The health belief model in the prediction of dietary compliance: a field experiment, *Journal of Health and Social Behaviour*, **18**, 348–66.

Becker, M.H., Kaback, M.M., Rosenstock, I.R. and Ruth, M. (1975) Some influences of public participation in a genetic screening program, *Journal of Community Health*, **1**, 3–14.

Becker, M.H. and Maiman, L.A. (1975). Sociobehavioural determinants of compliance with health and medical care recommendations. *Medical Care*, **13**, 10–24.

Becker, M.H., Radius, S.M. and Rosenstock, I.M. (1978) Compliance with a medical regimen for asthma: a test of the health belief model, *Public Health Reports*, **93**, 268–77.

Bentler, P.M. and Speckart, G. (1979) Models of attitude-behaviour relations, *Psychological Review*, **86**, 452–64.

Berkanovich, E., Telesky, C. and Reeder, S. (1981) Structural and social psychological factors on the decision to seek medical care for symptoms, *Medical Care*, **19**, 693–709.

Boldero, J., Moore, S. and Rosenthal, D. (1992) Intention, context, and safe sex: Australian adolescents' responses to AIDS, *Journal of Applied Social Psychology*, **22**, 1374–98.

Bollin N.W. and Hart, L.K. (1982) The relationship of health belief motivations, health focus of control and health valuing to dietary compliance of haemodialysis patients, *American Association of Nephrology Nurses and Technicians Journal*, **9**, 41–7.

Boyer, C.B. and Kegeles, S.M. (1991) AIDS risk and prevention among adolescents, *Social Science and Medicine*, **33**, 11–23.

Bradley, C., Gamsu, D.S. and Moses S.L. (1987) The use of diabetes-specific perceived control and health belief measures to predict treatment choice and efficacy in a feasibility study of continuous subcutaneous insulin infusion pumps, *Psychology and Health*, **1**, 133–46.

Breakwell, G.M., Millward, L.J. and Fife-Schaw, C. (1994) Commitment to 'safer' sex as a predictor of condom use among 16–20 year olds, *Journal of Applied Social Psychology*, **24**, 189–217.

Brown, L.K., DiClemente, R.J. and Reynolds, L.A. (1991) HIV prevention for adolescents: the utility of the health belief model, *AIDS Education and Prevention*, **3**, 50–9.

Brownlee-Duffeck, M., Peterson, L. and Simonds, J.F. (1987) The role of health beliefs in the regimen adherence and metabolic control of adolescents and adults with diabetes mellitus, *Journal of Consulting and Clinical Psychology*, **55**, 139–44.

Calnan, M. (1984) The health belief model and participation in programmes for the early detection of breast cancer: a comparative analysis, *Social Science and Medicine*, **19**, 823–30.

Calnan, M. (1985) An evaluation of the effectiveness of a class teaching breast self-examination, *British Journal of Medical Psychology*, **53**, 317–29.

Casey, R., Rosen, B., Glowasky, A. and Ludwig, S. (1985) An intervention to improve follow-up of patients with otitis media, *Clinical Pediatrics*, **24**, 149–52.

Cerkoney, K.A. and Hart, K.L. (1980) The relationship between the health belief model and compliance of persons with diabetic regimens, *Diabetes Care*, 3, 594–8.

Champion, V.L. (1984) Instrument development for health belief model constructs, *Advances in Nursing Science*, 6, 73–85.

Charney, E., Bynum, R. and Eldridge, D. (1967) How well do patients take oral penicillin? A collaborative study in private practice, *Journal of Pediatrics*, 40, 188.

Chen, M. and Land, K.C. (1986) Testing the Health Belief Model: LISREL analysis of alternative models of causal relationships between health beliefs and preventive dental behaviour, *Social Psychology Quarterly*, 49, 45–60.

Chen, M. and Land, K.C. (1990) Socioeconomic status (SES) and the health belief model: LISREL analysis of unidimensional versus multidimensional formulations, *Journal of Social Behaviour and Personality*, 5, 263–84.

Chen, M. and Tatsuoka, M. (1984) The relationship between American women's preventive dental behaviour and dental health beliefs, *Social Science and Medicine*, 19, 971–8.

Connelly, C.E. (1984) Compliance with outpatient lithium therapy, *Perspectives in Psychiatric Care*, 22, 44–50.

Connelly, C.E., Davenport, Y.B. and Nurnberger, J.I. (1982) Adherence to treatment regimen in a lithium carbonate clinic, *Archives of General Psychiatry*, 39, 585–8.

Conner, M. (1993) Pros and cons of social cognition models in health behaviour, *Health Psychology Update*, 14, 24–30.

Cooper, H.M. (1986) *Integrating Research: a Guide for Literature Reviews*. London: Sage.

Cummings, K.M., Becker, M.H. and Kirscht, J.P. (1982) Psychosocial factors affecting adherence to medical regimens in a group of haemodialysis patients, *Medical Care*, 20, 567–79.

Cummings, K.M., Jette, A.M. and Brock, B.M. (1979) Psychological determinants of immunization behaviour in a Swine Influenza campaign, *Medical Care*, 17, 639–49.

Eisen, M., Selman, G.L. and McAlister, A.L. (1985) A health belief model to adolescents' fertility control: some pilot program findings, *Health Education Quarterly*, 12, 185–210.

Emmons, C., Joseph, J., Kessler, R.C., Wortman, C.B., Montgomery, S.B. and Ostrow, D. (1986) Psychosocial predictors of reported behaviour change in heterosexual men at risk for AIDS, *Health Education Quarterly*, 13, 331–45.

Feather, N.T. (1982) *Expectations and Actions: Expectancy-value Models in Psychology*. Hillsdale, NJ: Erlbaum.

Fincham, J.E. and Wertheimer, A.L. (1985) Using the health belief model to predict initial drug therapy defaulting, *Journal of Psychology*, 118, 101–5.

Fisher, J.D., Misovich, S.J. and Fisher, W.A. (1992) Impact of perceived social norms on adolescents' AIDS-risk behaviour and prevention. In R.J. DiClemente (ed.) *Adolescents and AIDS: a Generation in Jeopardy*. Newbury Park, CA: Sage, 17–136.

Gerrard, M. and Warner, T.D. (1991) Antecedents of pregnancy among women Marines, *Journal of the Washington Academy of Sciences*, 80, 1015.

Gianetti, V.J., Reynolds, J. and Rihen, T. (1985) Factors which differentiate smokers from ex-smokers among cardiovascular patients: a discriminant analysis, *Social Science and Medicine*, 20, 241–5.

Gochman, D.S. and Parcel, G.S. (eds) (1982) Children's health beliefs and health behaviours, *Health Education Quarterly*, 9, 104–270.

Gollwitzer, P.M. (1993) Goal achievement: the role of intentions, *European Review of Social Psychology*, 4, 142–85.

Gordis, L., Markowitz, M. and Lilienfeld, A.M. (1969) Why patients don't follow medical advice: A study of children on long-term antistreptococcal prophylaxis, *Journal of Pediatrics*, 75, 957–68.

Gottleib, N.H. and Baker, J.A. (1986) The relative influence of health beliefs, parental and peer behaviours and exercise program participation on smoking, alcohol use and physical activity, *Social Science and Medicine*, 22, 915–27.

Grady, K.E., Kegeles, S.S., Lund, A.K., Wolk, C.H. and Farber, N.J. (1983) Who volunteers for a breast self-examination program? Evaluating the bases for self-selection, *Health Education Quarterly*, 10, 79–94.

Haefner, D.P. (1974) The health belief model and preventive dental behavior. In M.H. Becker (ed.) *The Health Belief Model and Personal Health Behavior*. Thorofare, NJ: Slack, 93–105.

Haefner, D.P. and Kirscht, J.P. (1970) Motivational and behavioural effects of modifying health beliefs, *Public Health Reports*, 85, 478–84.

Hallal, J.C. (1982) The relationship of health beliefs, health locus of control, and self concept to the practice of breast self-examination in adult women, *Journal of Nursing Research*, 31, 127–42.

Halper, M., Winawer, S. and Body, R. (1980) Issues of patient compliance. In S. Winawer, D. Schottenfeld and P. Sherlock (eds) *Colorectal Cancer: Prevention, Epidemiology and Screening*. New York: Raven Press, 299–310.

Harris, D.M. and Guten, S. (1979) Health protective behaviour: an exploratory study, *Journal of Health and Social Behaviour*, 20, 17–29.

Harris, R. and Lynn, M.W. (1985) Health beliefs, compliance and control of diabetes mellitus, *Southern Medical Journal*, 2, 162–6.

Harrison, J.A., Mullen, P.D. and Green, L.W. (1992) A meta-analysis of studies of the health belief model with adults, *Health Education Research*, 7, 107–16.

Hartman, P.E. and Becker, M.H. (1978) Non-compliance with prescribed regimen among chronic haemodialysis patients, *Journal of Dialysis and Transplantation*, 7, 978–85.

Heinzelmann, F. (1962) Factors in prophylaxis behaviour in treating rheumatoid fever: an exploratory study, *Journal of Health and Human Behaviour*, 3, 73.

Herold, E.S. (1983) The health belief model: can it help us to understand contraceptive use among adolescents, *Journal of School Health*, 53, 19–21.

Hershey, J.C., Morton, B.G., Davis, J.R. and Reichgolt, M.J. (1980) Patient compliance with antihypertensive medication, *American Journal of Public Health*, 70, 1081–9.

Hester, N.R. and Macrina, D.M. (1985) The health belief model and the contraceptive behaviour of college women: implications for health education, *Journal of American College Health*, 33, 245–52.

Hingson, R.W., Strunin, L., Berlin, B.M. and Heeren, T. (1990) Beliefs about AIDS, use of alcohol and drugs, and unprotected sex among Massachusett's adolescents, *American Journal of Public Health*, 80, 372–77.

Hochbaum, G.M. (1958) *Public Participation in Medical Screening Programs: a Socio-Psychological Study*. Public Health Service Publication No 572. Washington, DC: United States Government Printing Office.

Holland, J., Ramazanoglu, C., Scott, S., Sharpe, S. and Thomson, R. (1990) Sex, gender and power: young women's sexuality in the shadow of AIDS, *Sociology of Health and Illness*, **12**, 336–50.

Hoogewerf, P.E., Hislop, T.G., Morrison, B.J., Burns, S.D. and Sitzo, R. (1990) Health belief and compliance with screening for faecal occult blood, *Social Science and Medicine, 30*, 721–6.

Janz, N. and Becker, M.H. (1984) The health belief model: a decade later, *Health Education Quarterly*, **11**, 1–47.

Jones, P.K., Jones, S.L. and Katz, J. (1987) Improving compliance for asthma patients visiting the emergency department using a health belief model intervention, *Journal of Asthma*, **24**, 199–206.

Joseph, J., Montgomery, S.B., Emmons, C., Kessler, R.C., Ostrow, D., Wortman, C.B., O'Brien, K., Eller, M. and Eshleman, L. (1987) Magnitude and determinations of behavioural risk reduction: longitudinal analysis of a cohort at risk for AIDS, *Psychology and Health*, **1**, 73–96.

Keesling, B. and Friedman, H.S. (1987) Psychological factors in sunbathing and sunscreen use, *Health Psychology*, **6**, 477–93.

Kegeles, S.S. (1963) Why people seek dental care: a test of a conceptual framework, *Journal of Health and Human Behaviour, 4*, 166.

Kelly, G.R., Mamon, A. and Scott, E. (1987) Utility of the health belief model in examining medication compliance among psychiatric outpatients, *Social Science and Medicine*, **25**, 1205–11.

Kelly, H.H. (1967) Attribution theory in social psychology. In D. Levine (ed.) *Nebraska Symposium on Motivation*. Lincoln: University of Nebraska Press, 192–241.

King, J.B. (1982) The impact of patients' perceptions of high blood pressure on attendance at screening: an extension of the health belief model, *Social Science and Medicine*, **16**, 1079–91.

King, J.B. (1984) Illness attributions and the health belief model, *Health Education Quarterly*, **10**, 287–312.

Kirscht, J.P., Becker M.H. and Eveland, P. (1976) Psychological and social factors as predictors of medical behaviour, *Journal of Medical Care*, **14**, 422–31.

Kirscht, J.P. and Rosenstock, I.M. (1977) Patient adherence of antihypertensive medical regimens, *Journal of Community Health*, **3**, 115–24.

Kirscht, J.P. Becker, M.H., Haefner, D.P. and Maiman, L.A. (1978) Effects of threatening communications and mothers' health beliefs on weight change in obese children, *Journal of Behavioural Medicine*, **1**, 147–57.

Kristiansen, C.M. (1985) Value correlates of preventive health behaviour, *Journal of Personality and Social psychology*, **49**, 748–58.

Kruglanski, A.W. and Klar, Y. (1985) Knowing what to do: on the epistemology of actions. In J. Kuhl and J. Beckmann (eds) *Action Control: From Cognition to Behaviour*. Berlin: Springer-Verlag, 41–60.

Langlie, J.K. (1977) Social networks, health beliefs and preventive health behaviour, *Journal of Health and Social Behaviour*, **18**, 244–60.

Larson, E.B., Bergman, J. and Heidrich, F. (1982) Do postcard reminders improve influenza vaccination compliance?, *Journal of Medical Care*, **20**, 639–48.

Leavitt, F. (1979) The health belief model and utilization of ambulatory care services, *Social Science and Medicine*, **13**, 105–12.

Lewin, R.W. (1951) *Field Theory in Social Science*. Harper: New York.

Lewis, K.S. (1994) An examination of the health belief model when applied to diabetes mellitus, unpublished Doctoral Dissertation, University of Sheffield.

Lowe, C.S. and Radius, S.M. (1987) Young adults' contraceptive practices: An investigation of influences, *Adolescence*, 22, 291–304.

Maddux, J.E. and Rodgers, R.W. (1983), Protection motivation and self-efficacy: A revised theory of fear appeals and attitude change, *Journal of Experimental Social Psychology*, 19, 469–79.

Maiman, L.A., Becker, M.H., Kirscht, J.P., Haefner, D.P. and Drachman, R.H. (1977) Scales for measuring health belief model dimensions: a test of predictive value, internal consistency and relationships among beliefs, *Health Education Quarterly*, 4, 215–31.

McCuskar, J., Stoddard, A.M., Zapka, J.G., Zorn, M. and Mayer, K.H. (1989a) Predictors of AIDS-preventive behaviour among homosexually active men: a longitudinal analysis, *AIDS*, 3, 443–8.

McCuskar, J., Zapka, J.G., Stoddard, A.M. and Mayer, K.H. (1989b) Responses to the AIDS epidemic among homosexually active men: factors associated with preventive behaviour, *Patient Education and Counselling*, 13, 15–30.

Miller, L.C., Bettencourt, B.A., DeBro, S.C. and Hoffman, V. (1993) Negotiating safer sex; interpersonal dynamics. In J. B. Pryor and G. D. Reeder (eds) *The Social Psychology of HIV Infection*. Hillsdale, NJ: Erlbaum, 85–123.

Montgomery, S.B., Joseph, J.G., Becker, M.H., Ostrow, D.G., Kessler, R.C. and Kirscht, J.P. (1989) The health belief model in understanding compliance with preventive recommendations for AIDS: how useful?, *AIDS Education and Prevention*, 1, 303–23.

Mullen, P.D., Hersey, J.C. and Iversen, D.C. (1987) Health behaviour compared, *Social Science and Medicine*, 24, 973–81.

Nelson, E.C., Stason, W.B. and Neutra, R.R. (1978) Impact of patients' perceptions on compliance with treatment for hypertension, *Journal of Medical Care*, 16, 893–906.

Norman, P. and Conner, M. (1993) The role of social cognition models in predicting attendance at health checks, *Psychology and Health*, 8, 447–62.

Ogionwo, W. (1973) Socio-psychological factors in health behaviour: an experimental study of methods and attitude change, *International Journal of Health Education*, 16 (supplement), 1–14.

Oliver, R.L. and Berger, P.K. (1979) A path analysis of preventive care decision models. *Journal of Consumer Research*, 6, 113–22.

Orbell, S, Crombie, I. and Johnston, G. (1995) Social cognition and social structure in the prediction of cervical screening uptake, *British Journal of Clinical Psychology*.

Otten, W. and van der Pligt, J. (1992) Risk and behaviour: the mediating role of risk appraisal, *Acta Psychologia*, 80, 325–46.

Owens, R.G., Daly, J., Heron, K. and Lemster, S.J. (1987) Psychological and social characteristics of attenders for breast screening, *Psychology and Health*, 1, 303–13.

Pan, P. and Tantam, D. (1989) Clinical characteristics, health beliefs and compliance with maintenance treatment: a comparison between regular and irregular attenders at a depot clinic, *Acta Psychiatrica Scandinavica*, 79, 564–70.

Penderson, L.L., Wanklin, J.M. and Baskerville, J.C. (1982) Multivariate statistical models for predicting change in smoking behaviour following physician advice to stop smoking, *Journal of Preventive Medicine*, 11, 536–49.

Petosa, R. and Kirby, J. (1991) Using the health belief model to predict safer sex intentions among adolescents, *Health Education Quarterly*, 18, 463–76.

Portnoy, B. (1980) Effects of a controlled usage alcohol education program based on the health belief model, *Journal of Drug Education*, 10, 181.

Prentice-Dunn, S. and Rogers, R.W. (1986) Protection motivation theory and preventive health; beyond the health belief model, *Health Education Research: Theory and Practice*, 3, 153–61.

Rayant, G.A. and Sheiham, A. (1980) An analysis of factors affecting compliance with tooth-cleaning recommendations, *Journal of Clinical Periodontology*, 7, 289–99.

Rees, D.W. (1986) Changing patients' health beliefs to improve compliance with alcohol treatment: a controlled trial, *Journal of Studies of Alcohol*, 47, 436.

Richard, R. and van der Pligt, J. (1991) Factors affecting condom use among adolescents. *Journal of Community and Applied Social Psychology*, 1, 105–16.

Richard, R., van der Pligt, J. and De Vries, N. (1995) Anticipated affective reactions and prevention of AIDS, *British Journal of Social Psychology*, 34, 9–21.

Rogers, R.W. (1983) Cognitive and physiological processes in fear appeals and attitude change: a revised theory of protection motivation. In J. Cacioppo and R. Petty (eds) *Social Psychophysiology*. New York: Guilford, 153–76.

Rogers, R.W. and Mewborn, C.R. (1976) Fear appeals and attitude change: Effects of a threat's noxiousness, probability of occurrence and the efficacy of coping responses. *Journal of Personality and Social Psychology*, 34, 54–61.

Ronis, D.L. and Harel, Y. (1989) Health beliefs and breast examination behaviours: analysis of linear structural relations, *Journal of Psychology and Health*, 3, 259–85.

Rosenstock, I.M. (1966) Why people use health services, *Milbank Memorial Fund Quarterly*, 44, 94–124.

Rosenstock, I.M. (1974) Historical origins of the health belief model, *Health Education Monographs*, 2, 1–8.

Rosenstock, I.M., Strecher, V.J. and Becker, M.H. (1988) Social learning theory and the health belief model, *Health Education Quarterly*, 15, 175–83.

Rosenthal, D., Moore, S. and Flynn, I. (1991) Adolescent self-efficacy, self-esteem, and sexual risk taking, *Journal of Community and Applied Social Psychology*, 1, 77–88.

Rosenthal, D., Hall, C. and Moore, S.M. (1992) AIDS, adolescents and sexual risk taking: a test of the health belief model, *Australian Psychologist*, 27, 166–71.

Rosenthal, R. (1984) *Meta-analysis Procedures for Social Research*. Beverly Hills, CA: Sage.

Rotter, J.B. (1966) Generalized expectancies for internal versus external control of reinforcement, *Psychological Monographs*, 80, whole no. 609.

Rundall, T.G. and Wheeler, J.R. (1979) The effect of income on use of preventive care: an evaluation of alternative explanations, *Journal of Health and Social Behaviour*, 20, 397–406.

Rust, J. and Golombok, S. (1990) *Modern Psychometrics*. London: Routledge.

Sackett, D.L., Becker, M.H. and MacPherson, A.S. (1974) *The Standardized Compliance Questionnaire*. Hamilton, Ontario: McMaster University.

Salloway, J.C., Pletcher, W.R. and Collins, J.J. (1978) Sociological and social psychological models of compliance with prescribed regimen: in search of a synthesis, *Sociological Symposium*, 23, 100–21.

Schaalma, H., Kok, G. and Peters, L. (1993) Determinants of consistent condom use by adolescents: the impact of experience of sexual intercourse, *Health Education Research: Theory and Practice*, 8, 255–69.

Schwarzer, R. (1992) Self-efficacy in the adoption and maintenance of health behaviours: theoretical approaches and a new model. In R. Schwarzer (ed.) *Self-efficacy: Thought Control of Action*. Washington, DC: Hemisphere, 217–42.

Sheeran, P. and Orbell, S. (1995) How confidently can we infer health beliefs from questionnaire responses?, *Psychology and Health*.

Siegel, K., Mesagno, F.P., Chen, J. and Christ, G. (1989) Factors distinguishing homosexual males practising risky and safer sex, *Social Science and Medicine*, **28**, 561–9.

Simon, K.J. and Das, A. (1984) An application of the health belief model toward educational diagnosis for VD education, *Health Education Quarterly*, **11**, 403–18.

Slovic, P., Fischoff, B. and Lichtenstein, S. (1977) Behavioral decision theory, *Annual Review of Psychology*, **28**, 1–39.

Smith Klohn, L. and Rogers, R.W. (1991) Dimensions of severity of health threat: the persuasive effects of visibility, time of onset and rate of onset on young women's intentions to prevent osteoporosis, *Health Psychology*, **10**, 323–9.

Stacy, R.D. and Lloyd, B.H. (1990) An investigation of beliefs about smoking among diabetes patients: information for improving cessation efforts, *Journal of Patient Education and Counselling*, **15**, 181–9.

Stillman, M. (1977) Women's health beliefs about breast cancer and breast self-examination, *Nursing Research*, **26**, 121–7.

Sutton, S.R. (1994) The past predicts the future: interpreting behaviour-behaviour relationships in social-psychological models of health behaviours. In D.R. Rutter and L. Quine (eds) *Social Psychology and Health: European Perspectives*. Aldershot: Avebury Press, 71–88.

Taylor, D.W. (1979) A test of the health belief model in hypertension. In R.B. Haynes, D.W. Taylor and K.L. Sackett (eds) *Compliance in Health Care*. Baltimore, MD: Johns Hopkins University Press, 103–9

Thompson, R.S., Michnich, M.E., Gray, J., Friedlander, L. and Gilson, B. (1986) Maximizing compliance with hemoccult screening for colon cancer in clinical practice, *Medical Care*, **24**, 904–14.

Tversky, A. and Kahneman, D. (1981) The framing of decisions and the psychology of choice, *Science*, **211**, 453–8.

van der Pligt, J., Otten, W., Richard, R. and van der Velde, F. (1993) Perceived risk of AIDS: Unrealistic optimism and self-protective action. In J.B. Prior and G.D. Reeder (eds) *The Social Psychology of HIV Infection*. Hillsdale, NJ: Erlbaum, 39–58.

Wagner, P.J. and Curran, P. (1984) Health beliefs and physician identified 'worried well', *Health Psychology*, **3**, 459–74.

Wallston, K.A. and Wallston, B.S. (1982) Who is responsible for your health? The construct of health locus of control. In G.S. Sanders and J. Suls (eds) *The Social Psychology of Health and Illness*. Hillsdale, NJ: Erlbaum, 65–95.

Warwick, P., Terry, D. and Gallois, C. (1993) Extending the theory of reasoned action: the role of health beliefs. In D.J. Terry, C. Gallois and M. McCamish (eds) *The Theory of Reasoned Action: Its Application to AIDS-preventive Behaviour*. Oxford: Pergamon Press, 117–34.

Warshaw, P.R. and Davis, F.D. (1985) Disentangling behavioral intention and behavioral expectation, *Journal of Experimental Social Psychology*, **21**, 213–28.

Weinberger, M., Green, J.Y. and Mandin, J.J. (1981) Health beliefs and smoking behaviour, *American Journal of Public Health*, **71**, 1253–5.

Weinstein, N.D. (1980) Unrealistic optimism about future life events, *Journal of Personality and Social Psychology*, **39**, 806–20.

Weinstein, N.D. (1982) Unrealistic optimism about susceptibility to health problems, *Journal of Behavioural Medicine*, **5**, 441–60.

Weinstein, N.D. (1984) Why it won't happen to me: perceptions of risk factors and illness susceptibility, *Health Psychology*, **3**, 431–57.

Weinstein, N.D. (1988) The precaution adoption process, *Health Psychology*, **7**, 355–86.

Weinstein, N.D. and Nicolich, M. (1993) Correct and incorrect interpretations of correlations between risk perceptions and risk behaviours, *Health Psychology*, **12**, 235–45.

Werch, C.E. (1990) Behavioural self-control strategies for deliberately limiting drinking among college students, *Journal of Addictive Behaviours*, **15**, 119–28.

Wolcott, D.L., Sullivan, G. and Klein, D. (1990) Longitudinal change in HIV transmission risk behaviours by gay male physicians, *Journal of Psychosomatics*, **31**, 159–67.

3 PAUL NORMAN AND PAUL BENNETT

HEALTH LOCUS OF CONTROL

1 General background

Psychologists have long been interested in the beliefs that underlie people's health behaviour, with particular attention being focused on perceptions of control over health. It is generally assumed that those who believe that they have control over their health will be more likely to perform a range of health promoting behaviours (Strickland 1978; Wallston and Wallston 1981) and, as a result, have better health status (Seeman and Seeman 1983; Marshall 1991). As Allison (1991) notes, this assumption is mirrored in many health promotion interventions, ranging from 'internality training' (Wallston and Wallston 1978) to programmes which attempt to overcome the barriers to control (Green and Raeburn 1988). Moreover, it is an explicit feature of the *Ottawa Charter for Health Promotion* (World Health Organization 1986), which defines health promotion as 'the process of enabling people to increase control over, and to improve, their health'. In the UK, it is also an implicit feature of preventive care in primary health care where general practitioners are now under an obligation to give patients advice 'about the significance of diet, the use of tobacco, the consumption of alcohol and the misuse of drugs' in relation to their health (Department of Health 1989). In short, people are increasingly being encouraged to take responsibility for their health through the adoption of 'healthy' behaviours. Against this background, it is not surprising that health locus of control (HLC) is one of the most widely researched constructs in relation to the prediction of health behaviour (Wallston 1992).

The origins of the HLC construct can be traced back to Rotter's (1954) social learning theory. The main tenet of social learning theory is that the likelihood of a behaviour occurring in a given situation is a function of (a) the individual's expectancy that the behaviour will lead to a particular reinforcement, and (b) the extent to which the reinforcement is valued. Rotter (1954) proposed that the theory could operate on a general as well as a specific level. So, in addition to having expectancy beliefs for particular situations, individuals are also believed to have generalized expectancies that cut across situations. It was from this perspective that the notion of locus of control was introduced, as a generalized expectancy relating to the perceived relationship between one's actions and experienced outcomes. In particular, Rotter made the distinction between internal and external locus of control belief orientations: 'internals' are seen to believe that events are a consequence of their own actions and thereby under personal control, whereas 'externals' are seen to believe that events are unrelated to their actions and thereby determined by factors beyond their personal control.

The locus of control construct has similarities with many other constructs which emphasize the importance of perceptions of control, including mastery (Pearlin and Schoder 1978), self-efficacy (Bandura 1982), personal causation (deCharms 1976), personal competence (Harter and O'Connell 1984) and perceived competence (Smith *et al.* 1991). Its main overlap is with constructs that focus on the causes of events, such as explanatory style (Peterson *et al.* 1982). However, while Furnham and Steele (1993) have argued that locus of control beliefs are, to some extent, based on causal attributions, there is a clear conceptual distinction between locus of control beliefs and causal beliefs. Causal beliefs focus on the *causes of past events*, while locus of control beliefs focus on *expectancies for future events*. While there has been a good deal of work looking at causal attributions in response to serious illnesses such as cancer (Taylor *et al.* 1984), coronary heart disease (Affleck *et al.* 1987), diabetes (Tennen *et al.* 1984) and end stage renal failure (Witenberg *et al.* 1983), there has been little work applying attributional theories to the prediction of health behaviour among healthy populations (e.g. King 1982). This chapter therefore focuses exclusively on the large amount of research with the locus of control construct as a predictor of health behaviour.

Locus of control, as a generalized expectancy that one's actions are instrumental to goal attainment, was first measured in Rotter's (1966) internal–external scale. This scale has since become one of the most widely employed individual difference measures (Rotter 1990; Lefcourt 1991). Reviews of early work with this scale (Phares 1976; Strickland 1978) reported that, compared with externals, internals were more likely to exert efforts to control their environment, to take responsibility for their actions, to seek out and process relevant information, to exhibit better learning and to show more autonomous decision-making. Applying such findings to the question of health behaviour, it was predicted that internals would take a more active responsibility for their health and, as a result, would be more likely to engage in health-promoting activities. Early work applying the internal-external scale to the prediction of health behaviour met with some success (Strickland 1978; Wallston and Wallston 1978), although two main criticisms were increasingly levelled at its use.

First, the amount of variance in health behaviour explained by the internal-external scale was typically low, and this led to a call for, and development of, situation- or domain-specific locus of control measures. This is in line with Rotter's (1975) view that when the individual has some prior experience in a given situation, situation-specific expectancy beliefs will be more predictive of behaviour. Second, the scale was criticized by a number of researchers for conceptualizing locus of control as a uni-dimensional construct (Gurin *et al.* 1969; Mirels 1970; Collins 1974; Levenson 1974). In particular, Levenson (1974) called for the development of multidimensional locus of control measures, arguing that internal locus of control beliefs are orthogonal to external locus of control beliefs and that within external locus of control beliefs it is possible to distinguish between external control exerted by powerful others and the influence of chance or fate. Wallston *et al.* (1978) responded to these two criticisms by developing the multidimensional health locus of control (MHLC) scale, which has since become the most popular locus of control measure in research on health behaviour (Wallston 1992).

2 Description of the model

The MHLC scale (Wallston *et al.* 1978) measures generalized expectancy beliefs with respect to health along three dimensions. The first dimension measures the extent to which individuals believe their health is the result of their own actions (internal HLC), the second measures the extent to which individuals feel their health is under the control of powerful others (powerful others HLC), and the third measures the extent to which individuals believe their health is owing to chance or fate (chance HLC).

The main prediction from HLC theory is that internals on the MHLC scale should be more likely to engage in health-promoting activities. As Allison (1991) notes, there is an implicit assumption in much of the literature that internality is good. In relation to powerful others HLC, there are some situations when having a strong belief in the role of powerful others may be advantageous, particularly during acute or chronic illness (Wallston 1989). In addition, strong powerful others HLC beliefs may be predictive of health behaviour when recommended by a health professional. For self-initiated behaviour change though, powerful others HLC beliefs may be unrelated to health behaviour. Considering chance HLC, in situations when there is little anyone could do to change his or her health status, having moderately strong chance HLC beliefs may be adaptive (Burish *et al.* 1984). However, it is generally assumed that chance HLC beliefs merely provide a mirror reflection of the internality dimension (Wallston 1992), such that individuals with strong chance HLC beliefs should be less likely to engage in health-related behaviour.

According to social learning theory, the above relationships should only hold for individuals who value their health, as behaviour is a function of expectancy beliefs and the value attached to certain goals. However, as Wallston (1991) notes, the majority of research using the HLC construct does so without measuring the value people place on their health. HLC beliefs are simply related to health behaviour without reference to health value. The failure of most studies to consider health value may stem from a lack of appreciation of the complexity of social learning theory, in which health locus of control is embedded (Wallston 1991), or may stem from an unchallenged assumption that all people value their health (Lau *et al.* 1986).

This chapter first reviews research that has looked at the relationship between HLC beliefs and health behaviour, as this represents the majority of work with the HLC construct. In line with earlier reviews of research with the HLC construct (Wallston and Wallston 1981; Wallston 1992), this chapter primarily focuses on the relationship between internal HLC beliefs and health behaviour. This is for three main reasons (Wallston 1992). First, most research interest has focused on the relationship between internal HLC beliefs and the performance of health behaviour. Second, powerful others HLC beliefs have rarely been found to predict health behaviour in healthy populations and may be more relevant to illness behaviour. Third, chance HLC beliefs are indicative of a perceived lack of control and may therefore simply complement the other dimensions.

3 Summary of research

The main way in which the HLC construct has been used by health psychologists is as a predictor of preventive health behaviour. Internals are believed to take an active responsibility for their health, and so it is predicted that there should be a strong correlation between internal HLC beliefs and the performance of preventive health behaviour. In this section we consider studies which have examined the relationship between HLC and the performance of preventive health behaviour on a general level and for specific behaviours. Given that the HLC construct focuses on generalized expectancy beliefs with respect to health, Wallston (1992) has argued that internal HLC beliefs should show stronger correlations with the performance of preventive health behaviour on a general level (i.e. global indices) than with specific behaviours.

3.1 Preventive health behaviours

Studies linking internal HLC beliefs to the performance of preventive health behaviour on a general level have produced a mixed set of results. For example, some studies have found a positive relationship between internal HLC beliefs and indices of preventive health behaviour (Mechanic and Cleary 1980; Seeman and Seeman 1983; Rauckhorst 1987; Duffy 1988; Weiss and Larsen 1990; Waller and Bates 1992). In contrast, other studies have failed to find such a relationship (Winefield 1982; Brown *et al.* 1983; Muhlenkamp *et al.* 1985; Wurtele *et al.* 1985; Steptoe *et al.* 1994;

Norman 1995), although some studies have found a negative relationship between chance HLC and preventive health behaviour (Brown *et al.* 1983; Muhlenkamp *et al.* 1985; Steptoe *et al.* 1994). Overall, the evidence linking internal HLC beliefs with global indices of preventive health behaviour has been weak. In fact, Wallston and Wallston (1981, 1982, 1984) have drawn a number of pessimistic conclusions about the ability of the HLC construct to predict preventive health behaviour.

3.2 Exercise

Research which has focused on the relationship between HLC beliefs and participation in physical activity has produced inconclusive results. A number of studies have found some evidence to link internal HLC beliefs and exercise. For example, Slenker *et al.* (1985) compared the HLC beliefs of joggers and non-joggers and found the joggers to be more internal. Similarly, Carlson and Petti (1989) found that college students with strong internal HLC beliefs were more likely to participate in a range of physical activities high in caloric expenditure. Internal HLC beliefs have also been linked to attendance at work-site fitness programmes (O'Connell and Price 1982). However, a number of studies have found either only a weak relationship or no relationship between internal HLC beliefs and exercise behaviour (Laffrey and Isenberg 1983; Calnan 1989; Norman 1990; Rabinowitz *et al.* 1992).

3.3 Alcohol

There have been a number of studies which have examined the locus of control construct in relation to alcoholism, comparing alcoholics with non-alcoholics. However, these have produced conflicting results, with both internality (Gozali and Sloan 1971; Costello and Manders 1974) and externality (Butts and Chotlas 1973; Krampen 1980; Huckstadt 1987) being associated with alcoholism. Research with non-alcoholic populations has also produced mixed results, with some studies reporting a relationship between externality and increased drinking (Segal 1974; Naditch 1975; Aopoa and Damon 1982) and other studies failing to find such a relationship (Chess *et al.* 1971; Carman 1974; Drasgow *et al.* 1974; Donovan and O'Leary 1975; Schilling and Carman 1978). Similar mixed findings have been reported with more recent research using the HLC construct. For example, both Norman (1990) and Dean (1991) found no relationship between HLC beliefs and drinking behaviour while Calnan (1989) only found evidence for weak negative correlations between powerful others and chance HLC beliefs and alcohol consumption. Finally, Oziel *et al.* (1972) developed a unidimensional drinking-related locus of control measure which has shown alcoholics to be more external than non-alcoholic controls (Donovan and O'Leary 1978; Huckstadt 1987).

3.4 AIDS-related behaviour

In relation to AIDS-related behaviour, a positive relationship between internal HLC and the performance of safe sexual practices is expected. A number of studies have examined the relationships between HLC beliefs and AIDS-related behaviour, and have produced results which are generally in line with expectations. St Lawrence (1993) used the HLC construct to examine condom use behaviour among a sample of African-American adolescents and found a negative relationship between external HLC beliefs and frequency of condom use, but no relationship between internal HLC beliefs and condom use. Considering the AIDS-related behaviour of gay men, Price-Greathouse and Trice (1986) also found that those men who held strong chance HLC beliefs were less likely to attend AIDS education sessions, although no relationship was found with internal HLC beliefs. Finally, Kelley *et al.* (1990) found that gay men who reported having unprotected anal intercourse were less likely to have internal AIDS-related HLC beliefs and more likely to believe that the likelihood of infection with HIV was owing to chance factors.

3.5 Breast self-examination

A number of studies have examined the relationship between HLC and breast self-examination among women. Redeker (1989) found that women who practised breast self-examination at least three times a year had stronger internal HLC beliefs. However, other studies have failed to find any relationship between HLC beliefs and the performance of breast self-examination (Seeman and Seeman 1983; Lau *et al.* 1986; Smith *et al.* 1990). Both Hallal (1982) and Nemeck (1990) found that women who practised breast self-examination were less likely to believe in the role of powerful others in controlling their health, but no relationships were found for internal and chance HLC. As Nemeck (1990) argues, the negative relationship with powerful others HLC beliefs may be owing to those who did not practise breast self-examination, believing that breast examination was the responsibility of health professionals. Supporting this argument, Bundek *et al.* (1993) found a positive relationship between powerful others HLC beliefs and the recency of gynaecological screening including *physician* breast examination, while a positive relationship was found between internal HLC beliefs and *self* breast examination.

3.6 Smoking cessation

A number of studies have examined the role of HLC beliefs in predicting smoking cessation. As with other forms of behaviour change, it is generally assumed that smokers who perceive that they have personal control over their health will be more likely to initiate and maintain changes in their smoking behaviour. However, it also possible to put forward the argument that a belief in the role of powerful others may be conducive to smoking-related behaviour change, as for many people the initial impetus for change comes from a health professional's advice to change, or from attendance at a formal smoking cessation programme.

There is some evidence supporting the position that internal HLC beliefs may be predictive of smoking-related behaviour change. For example, Rosen and Shipley (1983) examined self-initiated smoking reduction and found that internal HLC beliefs were important in predicting successful maintenance of smoking reduction. Similarly, Shipley (1981) found that smokers attending a smoking cessation programme with an internal HLC orientation were more likely to have successfully quit smoking six months later. However, a number of non-significant results have been reported in the literature (Kaplan and Cowles 1978; Horwitz *et al.* 1985; Wojcik 1988; Segall and Wynd 1990). Overall, these results suggest that while internal HLC beliefs may have some role to play in encouraging smoking-related behaviour change, their influence is a weak one.

There is little evidence to support the view that smokers with a strong belief in the role of powerful others are more successful in quitting after attending a smoking cessation programme. In fact, a couple of studies suggest the opposite. Wojcik (1988) found that smokers with strong powerful others HLC beliefs attending formal treatment programmes were more likely to have relapsed at three months. Similarly, Segall and Wynd (1990) followed up smokers who had attended an eight-week quit smoking programme six months earlier and found relapsers to have a stronger belief in the role of powerful others than abstainers. One possible interpretation of these results is that while a belief in the role of powerful others may be important in initiating attempts to quit smoking, it is not sufficient to encourage and support the maintenance of long-term cessation.

3.7 Weight loss

As with research looking at the relationship between HLC and smoking cessation it is possible to put forward the argument that successful weight loss may be dependent on both internal and powerful others HLC beliefs. Internals are expected to be successful given that weight loss is to some extent dependent on the control of food intake and that internals are more likely to believe that they are able to control their food intake. However, a belief in the role of powerful others may be supportive of change given that relevant dietary advice is likely to be given by health professionals.

Studies examining the relationship between HLC beliefs and weight loss have produced inconclusive results. Schifter and Ajzen (1985) failed to find any relationships between HLC beliefs and weight loss over a six-week period. Moreover, Saltzer (1982) found HLC beliefs to be unrelated to completion of a six-week weight loss programme, and Gierszewski (1983) found no evidence that internals were more successful in losing weight following a worksite nutrition and weight control programme. However,

Zindler-Wernet and Weiss (1987) found that individuals who lost weight following a worksite screening session had higher internal HLC scores. Similarly, Chavez and Michaels (1980) found that internals in an obesity treatment programme lost more weight than externals.

4 Developments in health locus of control research

Research with the HLC construct has been criticized on a number of grounds. In this section, we consider two of the main criticisms which have highlighted important omissions from research with the construct. These criticisms have focused on the need to assess HLC of control in conjunction with health value and to develop behaviour-specific HLC scales.

4.1 Health value

A number of researchers have commented that many tests of the HLC construct have been inadequate because they have not paid attention to the value people place on their health (Lau *et al.* 1986; Weiss and Larsen 1990; Wallston 1992). According to social learning theory, behaviour is a function of expectancy beliefs (e.g. HLC) and the value attached to certain outcomes (e.g. health value). There is therefore a need to consider the influence of HLC beliefs in conjunction with the value placed on health. However, even when the influence of health value is considered, it is often considered in an additive, rather than multiplicative, fashion (Wallston 1991). Health value should be viewed as a moderator of the relationship between internal HLC beliefs and the performance of health behaviour. As Wallston and Wallston (1980) have argued, HLC beliefs should only predict health behaviour when people value their health; there is no theoretical reason to expect internal HLC beliefs to be related to the performance of health behaviour among individuals who place a low value on their health. As a result, it is predicted that internals who value their health should be the most likely to perform a range of health-related behaviours.

Studies which have tested for the predicted interaction between internal HLC beliefs and health value have generally produced positive results. For example, Weiss and Larsen (1990) found that for individuals who were classified as placing a high value on their health, a significant correlation was found between internal HLC beliefs and a health behaviour index. In contrast, the same correlation was non-significant for individuals placing a low value on their health. As a result, those individuals who had strong internal HLC beliefs and placed a high value on their health engaged in a greater number of health-promoting behaviours. Similar results have been found by a number of researchers (Wallston and Wallston 1980; Lau 1982; Seeman and Seeman 1983; Abella and Heslin 1984; Lau *et al.* 1986), although some studies have failed to find evidence for such an interaction (Wurtele *et al.* 1985; Norman 1995).

When considering the performance of specific health behaviours, a similar pattern of results emerges. Evidence for an interaction between internal HLC beliefs and health value has been found for dietary behaviour (Hayes and Ross 1987), smoking cessation (Kaplan and Cowles 1978), breast-self examination (Seeman and Seeman 1983; Lau *et al.* 1986) and information seeking (B.S. Wallston *et al.* 1976; K.A. Wallston *et al.* 1976). In each case, internals who placed a high value on their health were the most likely to perform the behaviour in question. However, some studies have failed to find such an interaction when considering cancer-related preventive behaviours (McCusker and Morrow 1979), information seeking (DeVito *et al.* 1982), leisure-time exercise (Laffrey and Isenberg 1983) and attendance at health checks (Norman 1991). Overall, though, the pattern of results points to the importance of considering health value as a moderator variable when using the HLC construct to predict health behaviour.

4.2 Behaviour-specific scales

A second criticism levelled at work with the HLC construct focuses on the issue of specificity. It is argued that one reason for the relatively weak relationship between HLC beliefs and the performance of health behaviour is that the MHLC scale measures generalized behaviour-reinforcement expectancy beliefs. In other words, while HLC is specific to a given goal (i.e. health), it cuts across many situations (smoking, diet, exercise, etc.). As a result, a number of researchers have sought to develop behaviour-specific HLC scales. There are a number of reasons for this development.

First, it is generally accepted that specific measures are likely to lead to better predictions of specific behaviours (Ajzen and Fishbein 1977). Second, it is likely that individuals may hold different control beliefs for different behaviours (Kirscht 1972). For example, a smoker may have external control beliefs when considering his or her smoking behaviour, but internal control beliefs in relation to taking regular exercise. It is therefore important to measure control beliefs that are relevant to the behaviour in question. Third, generalized control beliefs may only be important in determining behaviour in relatively novel situations (Wallston and Wallston 1981; Rotter 1982). In such situations, individuals will have little prior knowledge about the behaviour and will therefore be reliant on more general knowledge and beliefs. In contrast, in other situations, specific knowledge about the behaviour in question will be more relevant. The important point to make here is that most health behaviours are far from being novel behaviours, and as a result are unlikely to be predicted by general control beliefs. Instead, behaviour-specific control beliefs should be more predictive of behaviour.

There have been a number of attempts by researchers to develop behaviour-specific HLC scales. In general, these scales have been found to be useful in predicting health behaviour and have been found to be more predictive than the generalized MHLC scale. For example, Georgiou and Bradley (1992) developed a smoking-specific locus of control scale to examine smokers' beliefs about quitting. This scale was found to have greater predictive validity than the more general measure. For example, internals on the smoking locus of control scale were found to have quit for longer periods of time in previous attempts to quit. In contrast, no significant correlations were observed with the MHLC scale. Similarly, internals on the smoking locus of control scale were more likely to indicate that they wanted to quit and that they would be willing to try 'internal' methods of stopping in the future, whereas no such relationships were observed when the MHLC scale was used. Overall, Georgiou and Bradley (1992) concluded that the smoking locus of control scale showed stronger and more appropriate correlations with smokers' behaviours and intentions. Wallston and O'Connor (1987) have similarly developed a smoking-cessation locus of control scale to examine smoking cessation among cardiovascular risk patients, and have found the measure to be useful in predicting cigarette reduction at three months.

Kelley *et al.* (1990) developed an AIDS-specific HLC scale to examine high-risk behaviour among gay men and found that men who engaged in unprotected anal intercourse were more likely to believe that infection with HIV was a matter of luck. In contrast, those men who believed that personal control factors influenced the likelihood of infection were less likely to engage in such sexual behaviour. St Lawrence (1993) has similarly found the self-control subscale of the condom attitude scale (Sacco *et al.* 1991) to be predictive of frequency of condom use among a sample of African-American adolescents, with those adolescents who believed that they had self-control in sexual situations being more likely to use condoms.

Labs and Wurtele (1986) have developed a fetal health locus of control scale in order to look at the health-related behaviour of pregnant women. This scale examines the extent to which women believe the health of their child to be under the control of their own behaviour, powerful others or chance. In the initial validation study the internal dimension of the scale was found to be predictive of the womens' health-related behaviour. Internals on the scale were less likely to be smokers and to consume caffeine and more likely to hold strong intentions to attend childbirth classes to learn techniques to control pain during labour and delivery. In contrast, the internal dimension of the MHLC scale was unable to predict their health-related behaviour. Similarly, Tinsley and Holtgrave (1989) have linked mothers' neonatal health locus of control beliefs with the uptake of infant preventive services.

Saltzer (1982) has reported the development of a four-item (internal–external) weight locus of control scale to predict weight reduction behaviour. Internals on this scale were found to be more likely to complete a weight control programme. In contrast, the MHLC scale was unable to predict programme completion. Furthermore, Saltzer (1982) found that internals on the weight locus of control scale who also valued their health were the most successful in achieving their weight loss goals. Other researchers, though, have failed to report positive results with the weight locus of control scale. For example, Gierszewski (1983) found no evidence to link weight locus of control beliefs to successful weight reduction. Similarly, Groth-Marnat and Schumaker (1987–9) found the weight locus of control scale to be unrelated to weight control strategies among a sample of bulimics. More recently, Stotland and Zuroff (1990) have developed a dietary beliefs scale to examine locus of control beliefs in relation to weight loss goals and achievement.

Other situation-specific health locus of control scales have been developed for specific conditions including diabetes (Ferraro et al. 1987; Bradley et al. 1990), arthritis (Nicassio et al. 1985), heart and lung disease (Allison 1987), cancer (Prwun et al. 1988), hypertension (Stanton 1987) and alcoholism (Donovan and O'Leary 1978). Overall, studies using behaviour-specific HLC scales have tended to produce positive results (Lefcourt 1991). Moreover, these scales have been found to be more predictive of health behaviour than more general scales such as the MHLC scale. This is in line with Rotter's (1982) argument that when individuals have some prior experience in a situation, situation-specific expectancies will be more predictive of behaviour than generalized expectancies.

5 Operationalization of the model

In this section we introduce some of the most frequently used measures of health locus of control and health value.

5.1 Health locus of control

The most widely used measure of HLC, although it has a number of differing forms, is the MHLC scale. This scale was first developed by Wallston and colleagues in the late 1970s (Wallston et al. 1978). They originally developed a unidimensional measure (B.S. Wallston et al. 1976), in which a belief in ability to control one's own health was seen as at one end of the dimension (i.e. internal HLC), and a belief that one's health is beyond personal control at the other (i.e. external HLC). Levenson (1974) argued that internality and externality were, in fact, orthogonal and that within external locus of control beliefs it was possible to distinguish further between external control exerted by powerful others and the influence of chance or fate. Levenson (1974) developed a non-specific measure of locus of control incorporating these points. This was developed and made specific to health by Wallston et al. (1978). Their second questionnaire, the MHLC scale, measures three orthogonal dimensions: internal, powerful others and chance HLC. The internal HLC scale measures individuals' beliefs in their own ability to control their health, the powerful others HLC scale measures the extent to which people believe their health is controlled by health professionals and the chance HLC scale measures the extent to which people believe in chance or fate as determinants of their health.

Each of the three scales comprises six items measuring the strength of differing control beliefs, using a six-point Likert scale, ranging from 'strongly disagree' to 'strongly agree'. Two equivalent forms (A and B) of the MHLC scale, with matching items, were developed from responses of a sample of 115 persons over the age of 16 years randomly selected from people using a local internal American airport (Wallston *et al.* 1978). Items were selected from a larger pool of items using item analysis. Alpha reliabilities for the three derived health locus of control scales (forms A/ B) were 0.77/0.71 for the internal scale, 0.67/0.72 for the powerful others scale and 0.75/0.69 for the chance scale. The two forms of each scale were found to be highly correlated (internal, $r = 0.80$; powerful others, $r = 0.76$; chance, $r = 0.73$). When responses to forms A and B were combined, the internal and powerful others scales were found to be statistically independent, while the internal and chance scales were negatively correlated (-0.29, $p < 0.01$). Forms A and B of the MHLC scale are presented in Table 3.1.

No validation study was reported in Wallston's initial report, although a number have since been conducted (see Lefcourt 1991). These have generally confirmed the factor structure and the reliability of form A as satisfactory (e.g. Hartke and Kunce 1982; Marshall *et al.* 1990). Some (e.g. Cooper and Fraboni 1990) report higher Cronbach's alpha coefficients than the original report (0.87, internal; 0.68, powerful others; 0.76, chance) while lower alpha coefficients have been reported by Winefield (1982). In one of few studies examining the psychometric qualities of form B of the MHLC scale, Cooper and Fraboni (1990) found low item-by-item correlations ($r = 0.00$–0.69) between equivalent items of forms A and B of the MHLC scale. In addition, they found a five-factor structure for form A of the MHLC scale and a three-factor solution for form B, only the latter replicating the factor structure reported by Wallston and colleagues. However, the population studied was small ($n = 82$) and biased, comprising people attending a back injury clinic. As a result, Cooper and Fraboni's (1990) results must be viewed with some caution. Furthermore, earlier data from O'Looney and Barrett (1983) suggest that forms A and B of the MHLC scale are, in fact, parallel. Conducted on a sample of undergraduates (70 males, 77 females) they found correlations between the forms to be high, with a mean correlation between cross-form items of 0.48 and cross-scale correlations greater than 0.68. In addition, the factor structures obtained for forms A and B were found to be the same, although the predicted three-factor solutions were only found for females. For males, two-factor solutions were obtained, with the internal and chance items loading together.

Lau and Ware (1981) and Lau (1982) developed an alternative measure of HLC to the MHLC scale. This comprised four dimensions, three of which map on to those of the MHLC scale: self-control (internal), provider control (powerful others) and chance. In addition, the instrument included a four-item scale assessing general health threat; the extent to

Table 3.1   The multidimensional health locus of control scale (forms A and B)

Internal health locus of control
  1   If I get sick, it is my own behaviour which determines how soon I get well.
  6   I am in control of my health.
  8   When I get sick I am to blame.
 12   The main thing that affects my health is what I myself do.
 13   If I take care of myself, I can avoid illness.
 17   If I take the right actions, I can stay healthy.

Powerful others health locus of control
  3   Having regular contact with my physician is the best way for me to avoid illness.
  5   Whenever I don't feel well, I should consult a medically trained professional.
  7   My family has a lot to do with my becoming sick or staying healthy.
 10   Health professionals control my health.
 14   When I recover from an illness, it's usually because other people (for example, doctors, nurses, family, friends) have been taking good care of me.
 18   Regarding my health, I can only do what my doctor tells me to do.

Chance health locus of control
  2   No matter what I do, if I am going to get sick, I will get sick.
  4   Most things that affect my health happen to me by accident.
  9   Luck plays a big part in determining how soon I will recover from an illness.
 11   My good health is largely a matter of good fortune.
 15   No matter what I do, I'm likely to get sick.
 16   If it's meant to be, I will stay healthy.

Internal health locus of control
  1   If I become sick, I have the power to make myself well again.
  6   I am directly responsible for my health.
  8   Whatever goes wrong with my health is my own fault.
 12   My physical well-being depends on how well I take care of myself.
 13   When I feel ill, I know it is because I have not been taking care of myself properly.
 17   I can pretty much stay healthy by taking good care of myself.

Powerful others health locus of control
  3   If I see an excellent doctor regularly, I am less likely to have health problems.
  5   I can only maintain my health by consulting health professionals.
  7   Other people play a big part in whether I stay healthy or become sick.
 10   Health professionals keep me healthy.
 14   The type of care I receive from other people is what is responsible for how well I recover from an illness.

Table 3.1 cont'd

18 Following doctor's orders to the letter is the best way for me to stay healthy.

Chance health locus of control
2 Often I feel that no matter what I do, if I am going to get sick, I will get sick.
4 It seems that my health is greatly influenced by accidental happenings.
9 When I am sick, I just have to let nature run its course.
11 When I stay healthy, I'm just plain lucky.
15 Even when I take care of myself, it's easy to get sick.
16 When I become ill, it's a matter of fate.

Note: English versions of the scales usually replace 'sick' with 'ill'.

which individuals regard health outcomes as threatening. These combine to form a 36-item questionnaire, with items answered using a six-point Likert scale. Marshall *et al.* (1990) assessed the convergent validity, internal reliability and factor structure of the Lau (1982) and Wallston *et al.* (1978) questionnaires using data from 181 medical outpatients. Only minimal evidence of convergence was found between the corresponding scales of the two instruments, with correlations varying between $r = 0.32$ and $r = 0.38$. Although significant, these correlations are lower than would be expected if the measures were tapping the same latent variables. The estimates of reliability were satisfactory for the Wallston *et al.* (1978) scale, but not the Lau (1982) scale, suggesting that some of the low convergence may be attributable to this low internal consistency. Finally, the factor structure of the Wallston, but not the Lau, scale was supported using a principal components, factor analytic, procedure. The authors conclude that the psychometric superiority of the Wallston instrument makes this the instrument of choice.

A number of further developments from the original MHLC scale have been reported. First, K.A. Wallston has developed a questionnaire (MHLC form C) which is diagnosis or disease specific. Form C comprises a 24-item questionnaire (eight items per scale), with each question designed so that the question can be made appropriate to the medical condition the patient has (e.g. 'If my condition (diabetes, renal disease, etc.) worsens, it is my own behaviour which determines how soon I shall feel better again'). Second, McCallum *et al.* (1988) reported an attempt to simplify the administration of the MHLC scale by reducing the response format to a two-point response scale (agree–disagree). In a sample of 54 college students, they found correspondence between classification of subjects into high–low categories (based on a median split) on each of the full and shortened response scales to vary between 75 and 83 per cent. However, McCallum *et al.*'s (1988) version was found to have lower levels of internal consistency. Nevertheless, the authors note that their results suggest that this format may be sufficiently valid to warrant its use under conditions where use of the full

questionnaire may be difficult or unwarranted, such as telephone interviews, or where respondents lack motivation or have limited intellectual
capacity.

Third, Anderson *et al*. (1994) have further investigated the use of different response formats. In doing so, they questioned whether the MHLC
Scale measures expectancies about control or desires for control, given that
studies including both the MHLC scale and measures of desire for control
have found the two to correlate (Wallston and Wallston 1982; Wallston
et al. 1983). A sample of 237 adults completed three versions of the
MHLC scale. In addition to completing the original version with response
scales of strongly disagree to strongly agree, subjects also completed an
expectancy version (response formats: I strongly *believe* this is *not* true for
me – I strongly *believe* this is true for me) and a desire for control version
(response formats: I strongly *don't want* to believe this is true for me – I
strongly *want* to believe this is true for me). They found the original
version to correlate more highly with the expectancy version than with
the desire version, suggesting that the original scale is primarily tapping
expectancies about control. The expectancy version was found to have
higher internal consistency than the original version, although Anderson
et al. (1994) suggest that further validation of the expectancy version is
required before it is widely used.

Fourth, Marshall (1991) has questioned the extent to which internal
HLC beliefs are unidimensional. A principal components factor analysis of
internal HLC items from a number of sources (Wallston *et al*. 1978; Lau
and Ware 1981) identified four empirically distinct dimensions. Marshall
(1991) identified internal HLC beliefs in relation to self-mastery (e.g. 'If I
become ill, I have the power to make myself well again'), illness prevention
(e.g. 'If I take care of myself, I can avoid illness'), illness management (e.g.
'If I get ill, it is my own behaviour that determines how soon I will get well
again') and self-blame (e.g. 'Whatever goes wrong with my health is my
own fault'). Only the self-mastery dimension was found to be an independent
predictor of self-report health status. Marshall's (1991) approach may
have considerable potential for predicting different kinds of health-related
behaviour.

Finally, Wallston (1989) has developed a shorter version of the MHLC
scale for use in large-scale epidemiological studies, where competing demands
for questionnaire space require each scale to use a minimum of items to
measure the construct in question. The development and use of this short
version of the MHLC scale is reported in more detail in Section 6.1.

5.2 Health value

As we have previously noted, health behaviour is best predicted by an
interaction of HLC and health value. Two measures of health value have
been particularly prominent (Rokeach 1973, 1979; Lau *et al*. 1986). Both
take a different approach to the measurement of health value.

The first approach to the assessment of health value measures the value placed on health as an *absolute* value (Lau *et al.* 1986). The Lau *et al.* (1986) scale asks respondents to rate the importance they place on health without placing such questions in any context or asking them to make comparisons with the value they would place on any other factor. The scale comprises four items, measured using a six-point Likert scale ranging from 'strongly agree' (6) to 'strongly disagree' (1): 'If you don't have your health, you don't have anything', 'There are many things I care about more than my health', 'Good health is only of minor importance in a happy life' and, 'There is nothing more important than good health'. The second and third items are reverse coded and the sum of the four scores provides an overall measure of health value, with scores ranging from 4 to 24. Lau *et al.* (1986) report satisfactory levels of internal consistency (0.63 to 0.72) for their scale across different populations.

The second approach to the measurement of health value is a variant of Rokeach's (1973) health value survey (e.g. K.A. Wallston *et al.* 1976; Kaplan and Cowles 1978; Saltzer 1978; Ware and Young 1979; Abella and Heslin 1984; Kristiansen 1985; Lau *et al.* 1986). The health value survey asks respondents to rank 18 terminal values in order of importance, by placing a 1 next to the value considered to be the most important through to 18 for the least important value (see Table 3.2). A number of researchers have used a variant of this procedure to measure health value through including health in the list of 18 terminal values or a reduced set of values. In later versions of the health value survey Rokeach has actually replaced the terminal value 'Happiness (contentedness)' with 'Health (physical and mental well-being)'. The advantage of this approach is that health is ranked in

Table 3.2 The health value survey (terminal values)

A comfortable life (a prosperous life)	Inner harmony (freedom from inner conflict)
An exciting life (a stimulating, active life)	Mature love (sexual and spiritual intimacy)
A sense of accomplishment (lasting contribution)	National security (protection from attack)
A world at peace (free of war and conflict)	Pleasure (an enjoyable, leisurely life)
A world of beauty (beauty of nature and the arts)	Salvation (saved, eternal life)
Equality (brotherhood, equal opportunity for all)	Self-respect (self-esteem)
Family security (taking care of loved ones)	Social recognition (respect, admiration)
Freedom (independence, free choice)	True friendship (close companionship)
Happiness (contentedness)	Wisdom (a mature understanding of life)

order of importance against other potentially desirable outcomes. The instrument therefore measures the *relative value* of health. It has been argued that this method of assessment may be particularly applicable to health behaviours in that they frequently involve a choice between 'unhealthy' behaviours which may appear more glamorous or thrilling, or healthier actions which may require considerably more persistent effort (Rotter 1982; Kristiansen 1985). However, concerns have been raised about the reliability of the health value survey (Braithwaite and Scott 1991).

Direct comparisons of the two methods (e.g. Wurtele *et al.* 1985) suggest that they vary little in predictive utility either alone or in interaction with HLC dimensions. Given space demands within questionnaires, Lau's shorter scale is currently the most frequently used measure of health value.

6 An application of health locus of control to dietary choice

The excessive consumption of nutrients such as fat, sugar and salt has been linked to conditions such as obesity and diseases such as coronary heart disease and some cancers (e.g. World Health Organization 1982; Shaper 1988). Against this backdrop, a number of health promotion initiatives have been established to encourage the consumption of a healthy diet in the general population (e.g. Directorate of the Welsh Heart Programme 1985; Farquhar *et al.* 1985; Puska *et al.* 1985; Department of Health 1992). For example, the Health of the Nation White Paper for England (Department of Health 1992) sets outs a number of targets to be achieved by the beginning of the twenty-first century, including reductions in the percentage of food energy derived from total fat. Interventions have therefore advocated a decreased consumption of dairy fats and an increased consumption of fish, lean meats, fruit, vegetables, whole grain rice and bread.

6.1 Study details

The study reported in this section focuses on the relationship between HLC and dietary choice. It forms part of a survey evaluating a major health promotion programme, Heartbeat Wales (Directorate of the Welsh Heart Programme 1985), conducted on a representative population of approximately 13 000 people. A more detailed description of the study can be found in Bennett *et al.* (1995). Given that the study variables were part of a larger questionnaire assessing health and lifestyle factors, it was important that the psychological measures were as short as was reasonably possible.

To achieve the required brevity, a short-form version of the MHLC scale was developed. This comprised three questions for each of the three subscales (items 2, 3, 5, 10, 11, 12, 13, 16 and 17 from form A of the MHLC scale; see Table 3.1). Selection of items was derived from analyses conducted on data derived from an analysis of 2260 responses to the full MHLC scale completed as part of a previous survey of adults in Wales

(Wallston 1989). In the present data set, values for all three scales ranged from 3 to 18. The mean value for the internal HLC scale was 13.78 (SD = 2.31), and Cronbach's alpha was 0.58; for the powerful others HLC scale the mean was 8.41 (SD = 2.89), alpha 0.61; and for the chance HLC scale the mean was 8.92 (SD = 3.27), with an alpha of 0.69. These internal reliability coefficients compare favourably with findings from previous analyses of the full MHLC scale. In addition to the health locus of control questions, the four-item health value scale of Lau *et al.* (1986) was used, as described earlier. The health value scale had a mean of 18.78 (SD = 3.56), and Cronbach's alpha was 0.65.

Dietary choice was measured using two instruments. The first, the dietary frequency questionnaire, involved measures of the frequency of consumption of 16 foodstuffs. Respondents were requested to tick a box indicating whether they usually ate each type of food 'most days', '4 or 5 days a week', '2 or 3 days a week', 'about once a week', 'about once or twice a month' or 'rarely or never'. Dietary grouping variables were derived from a factor analysis of the frequency of consumption of the 16 food items. The factor analysis used principal components analysis and varimax factor rotation. A four-factor solution was selected, which accounted for 46.4 per cent of the variance in the food frequency items: fruit and vegetables, pasta and rice, high fat foods and snacks. The first two factors characterize a generally healthy diet, while the latter may be considered less healthy.

A second measure, the food choice questionnaire, asked respondents to make forced choices, reflecting their typical dietary choices, between similar foodstuffs. Three of these questions asked whether the respondent usually used: wholemeal, brown, white or other types of bread; skimmed, semi-skimmed, ordinary whole milk or other types of milk; butter, polyunsaturated margarine or other types of margarine. Categories for non-use of these foods were also available, where applicable. The fourth question asked whether the respondent usually salted meals only after tasting, before tasting or not at all. Each dietary choice was rated for its 'healthiness', and scores from each of the items were summed to produce the healthy diet habits score. This had a mean score of 5.59 (SD = 2.59) and ranged from 1 to 12 with high scores indicating a healthier choice of foodstuffs.

6.2 Results

The first stage of analysis involved simple correlations between the MHLC scales and the dietary choice measures. This type of analysis was chosen as an example of the simplest, and most common, analysis in the health locus of control literature. Because the number of subjects used in this analysis was extremely high (n = 11 896), only where statistical significance achieved $p < 0.0001$ is it reported. A majority of the correlations were significant (see Table 3.3). The internal HLC scale correlated positively with the consumption of fruit/vegetables and pasta/rice and the healthy

Table 3.3 Correlations between the health locus of control, health value and dietary choice

	Fruit/vegetables	Pasta/rice	High-fat foods	Snacks	Healthy diet score
Internal HLC	0.04*	0.08*	−0.02	−0.03	0.08*
Powerful others HLC	−0.01	−0.11*	0.03	−0.06*	−0.08*
Chance HLC	−0.08*	−0.14*	0.09*	0.02	−0.18*
Health value	0.10*	−0.07*	−0.07*	−0.04*	0.05*

Note: * p < 0.0001.

Table 3.4 Correlations between the MHLC scales and the dietary choice measures for low and high health value respondents

	Fruit/vegetables	Pasta/rice	High-fat foods	Snacks	Healthy diet score
Low HV group					
Internal HLC	0.03	0.08*	0.01	−0.01	0.08*
Powerful others HLC	−0.01	−0.08*	0.06*	−0.04	−0.09*
Chance HLC	−0.11*	−0.14*	0.09*	0.01	−0.22*
High HV group					
Internal HLC	0.03	0.08*	−0.03	−0.04	0.06*
Powerful others HLC	−0.04	−0.12*	0.01	−0.06	−0.08*
Chance HLC	−0.08*	−0.16*	0.10*	0.04	−0.17*

Note: * p < 0.0001.

diet score. Powerful others HLC beliefs correlated negatively with the consumption of pasta/rice, snacks and the healthy diet score. Chance HLC beliefs correlated positively with the consumption of high fat foods and negatively with the consumption of fruit/vegetables and pasta/rice and the healthy diet score. Finally, health value correlated negatively with the consumption of high fat foods, snacks and pasta/rice, and positively with the consumption of fruit/vegetables and the healthy diet score. While these correlations are generally in line with expectations, their absolute values are low.

As we have noted previously, the above correlations fail to take into account variations in health value, and as a result are theoretically unsound. Accordingly, a second series of correlations were conducted among respondents within the upper (*n* = 3959) and lower (*n* = 3923) third of health value scores. (Again, only where statistical significance achieved *p* < 0.0001 is it reported). As can be seen from Table 3.4, a similar pattern

Table 3.5 Regression analyses for low and high health value respondents (beta values)

	Fruit/vegetables	Pasta/rice	High-fat foods	Snacks	Healthy diet score
Low HV group					
Internal HLC	0.02	0.07*	0.01	−0.01	0.06
Powerful others HLC	0.03	−0.06	0.04	−0.05	−0.05
Chance HLC	−0.11*	−0.12*	0.08*	0.02	−0.19*
R^2	0.012	0.027	0.010	0.002	0.051
High HV group					
Internal HLC	0.02	0.05	−0.01	−0.02	0.02
Powerful others HLC	−0.03	−0.11*	−0.03	−0.06	−0.06
Chance HLC	−0.07	−0.13*	0.10*	0.05	−0.15*
R^2	0.007	0.039	0.010	0.007	0.031

Note: * $p < 0.0001$.

of correlations was found for both high and low health value respondents which mirrored the correlations obtained for the full sample. Furthermore, when the correlations were transformed to Fisher's z scores to test the significance of the differences between correlations in the high and low health value groups, no significant differences were found. Thus, the hypothesis that the correlations within the high health value group would be significantly greater than those within the low health value group was not supported.

Multiple regression analyses were conducted to identify the amount of variance in dietary choice accounted for by the MHLC scales among low and high health value respondents respectively. Multiple regression analyses were therefore conducted within the two groups defined by health value for each of the dependent variables. The independent variables were the three MHLC scales. As in previous analyses, it was hypothesized that the percentage of variance in dietary choice explained by the HLC dimensions would be greater in the analysis conducted on high health value respondents.

The results of the regression analyses are presented in Table 3.5. Three main findings are worth noting. First, a similar pattern of results was found among the two groups, both in terms of significance of the beta weights and in terms of the amount of variance explained in dietary choice. Second, with only one exception, the internal HLC dimension failed to emerge as a significant independent predictor of dietary choice. Rather, the chance HLC dimension emerged as the most important predictor. Third, the HLC dimensions accounted for less than 5 per cent of the variance in dietary choice. Only the healthy diet score exceeded this level, and this was only in the model for respondents with low health value.

6.3 Discussion

The findings of this study provide only modest support for the hypothesis that frequency of consumption of healthier and less healthy diets is mediated by an interaction between locus of control beliefs and the value placed on health. While virtually all the associations between the locus of control dimensions and frequency of food consumption were in the predicted direction, the strength of the associations was weak and the model only accounted for a small proportion of the variance in consumption. In addition, taking account of the value placed on health added little to the explanatory power of the HLC construct.

The strongest relationship between HLC and health value and dietary choice was found on the healthy diet score, where it was possible to account for 5 per cent of the variance. This finding may be of particular importance. All other dietary scales measured frequency of consumption of foodstuffs, a measure complicated by total energy expenditure and requirements, and the possibility of eating both healthier and less healthy foodstuffs as part of overall caloric intake. Because the items of the healthy diet score force participants to identify choices between *similar* foodstuffs (bread, spreads, etc.), these scores may be more indicative of the 'healthy' versus 'unhealthy' choices people make.

This result, in particular, suggests that the HLC construct may have some utility in predicting some dietary choices at a population level (Booth-Kewley and Friedman 1987). In addition, the extent of dietary changes potentially mediated by changes in HLC and health value may be sufficient to warrant population-based health promotion interventions targeted at changing these dimensions, particularly in Western populations where small changes in diet may impact strongly on population levels of disease.

A number of factors may have lessened the apparent relationship between locus of control and dietary choice found in the study. In particular, it was not clear whether respondents acknowledged an association between diet and long-term health. Indeed, there are data to suggest that many people are not convinced of such an association; only half the respondents to a survey conducted in Wales reported that diet affected long-term health (Directorate of the Welsh Heart Programme 1986). Issues of HLC or the value attached to health may be of little relevance with regard to dietary choice in this population. Social cognitive theory (Bandura 1986) may also contribute a partial explanation to this finding. The long-term health consequences of diet are distal and probabilistic. Immediate or shorter-term outcomes may be more powerful in determining food choice. In particular, concerns about weight control and appearance may be more important influences on dietary choice than longer-term health gains (Hayes and Ross 1987).

7 Future directions

The results of the study presented in this chapter coincide with a number of recent reviews which have concluded that the health locus of control construct is a weak predictor of health behaviour, even when its inter-action with health value is considered (Wallston 1991, 1992). Responses to this position have been three-fold. First, Wallston and Wallston (1982) have suggested alternative ways in which health locus of control scores can be analysed. Second, the nature of health value and the way in which it is measured has been questioned (Wurtele *et al.* 1985; Lau *et al.* 1986; Kristiansen 1987). Third, some researchers have pointed to a number of neglected variables in social learning theory and have called for a consid-eration of other types of expectancy beliefs (Kristiansen 1987; Wallston 1989, 1991, 1992; Norman 1991). Other researchers have gone further and have questioned the sufficiency of social learning theory, arguing for the inclusion of variables from other theoretical approaches (Wurtele *et al.* 1985). Each of these responses, and their implications for future research, will be considered in turn.

7.1 The analysis of HLC scores

Wallston and Wallston (1982) have questioned the way in which health locus of control scores are typically analysed. They challenged the assump-tion of a linear relationship between HLC beliefs and health behaviour and have suggested that the possibility of non-linear relationships be ex-amined. However, it is unlikely that the failure of researchers to consider non-linear relationships is hiding potentially strong relationships. For ex-ample, Steptoe *et al.* (1994) divided their sample into quartiles on the basis of their scores on a health behaviour index and examined the possibility of non-linear associations with health locus of control through the use of analysis of variance. They concluded that there was no evidence for such associations. Moreover, there is little theoretical justification for expect-ing non-linear relationships if one keeps within a social learning theory framework.

Wallston and Wallston (1981, 1982) have also argued that in some situations it may be advantageous to have particular mixtures of health locus of control beliefs. For example, when individuals are being advised by health professionals to change their health behaviour (e.g. dietary change, smoking cessation), a belief in the role of powerful others *and* strong internal HLC beliefs may be particularly supportive of change. Having strong powerful others HLC beliefs may allow one to be receptive to the health message, but also holding internal HLC beliefs may mean that the advice is translated into behaviour change. Wallston and Wallston (1981) have therefore suggested a multidimensional ($2 \times 2 \times 2$) typology based on median splits on the three HLC dimensions (see also Waller and Bates 1992). Of particular interest are 'believers in control' who score above the median on the internal and powerful others dimensions, but below the median on the chance dimension. Roskam (1986) used this approach to examine the reactions of patients with rheumatoid arthritis when their arthritis flared up. Compared to other types, 'believers in control' were less likely to report increases in depression following such flare ups. While this approach has some promise, its utility may be limited. In particular, it may produce results which are difficult to interpret given that the proposed typology may lead to comparisons between eight different 'types'. If health value is also considered, then this may lead to four-way interactions. Clearly, such interactions may be difficult to explain.

7.2 Measurement of health value

A number of researchers have considered the way in which health value is measured in more detail. Ware (1976) has argued that it is possible to distinguish between physical, mental and social aspects of health. As a result, researchers cannot be sure which aspects of health respondents are considering when they complete health value items. However, given the way in which health value has been used to predict health behaviour it is likely that respondents are primarily considering the value attached to their physical health (Ware and Young 1979; Lau *et al.* 1986).

As outlined earlier, other researchers have argued for the need to consider health value in relation to other values. In deciding whether or not to perform a specific health behaviour (e.g. sensible drinking), individuals are often faced with a range of potentially more exciting or rewarding alternatives. As a result, values other than the value placed on health may be important in determining behaviour. Kristiansen (1987) has advocated the need to measure 'relative health value', in which the value of health is assessed through a ranking procedure. This is generally achieved by employing a modified version of Rokeach's (1973) value survey where health is rank ordered in importance against other potentially desirable outcomes. This can be contrasted with the approach taken by other researchers, in which a health value index is used (e.g. Seeman and Seeman 1983; Lau *et al.* 1986; Norman 1991). Kristiansen (1986) found that measuring health value relative to the value of an exciting life accounted for more of the variance in the preventive health behaviour of young people than a standard health value index. One reason for this may come from research which has shown that values which are salient to people are more likely to guide their behaviour; and for young people leading an exciting life may be more salient to them than longer-term health gains. However, Wurtele *et al.* (1985) found the opposite pattern of results in a sample of female students, with the health value index being the only measure of health value to correlate with preventive health behaviour. Clearly, there is a need for more research comparing different measures of health value, particularly as Wurtele *et al.* (1985) reported that the two measures they employed were only weakly correlated.

7.3 Other expectancy beliefs

Some researchers have pointed to the need to consider other expectancy beliefs (Kristiansen 1987; Calnan 1989; Wallston 1989, 1991, 1992;

Norman 1991). As argued earlier, HLC taps generalized expectancy beliefs with respect to health; it does not refer to expectancies about specific behaviours. To take the example of smoking, a male smoker may value his health, believe that it is under his control, but may or may not believe that quitting smoking would help his health. Concentrating purely on generalized expectancy beliefs would obscure any relationship between expectancy beliefs and behaviour. Examining behavioural efficacy beliefs may lead to a stronger prediction of behaviour. In short, a key variable may be the individual's beliefs about the efficacy of certain behaviours in promoting health. Evidence in support of this view has been presented by Norman (1991), who found that health value and HLC were unrelated to attendance at health checks, while these variables in conjunction with behavioural efficacy beliefs were able to predict attendance behaviour. Similar results have been reported by Kristiansen (1987) in relation to preventive health behaviour intentions. Thus, health behaviour may be best predicted by the extent to which individuals believe that certain behaviours are likely to facilitate their health and the extent to which their health is valued. This move towards considering behavioural efficacy beliefs is simply a move back towards applying Rotter's (1954) original social learning theory on a specific level.

Behavioural efficacy beliefs are concerned with outcome expectancies. However, as Rosenstock *et al.* (1988) have highlighted, it is also possible to consider expectancies concerned with one's perceived competence to perform the behaviour in question, or self-efficacy beliefs (Bandura 1986). So, in addition to believing that a behaviour is likely to facilitate one's health, it is also important to believe that one can perform the behaviour in question. This may be particularly important when considering preventive health behaviours which may be difficult for many people to perform, such as quitting smoking. Mullen *et al.* (1987), for example, found that self-efficacy beliefs were predictive of reductions in the consumption of fried foods and of attempts to quit smoking over an eight-month period. In fact, Wallston (1989) has concluded that self-efficacy beliefs provide stronger predictions of health behaviours than HLC beliefs.

In an attempt to salvage the utility of the HLC construct, Wallston (1989, 1992) has put forward a 'modified social learning theory' in which internal HLC beliefs are a necessary, but not sufficient, condition for performing a health behaviour. In this version of social learning theory it is argued that health behaviour is a function of health value, HLC beliefs and self-efficacy beliefs. Thus, to perform a health behaviour individuals must value their health, believe that it is owing to their health-related actions and concurrently believe that they are capable of performing the behaviour in question. As a result, self-efficacy beliefs should only predict health behaviour when the individual values his or her health and has an internal HLC orientation. To date, there have been no formal tests of Wallston's modified social learning theory. One question which is open to further research is the extent to which it is necessary to hold on to the

HLC construct when predicting health behaviour. Even in the modified social learning theory there is a good case to be made for simply replacing the HLC construct with behavioural efficacy beliefs. Thus, to perform a health behaviour, individuals would have to value their health, believe that the behaviour would facilitate their health and believe that they could perform the behaviour. Following such an approach would make the HLC construct redundant, although there may still be a case for considering HLC beliefs when attempting to predict health behaviour on a general level (i.e. a health behaviour index). This would also require the measurement of generalized self-efficacy beliefs, as Pender *et al.* (1990) have done to predict the performance of health-promoting behaviours.

7.4 Concluding remarks

The role of HLC in predicting health behaviour is a weak one. As Wallston (1991, 1992) has concluded, the amount of variance explained by the HLC construct, even in conjunction with health value, is low. However, it would be surprising if any one construct was able to provide the 'silver bullet' to predict health behaviour fully (Wallston 1989). In short, health behaviour is complex and multidetermined. As a result, HLC theory may simply be too narrow to explain health behaviour adequately (Wurtele *et al.* 1985). The need to consider variables from other theoretical approaches is apparent, and Wallston's (1989, 1992) move towards considering the HLC construct as part of a modified social learning theory is clearly an encouraging development.

References

Abella, R. and Heslin, R. (1984) Health locus of control, values and the behaviour of families and friends. An integrated approach to understanding preventive health behaviour, *Basic and Applied Social Psychology*, 5, 283–93.

Affleck, G., Tennen, H., Croog, S. and Levine, S. (1987) Causal attribution, perceived control, and recovery from a heart attack, *Journal of Social and Clinical Psychology*, 5, 356–64.

Ajzen, I. and Fishbein, M. (1977) Attitude-behavior relations: a theoretical analysis and review of empirical research, *Psychological Bulletin*, 84, 888–918.

Allison, K.R. (1987) Perceived control as a determinant of preventive health behaviour for heart disease and lung cancer, unpublished PhD dissertation, University of Toronto.

Allison, K.R. (1991) Theoretical issues concerning the relationship between perceived control and preventive health behaviour, *Health Education Research*, 6, 141–51.

Anderson, L.A., DeVellis, R.F., Sharpe, P.A. and Marcoux, B. (1994) Multidimensional health locus of control scales: do they measure expectancies about control or desires for control?, *Health Education Research*, 9, 145–51.

Aopoa, W.K. and Damon, A.M. (1982) Locus of control and the quantity-frequency index of alcohol use, *Journal of Studies on Alcohol*, 43, 23–239.

Bandura, A. (1982) Self-efficacy mechanisms in human agency, *American Psychologist*, 37, 122–47.

Bandura, A. (1986) *Social Foundations of Thought and Action*. Englewood Cliffs, NJ: Prentice-Hall.

Bennett, P., Moore, L., Smith, A., Murphy, S. and Smith, C. (1995) Health locus of control and value for health as predictors of dietary behaviour, *Psychology and Health*.

Booth-Kewley, S. and Friedman, H.S. (1987) Psychological predictors of heart disease: a quantitative review, *Psychological Bulletin*, 101, 343–62.

Bradley, C., Lewis, K., Jennings, A. and Ward, S. (1990) Scales to measure perceived control developed specifically for people with tablet-treated diabetes, *Diabetic Medicine*, 7, 685–94.

Braithwaite, V.A. and Scott, W.A. (1991) Values. In J.P. Robinson, P.R. Shaver and L.S. Wrightsman (eds) *Measures of Personality and Social Psychological Attitudes*. New York: Academic Press, 661–753.

Brown, N., Muhlenkamp, A., Fox, L. and Osborn, M. (1983) The relationship among health beliefs, health values, and health promotion activity, *Western Journal of Nursing Research*, 5, 155–63.

Bundek, N.I., Marks, G. and Richardson, J.L. (1993) Role of health locus of control beliefs in cancer screening of elderly Hispanic women, *Health Psychology*, 12, 193–9.

Burish, T.G., Carey, M.P., Wallston, K.A., Stein, M.J., Jamison, R.N. and Lyles, J.N. (1984) Health locus of control and chronic disease: an external orientation may be advantageous, *Journal of Clinical and Social Psychology*, 2, 326–32.

Butts, S.V. and Chotlas, J.A. (1973) A comparison of alcoholics and nonalcoholics on perceived locus of control, *Quarterly Journal of Studies on Alcohol*, 34, 1327–32.

Calnan, M. (1989) Control over health and patterns of health-related behaviour, *Social Science and Medicine*, 29, 131–6.

Carlson, B. and Petti, K. (1989) Health locus of control and participation in physical activity, *American Journal of Health Promotion*, 3, 32–7.

Carman, R.S. (1974) Internal–external locus of control, alcohol use and adjustment among high school students in rural communities, *Journal of Community Psychology*, 2, 129–33.

Chavez, E.L. and Michaels, A.C. (1980) Evaluation of the health locus of control for obesity treatment, *Psychological Reports*, 47, 709–10.

Chess, S.B., Neuringer, C. and Goldstein, G. (1971) Arousal and field dependency in alcoholics, *Journal of General Psychology*, 85, 93–102.

Collins, B.E. (1974) Four separate components of the Rotter I–E scale: belief in a difficult world, a just world, a predictable world and a politically responsive world, *Journal of Personality and Social Psychology*, 29, 381–91.

Cooper, D. and Fabroni, M. (1990) Psychometric study of forms A and B of the multidimensional health locus of control scale, *Psychological Reports*, 66, 859–64.

Costello, R.M. and Manders, K.R. (1974) Locus of control and alcoholism, *British Journal of Addiction*, 69, 11–17.

Dean, K. (1991) Relationships between knowledge and belief variables and health maintenance behaviours in a Danish population over 45 years of age, *Journal of Ageing and Health*, 3, 386–406.

DeCharms, R. (1976) *Enhancing Motivation: Change in the Classroom*. New York: Irvington.

Department of Health (1992) *Health of the Nation.* London: HMSO.

Department of Health and Welsh Office (1989) *General Practice in the National Health Service: a New Contract.* London: HMSO.

DeVito, A.J., Bogdanowicz, J. and Reznikoff, M. (1982) Actual and intended health-related information seeking and health locus of control, *Journal of Personality Assessment*, **46**, 63–9.

Directorate of the Welsh Heart Programme (1985) *Take Heart. A Consultative Document on the Development of Community-based Heart Health Initiatives in Wales. Heartbeat Report No. 1.* Cardiff: Health Promotion Wales.

Directorate of the Welsh Heart Programme (1986) *Pulse of Wales. Preliminary Report of the Welsh Heart Health Survey, 1985. Heartbeat Report No. 4.* Cardiff: Health Promotion Wales.

Donovan, D.M. and O'Leary, M.R. (1975) Comparison of perceived and experienced control among alcoholics and nonalcoholics, *Journal of Applied Psychology*, **89**, 726–8.

Donovan, D.M. and O'Leary, M.R. (1978) The drinking-related locus of control scale, *Journal of Studies on Alcohol*, **39**, 759–84.

Drasgow, F., Palau, J., Taibi, R. and Drasgow, J. (1974) Levels of functioning and locus of control, *Journal of Clinical Psychology*, **30**, 365–9.

Duffy, M.E. (1988) Determinants of health promotion in midlife women, *Nursing Research*, **37**, 358–62.

Farquhar, J.W., Fortman, S.P., Maccoby, N., Haskell, W.L., Williams, P.T., Flora, J.A., Taylor, C.B., Brown, B.W., Solomon, D.S. and Hulley, S.B. (1985) The Stanford five city project: design and methods, *American Journal of Epidemiology*, **122**, 232–334.

Ferraro, L., Price, J., Desmond, S. and Roberts, S. (1987) Development of a diabetes locus of control scale, *Psychological Reports*, **61**, 763–70.

Furnham, A. and Steele, H. (1993) Measuring locus of control: a critique of general, children's, health- and work-related locus of control questionnaires, *British Journal of Psychology*, **84**, 443–79.

Georgiou, A. and Bradley, C. (1992) The development of a smoking specific locus of control scale, *Psychology and Health*, **6**, 227–40.

Gierszewski, S.A. (1983) The relationship of weight loss, locus of control, and social support, *Nursing Research*, **32**, 43–7.

Gozali, J. and Sloan, J. (1971) Control orientation as a personality dimension among alcoholics, *Quarterly Journal of Studies on Alcohol*, **32**, 159–61.

Green, L. and Raeburn, J. (1988) Health promotion. What is it? What will it become?, *Health Promotion*, **3**, 151–9.

Groth-Marnat, G. and Schumaker, J.F. (1987–9) Locus of control as a predictor of severity of weight-control strategies in bulimics, *Psychology and Human Development*, **2**, 61–6.

Gurin, P., Gurin, G., Lao, R.C. and Beattie, M. (1969) Internal–external control in the motivational dynamics of Negro youth, *Journal of Social Issues*, **25**, 29–53.

Hallal, J. (1982) The relationship of health beliefs, health locus of control, and self-concept to the practice of breast self-examination in adult women, *Nursing Research*, **31**, 137–42.

Harter, S. and O'Connell, J.P. (1984) A model of the relationships among children's academic achievement and their self-perceptions of competence, control, and motivational orientation. In J. Nicholls (ed.) *The Development of Achievement Motivation.* Greenwich, CT: JAI Press, 219–50.

Hartke, R.J. and Kunce, J.T. (1982) Multidimensionality of health-related locus-of-control items, *Journal of Consulting and Clinical Psychology*, 50, 594–5.

Hayes, D. and Ross, C.E. (1987) Concern with appearance, health beliefs and eating habits, *Journal of Health and Social Behaviour*, 28, 120–30.

Horwitz, M.B., Hindi-Alexander, M. and Wagner, T.J. (1985) Psychosocial mediators of abstinence, relapse, and continued smoking: a one-year follow-up of a minimal intervention, *Addictive Behaviors*, 10, 29–39.

Huckstadt, A. (1987) Locus of control among alcoholics, recovering alcoholics, and non-alcoholics, *Research in Nursing and Health*, 10, 23–8.

Kaplan, G.D. and Cowles, A. (1978) Health locus of control and health value in the prediction of smoking behavior, *Health Education Monographs*, 6, 129–37.

Kirscht, J.P. (1972) Perception of control and health beliefs, *Canadian Journal of Behavioral Science*, 4, 225–37.

Kelley, J.A., St. Lawrence, J.S., Brasfield, T.L., Lemke, A., Amidei, T., Roffman, R.E., Hood, H.V., Smith, J.E., Kilgore, H. and McNeill, C. (1990) Psychological factors that predict AIDS high-risk versus AIDS precautionary behavior, *Journal of Consulting and Clinical Psychology*, 58, 117–20.

King, J. (1982) The impact of patients' perceptions of high blood pressure on attendance at screening, *Social Science and Medicine*, 16, 1079–91.

Krampen, G. (1980) Generalized expectations of alcoholics: multidimensional locus of control, hopelessness, and Machiavellianism, *Journal of Clinical Psychology*, 36, 1022–3.

Kristiansen, C.M. (1985) Value correlates of preventive health behavior, *Journal of Personality and Social Psychology*, 49, 748–58.

Kristiansen, C.M. (1986) A two-value model of preventive health behaviour, *Basic and Applied Social Psychology*, 7, 173–84.

Kristiansen, C.M. (1987) Social learning theory and preventive health behaviour: some neglected variables, *Social Behaviour*, 2, 73–86.

Labs, S. and Wurtele, S. (1986) Fetal health locus of control: development and validation, *Journal of Consulting and Clinical Psychology*, 54, 814–19.

Laffrey, S.C. and Isenberg, M. (1983) The relationship of internal locus of control, value placed on health, perceived importance of exercise and participation in physical activity during leisure, *International Journal of Nursing Studies*, 20, 187–96.

Lau, R.R. (1982) Origins of health locus of control beliefs, *Journal of Personality and Social Psychology*, 42, 322–34.

Lau, R.R., Hartman, K.A. and Ware, J.E. (1986) Health as value: methodological and theoretical considerations, *Health Psychology*, 5, 25–43.

Lau, R.R. and Ware, J.E. (1981) Refinements in the measurement of health-specific locus-of-control beliefs, *Medical Care*, 19, 1147–58.

Lefcourt, H.M. (1991) Locus of control. In J.P. Robinson, P.R. Shaver and L.S. Wrightsman (eds) *Measures of Personality and Social Psychological Attitudes*. New York: Academic Press, 661–753.

Levenson, H. (1974) Multidimensional locus of control in psychiatric patients, *Journal of Consulting and Clinical Psychology*, 41, 397–404.

McCallum, D.M., Keith, B.R. and Wiebe, D.J. (1988) Comparison of response formats for multidimensional health locus of control scales: six levels versus two levels, *Journal of Personality Assessment*, 54, 732–6.

McCusker, J. and Morrow, G. (1979) The relationship of health locus of control to preventive health behaviors and health beliefs, *Patient Counselling and Health Education*, 1, 146–50.

Marshall, G. (1991) A multidimensional analysis of internal health locus of control beliefs: separating the wheat from the chaff, *Journal of Personality and Social Psychology*, **61**, 483–91.

Marshall, G.N., Collins, B.E. and Crooks, B.C. (1990) A comparison of two multidimensional health locus of control instruments, *Journal of Personality Assessment*, **54**, 181–90.

Mechanic, D. and Cleary, P.D. (1980) Factors associated with the maintenance of positive health behavior, *Preventive Medicine*, **9**, 805–14.

Mirels, H.L. (1970) Dimensions of internal versus external control, *Journal of Consulting and Clinical Psychology*, **34**, 226–8.

Muhlenkamp, A.F., Brown, N.J. and Sands, D. (1985) Determinants of health promotion activities in nursing clinic clients, *Nursing Research*, **34**, 327–33.

Mullen, P.D., Hersey, J.C. and Iverson, D.C. (1987) Health behaviour models compared, *Social Science and Medicine*, **24**, 973–81.

Naditch, M.P. (1975) Locus of control and drinking behavior in a sample of men in army basic training, *Journal of Consulting and Clinical Psychology*, **43**, 96.

Nemeck, M.A. (1990) Health beliefs and breast self-examination among black women, *Health Values*, **14**, 41–52.

Nicassio, P., Wallston, K., Callahan, L., Herbert, M. and Pincus, T. (1985) The measurement of helplessness in rheumatoid arthritis: the development of the arthritis helplessness scale, *Journal of Rheumatology*, **12**, 462–7.

Norman, P. (1990) Health locus of control beliefs and preventive health behaviours, *Journal of the Institute of Health Education*, **28**, 113–17.

Norman, P. (1991) Social learning theory and the prediction of attendance at screening, *Psychology and Health*, **5**, 231–9.

Norman, P. (1995) Heath locus of control and health behaviour: an investigation into the role of health value and behaviour-specific efficacy beliefs, *Personality and Individual Differences*, **18**, 213–8.

O'Connel, J.K. and Price, J.H. (1982) Health locus of control of physical fitness program participants, *Perceptual and Motor Skills*, **55**, 925–6.

O'Looney, B.A. and Barrett, P.T. (1983) A psychometric investigation of the multidimensional health locus of control questionnaire, *British Journal of Clinical Psychology*, **22**, 217–18.

World Health Organization (1986) *Ottawa Charter for Health Promotion*. Ottawa: Canadian Public Health Association.

Oziel, L.V., Obitz, F.W. and Keyson, M. (1972) General and specific perceived locus of control in alcoholics, *Psychological Reports*, **30**, 957–8.

Pearlin, L. and Schoder, C. (1978) The structure of coping, *Journal of Health and Social Behavior*, **19**, 2–21.

Pender, N.J., Walker, S.N., Sechrist, K.R. and Frank-Stromberg, M. (1990) Predicting health-promoting lifestyles in the workplace, *Nursing Research*, **39**, 326–32.

Peterson, C., Semmel, A., von Baeyer, C., Abramson, L.Y., Metalsky, G.I. and Seligman, M.E.P. (1982) The attributional style questionnaire, *Cognitive Therapy and Research*, **6**, 287–300.

Phares, E.J. (1976) *Locus of Control in Personality*. Morristown, NJ: General Learning Press.

Price-Greathouse, J. and Trice, A.D. (1986) Chance health-orientation and AIDS information seeking, *Psychological Reports*, **59**, 10.

Prwun, J., van der Borne, H., de Reuver, R., de Boer, M., Ter Pelkwijk, M. and de Jong, P. (1988) The locus of control scale for cancer patients, *Tijdscrift vour Sociale Gezondherdszong*, **66**, 404–8.

Puska, P., Nissinen, A., Tuomilheto, J., Salonen, J.T., Mcalister, A., Kottke, T.E., Maccoby, N. and Farquhar, J.W. (1985) The community-based strategy to prevent coronary heart disease: conclusions from the ten years of the North Karelia Project, *Annual Review of Public Health*, **6**, 147–93.

Rabinowitz, S., Melamed, S., Weisberg, E., Tal, D. and Ribak, J. (1992) Personal determinants of leisure-time exercise activities, *Perceptual and Motor Skills*, **75**, 779–84.

Rauckhorst, L.M. (1987) Health habits of elderly widows, *Journal of Gerontological Nursing*, **13**, 19–22.

Redeker, N.S. (1989) Health beliefs, health locus of control, and the frequency of practice of breast self-examination in women, *Journal of Obstetrics, Gynaecology and Neonatal Nursing*, **18**, 45–51.

Rokeach, M. (1973) *The Nature of Human Values*. New York: Free Press.

Rokeach, M. (1979) *Understanding Human Values: Individual and Societal*. New York: Free Press.

Rosen, T.J. and Shipley, R.H. (1983) A stage analysis of self-initiated smoking reductions, *Addictive Behaviors*, **8**, 263–72.

Rosenstock, I.M., Strecher, V.J. and Becker, M.H. (1988) Social learning theory and the health belief model, *Health Education Quarterly*, **15**, 175–83.

Roskam, S. (1986) Application of health locus of control typology toward predicting depression and medical adherence in rheumatoid arthritis, unpublished doctoral dissertation, Vanderbilt University, Nashville, TN.

Rotter, J.B. (1954) *Social Learning and Clinical Psychology*. Englewood Cliffs, NJ: Prentice-Hall.

Rotter, J.B. (1966) Generalized expectancies for internal and external control of reinforcement, *Psychological Monographs: General and Applied*, **80** (whole no. 609), 1–28.

Rotter, J.B. (1975) Some problems and misconceptions related to the construct of internal versus external control of reinforcement, *Journal of Consulting and Clinical Psychology*, **43**, 56–67.

Rotter, J.B. (1982) *The Development and Applications of Social Learning Theory: Selected Papers*. Brattleboro, VT: Praeger.

Rotter, J.B. (1990) Internal versus external control of reinforcement: a case history of a variable, *American Psychologist*, **45**, 489–93.

Sacco, W.P., Levine, B., Reed, D.I. and Thompsom, K. (1991) Attitudes about condom use as an AIDS-relevant behaviour: their factor structure and relation to condom use, *Psychological Assessment: Journal of Consulting and Clinical Psychology*, **3**, 265–72.

St Lawrence, J.S. (1993) African-American adolescents' knowledge, health-related attitudes, sexual behaviour, and contraceptive decisions: implications for the prevention of adolescent HIV infection, *Journal of Consulting and Clinical Psychology*, **61**, 104–12.

Saltzer, E.B. (1978) Locus of control and one's intention to lose weight, *Health Education Monographs*, **6**, 118–28.

Saltzer, E.B. (1982) The weight locus of control (WLOC) scale: a specific measure for obesity research, *Journal of Personality Assessment*, **46**, 620–8.

Schifter, D.B. and Ajzen, I. (1985) Intention, perceived control and weight loss: an application of the theory of planned behavior, *Journal of Personality and Social Psychology*, **49**, 843–51.

Schilling, M.E. and Carman, R.S. (1978) Internal-external control and motivations for alcohol use among high school students, *Psychological Reports*, **42**, 1088–90.

Seeman, M. and Seeman, T.E. (1983) Health behaviour and personal autonomy: a longitudinal study of the sense of control in illness, *Journal of Health and Social Behaviour*, **24**, 144–60.

Segal, B. (1974) Locus of control and drug and alcohol use in college students, *Journal of Alcohol and Drug Education*, **19**, 1–5.

Segall, M.E. and Wynd, C.A. (1990) Health conception, health locus of control, and power as predictors of smoking behavior change, *American Journal of Health Promotion*, **4**, 338–44.

Shaper, A.G. (1988) *Coronary Heart Disease: Risks and Reasons*. London: Current Medical Literature.

Shipley, R.H. (1981) Maintenance of smoking cessation: effect of follow-up letters, smoking motivation, muscle tension, and health locus of control, *Journal of Consulting and Clinical Psychology*, **49**, 982–4.

Slenker, S.E., Price, J.H. and O'Connell, J.K. (1985) Health locus of control of joggers and nonexercisers, *Perceptual and Motor Skills*, **61**, 323–8.

Smith, C.A., Dobbins, C. and Wallston, K.A. (1991) The mediational role of perceived competence in adaptation to rheumatoid arthritis, *Journal of Applied Social Psychology*, **21**, 1218–47.

Smith, I.K., Lancaster, C.J., Delbene, V.E. and Fleming, G.A. (1990) The relationship between medical students' locus of control and promotion of breast self-examination, *Medical Education*, **24**, 164–70.

Stanton, A. (1987) Determinants of adherence to medical regimens by hypertensive patients, *Journal of Behavioural Medicine*, **10**, 377–94.

Steptoe, A., Wardle, J., Vinck, J., Tuomisto, M., Holte, A. and Wickstrom, L. (1994) Personality and attitudinal correlates of healthy and unhealthy lifestyles in young adults, *Psychology and Health*, **9**, 331–43.

Stotland, S. and Zuroff, D. (1990) A new measure of weight locus of control: the dieting beliefs scale, *Journal of Personality Assessment*, **54**, 191–203.

Strickland, B.R. (1978) Internal–external expectancies and health-related behaviors, *Journal of Consulting and Clinical Psychology*, **46**, 1192–211.

Taylor, S.E., Lichtman, R.R. and Wood, J.V. (1984) Attributions, beliefs about control and adjustment to breast cancer, *Journal of Personality and Social Psychology*, **46**, 489–502.

Tennen, H., Affleck, G., Allen, D.A., McGrade, B.J. and Ratzan, S. (1984) Causal attributions and coping with insulin-dependent diabetes, *Basic and Applied Social Psychology*, **5**, 131–42.

Tinsley, B.J. and Holtgrave, D.R. (1989) Maternal health locus of control beliefs, utilization of childhood preventive health services, and infant health, *Journal of Developmental and Behavioral Paediatrics*, **10**, 236–41.

Waller, K.V. and Bates, R.C. (1992) Health locus of control and self-efficacy beliefs in a healthy elderly sample, *American Journal of Health Promotion*, **6**, 302–9.

Wallston, B.S. and Wallston, K.A. (1978) Locus of control and health: a review of the literature, *Health Education Monographs*, **6**, 107–17.

Wallston, B.S., Wallston, K.A., Kaplan, G.D. and Maides, S.A. (1976) Development and validation of the health locus of control (HLC) scale, *Journal of Consulting and Clinical Psychology*, **44**, 580–5.

Wallston, K.A. (1989) Assessment of control in health care settings. In A. Steptoe and A. Appels (eds) *Stress, Personal Control and Health*. London: Wiley, 85–105.

Wallston, K.A. (1991) The importance of placing measures of health locus of control beliefs in a theoretical context, *Health Education Research: Theory and Practice*, **6**, 251–2.

Wallston, K.A. (1992) Hocus-pocus, the focus isn't strictly on locus: Rotter's social learning theory modified for health, *Cognitive Therapy and Research*, **16**, 183–99.

Wallston, K.A., Maides, S. and Wallston, B.S. (1976) Health-related information seeking as a function of health-related locus of control and health value, *Journal of Research in Personality*, **10**, 215–22.

Wallston, K.A. and O'Connor, E. (1987) The initial development and validation of the smoking cessation locus of control scale, unpublished manuscript, Vanderbilt University, Nashville, TN.

Wallston, K.A., Smith, R.A., King, J.E., Forsberg, P.R., Wallston, B.S. and Nagy, V.T. (1983) Expectancies about control over health: relationship to desire for control of health care, *Personality and Social Psychology Bulletin*, **9**, 377–85.

Wallston, K.A. and Wallston, B.S. (1980) Health locus of control scales. In H. Lefcourt (ed.) *Advances and Innovations in Locus of Control Research*. New York: Academic Press, 198–234.

Wallston, K.A. and Wallston, B.S. (1981) Health locus of control scales. In H. Lefcourt (ed.) *Research with the Locus of Control Construct*, Vol. 1. New York: Academic Press, 189–243.

Wallston, K.A. and Wallston, B.S. (1982) Who is responsible for your health? The construct of health locus of control. In G. Sanders and J. Suls (eds) *Social Psychology of Health and Illness*. Hillsdale, NJ: Erlbaum, 65–95.

Wallston, K.A. and Wallston, B.S. (1984) Social psychological models of health behaviour: an examination and integration. In A. Baum, S. Taylor and J.E. Singer (eds) *Handbook of Psychology and Health*, Vol. IV: *Social Aspects of Health*. Hillsdale, NJ: Erlbaum, 23–53.

Wallston, K.A., Wallston, B.S. and DeVellis, R. (1978) Development of multidimensional health locus of control (MHLC) scales, *Health Education Monographs*, **6**, 160–70.

Ware, J.E. (1976) Scales for measuring general health perceptions, *Health Services Research*, **11**, 396–415.

Ware, J.E. and Young, J. (1979) Issues in the conceptualization and measurement of value placed on health. In S.J. Mushkin and D.W. Dunlop (eds) *Health: What Is It Worth?* New York: Pergamon, 141–66.

Weiss, G.L. and Larsen, D.L. (1990) Health value, health locus of control, and the prediction of health protective behaviors, *Social Behavior and Personality*, **18**, 121–36.

Winefield, H.R. (1982) Reliability and validity of the health locus of control scale, *Journal of Personality Assessment*, **46**, 614–19.

Witenberg, S.H., Blanchard, E.B., Suls, J., Tennen, H., McCoy, G. and McGoldrick, M.D. (1983) Perceptions of control and causality as predictors of compliance with hemodiakysis, *Basic and Applied Social Psychology*, **1**, 319–36.

Wojcik, J.V. (1988) Social learning predictors of the avoidance of smoking relapse, *Addictive Behaviors*, **13**, 177–80.

World Health Organization (1982).*Prevention of Coronary Heart Disease. Report of a WHO Expert Committee*. Technical Report Series No. 678. Geneva: WHO.

Wurtele, S.K., Britcher, J.C. and Saslawsky, D.A. (1985) Relationships between locus of control, health value and preventive health behaviors among women, *Journal of Research in Personality*, **19**, 271–8.

Zindler-Wernet, P. and Weiss, S.J. (1987) Health locus of control and preventive behaviour, *Western Journal of Nursing Research*, **9**, 160–79.

4

HENK BOER AND
ERWIN R. SEYDEL

PROTECTION MOTIVATION THEORY

1 General background

Protection motivation theory was originally (Rogers 1975) proposed to provide conceptual clarity to the understanding of fear appeals. A later revision of protection motivation theory (Rogers 1983) extended the theory to a more general theory of persuasive communication, with an emphasis on the cognitive processes mediating behavioural change.

Protection motivation theory was first developed within the framework of fear-arousing communication. In fear-arousing communication research a central issue has been whether fear-arousing communications can in themselves influence cognitions, attitudes, behavioural intentions and health behaviour, or whether the effects are of a more indirect nature. In the Yale Programme of Research on Communication and Attitude Change (Hovland *et al.* 1953) a systematic study was made of the way in which, and the conditions under which, communication is effective in changing beliefs, attitudes and behaviour. This research was based on the fear-drive model. The point of departure of the fear-drive model is that fear acts as a drive that motivates trial and error behaviour. If a message evokes fear in the receiver, the receiver is motivated to reduce this unpleasant emotional situation. If the message contains reassuring behavioural advice, following this advice is a way to reduce the threat. If execution of the advised behaviour leads to a reduction of fear, this behavioural response is reinforced and the chance of following the advised behaviour is enhanced. If the execution of the advised behaviour does not lead to a reduction of fear, maladaptive coping reactions, such as denial of the threat or avoidance of the fear-evoking message, may be used as ways of avoiding the fear arousal.

The fear-drive model assumes that a non-linear, parabolic relation exists between the level of evoked fear and preparedness to follow the advised, adaptive, behaviour (Janis 1967). A medium level of evoked fear leads to maximal adoption of the advised behaviour. At a medium level of evoked fear, cognitive responses that promote the adoption of the advised behaviour are more prominent than cognitive responses that promote the adoption of maladaptive cognitive responses, like denial of the threat. The balance between the adoption of adaptive and maladaptive responses in reaction to fear-arousing communications has been elaborated in the parallel response model (Leventhal 1970). In the parallel response model danger control is distinguished from fear control. Danger control refers to the process of selecting (behavioural) responses aimed at reducing the actual danger (e.g. adopting the advised behaviour), while fear control refers to the process of selecting responses aimed at reducing the emotional threat (e.g. avoiding threatening messages or denying the threat). In comparison to the fear-drive model, which assumes that in fear-arousing communications the level of evoked fear plays a direct role in the adoption of adaptive behaviours, in the parallel response model the cognitive reaction of the individual in terms of fear control or danger control plays a prominent role in the adoption of adaptive behaviours.

Results on the relation between fear-arousing communications and the adoption of adaptive responses has led to unequivocal results. Sutton (1982) has studied some assumptions from the fear-drive model by reviewing the results of 40 studies – from Janis and Feshbach (1953) to Mewborn and Rogers (1979) – on the effectiveness of fear-arousing communications. Sutton concludes that a linear relation exists between the level of evoked fear and the adoption of the advised behaviour. There is no evidence of a non-linear relation between level of evoked fear and adoption of the advised behaviour. Sutton concludes that enhancing the effectiveness of the advised behaviour enhances the adoption of the advised behaviour. Level of evoked fear and the judged effectiveness of the advised behaviour have an independent influence on the adoption of the advised behaviour.

2 Description of the model

The obtained results of various studies into the effectiveness of fear-arousing communications led to the conclusion that level of evoked fear has a linear relation with the adoption of adaptive responses. In fear-evoking health communications, level of fear arousal may lead to an enhancement of the perceived severity of the disease and the perceived vulnerability to the disease. This effect of fear-arousing communication is elaborated upon in protection motivation theory (PMT) (Rogers 1975). Since the original formulation protection motivation theory has been revised several times (Maddux and Rogers 1983; Rogers 1983; Tanner et al. 1991). A schematic representation of PMT is given in Figure 4.1.

Protection motivation theory (Rogers 1983) is partially based on the

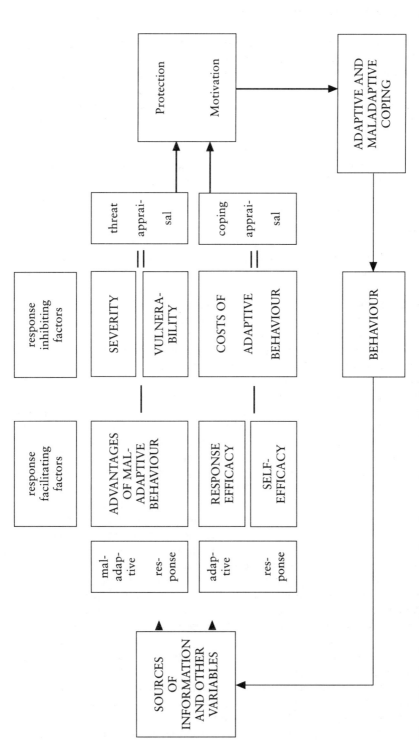

Figure 4.1 A schematic representation of protection motivation theory.

work of Lazarus (1966) and Leventhal (1970) and describes adaptive and maladaptive coping with a health threat as the result of two appraisal processes: a process of threat appraisal and a process of coping appraisal, in which the behavioural options to diminish the threat are evaluated. The appraisal of the health threat and the appraisal of the coping responses result in the intention to perform adaptive responses (protection motivation) or may lead to maladaptive responses. Maladaptive responses are those that place an individual at a health risk. They include behaviours that lead to negative consequences (e.g. smoking) and the absence of behaviours, which eventually may lead to negative consequences (e.g. not participating in breast cancer screening and thus missing the opportunity of early detection of a tumour).

According to PMT the threat appraisal process evaluates the components that are relevant for an evaluation of the threat. In the case of health behaviour these are, for example, estimates of the chance of contracting a disease (perceived vulnerability or susceptibility) and estimates of the seriousness of a disease (perceived severity). Perceived vulnerability and perceived severity of a disease are expected to inhibit the probability of maladaptive responses. Advantages of maladaptive behaviour (e.g. saving time by not participating in breast cancer screening) facilitate the probability of a maladaptive response. Fear arousal indirectly enhances the protection motivation by heightening perceived severity of the disease and perceived vulnerability to the disease.

The coping appraisal process evaluates the components that are relevant for the evaluation of the coping responses. These components are the individual's expectancy that carrying out recommendations can remove the threat (response efficacy) and the belief in one's ability to execute the recommended courses of action successfully (self-efficacy). Self-efficacy was added to the original model (Rogers 1975) in 1983 and is taken from the social learning theory of Bandura (1977, 1986). According to protection motivation theory, adaptive behaviour (protection motivation) is enhanced by the belief that the behaviour is effective in reducing the threat (response efficacy) and by the expectation that one can successfully execute the advised adaptive behaviour (self-efficacy). The costs of the adaptive behaviours limit the protection motivation.

Protection motivation is the result of the threat appraisal and the coping appraisal. Protection motivation is a mediating variable whose function is to arouse, sustain and direct protective health behaviour. It facilitates the adoption of adaptive behaviours and can best be measured by behavioural intentions. Not all components of the model are measured in all studies. The main components of the model that are used in most studies are shown in Table 4.1.

Originally, perceived severity, vulnerability and response efficacy were hypothesized to combine multiplicatively to arouse protection motivation (Rogers 1975). This multiplicative relation was proposed because no protection motivation would be aroused if the value of any of the three

Table 4.1 The main components of protection motivation theory

Severity	How severe are the consequences of the disease?
Vulnerability	How probable is it that I will contract the disease?
Response efficacy	How effective is the recommended behaviour in avoiding the negative consequences?
Self-efficacy	To what extent am I able to perform the recommended behaviour succesfully?
Protection motivation	Am I intending to perform the recommended behaviour?
Protective behaviour	Performing the recommended behaviour

components were zero. This combinatorial rule, however, failed repeatedly to receive empirical support (see Rippetoe and Rogers 1987, for an exception). In the revised version of the theory, Rogers (1983) rejected the multiplicative combinatorial rule in favour of an additive model, which included the main effects of severity, vulnerability, response efficacy and self-efficacy. Whether the multiplicative or additive model is correct under specific circumstances remains an empirical question.

3 Summary of research

PMT has been used as a framework for influencing and predicting various behaviours, such as persuading consumers to use less energy (Hass *et al.* 1975), promoting water conservation (Kantola *et al.* 1983), increasing intentions to engage in behaviours related to the prevention of nuclear war (Wolf *et al.* 1986), increasing assertive behaviour in interpersonal communication (Maddux *et al.* 1986), increasing precautionary measures to prevent burglary (Wiegman *et al.* 1992) and increasing earthquake preparedness (Mulilis and Lippa 1990).

PMT has also been widely applied to health-related behaviours. In these studies PMT has frequently been used as a framework for health education interventions designed to influence health behaviour. Typically various pamphlets are used, in which the content of the health education is varied on a number of dimensions, which, according to PMT, mediate adaptive, protective health behaviour. The main fields of application to date are reducing alcohol use, enhancing healthy lifestyles, enhancing diagnostic health behaviours and preventing disease.

3.1 Reducing alcohol use

Stainback and Rogers (1983) used PMT as a framework for the design of persuasive messages that described the unpleasant consequences of abusive drinking to junior high school students. Two components of PMT were varied in the messages by various descriptions of the severity of the consequences of drinking and the probability that these consequences will occur. The third component, efficacy of not drinking in preventing unfavourable consequences, was held constant across messages by stating that teenage abstinence was the best way to avoid the negative consequences of drinking. Manipulation checks revealed that the high-fear group (who received messages describing severe consequences and a high probability of occurrence) rated the severity of the consequences of drinking and the likelihood of experiencing these consequences as greater than the low-fear group (who received messages describing no severe consequences and a low probability of occurrence). Immediately after exposure to the information the high-fear condition produced stronger intentions to remain abstinent than the low-fear condition. Results were, however, short-lived because in the study the provision of a counter-argument significantly weakened the effects of the high-fear condition, resulting in equal intentions to abstain in both the high-fear and the low-fear groups.

The study of Stainback and Rogers (1983) does not provide information about the relative importance of PMT components in predicting intentions to abstain. Some clues about their relative importance in predicting alcohol drinking intentions are provided by the study of Runge *et al.* (1993). Responses of a community sample of elderly persons with no alcohol abuse problems were compared with responses of inpatients who had alcohol abuse problems. The results indicated that the hospital sample felt more vulnerable to the dangers of alcohol abuse than did the community sample. Hospitalized individuals reported lower response efficacy for moderate drinking than did their community counterparts. No differences were observed for the severity of consequences of alcohol abuse.

3.2 Enhancing healthy lifestyles

Stanley and Maddux (1986) investigated the usefulness of a combined protection motivation and self-efficacy theory as a framework for the design of persuasive messages aimed at promoting exercise behaviour. In a between-subjects factorial design, written persuasive communications were provided to undergraduate students. The persuasive communications varied (low versus high) on response efficacy, self-efficacy and outcome value. Manipulation checks revealed that the self-efficacy manipulation had a significant effect on self-efficacy expectation with respect to participation in the exercise programme, the response efficacy manipulation had a significant effect on the perceived response efficacy and the outcome manipulation had a significant effect on the perceived outcome value. Subjects in the high response efficacy condition reported stronger behavioural intentions to participate in the exercise programme than did the subjects in the low response efficacy condition. Subjects in the high self-efficacy condition reported stronger behavioural intentions to participate in the exercise programme than the subjects in the low self-efficacy condition. Response efficacy was the best single predictor of the intention to exercise ($R^2 = 0.26$), but self-efficacy was also a significant predictor of the intention to exercise ($R^2 = 0.17$) and it added significant predictability to response efficacy (R^2 total $= 0.35$).

Wurtele and Maddux (1987) used a factorial design to test the relative effectiveness of persuasive appeals for increasing exercise, which varied on four components of PMT (severity, vulnerability, response efficacy and self-efficacy). Manipulation checks revealed a significant main effect of components described in the persuasive appeals with regard to, respectively, the severity of the consequences of not exercising, the vulnerability to cardiovascular problems, the efficacy of exercising for preventing cardiovascular problems and the perceived ability to begin and continue with a regular programme of exercise. Analysis revealed a predicted main effect of perceived vulnerability and a predicted main effect of perceived self-efficacy on intentions to exercise. Perceived severity of the consequences of not exercising and perceived response efficacy were not related to exercise intentions and behaviour. Self-efficacy expectancy emerged from multiple regression analysis as the most powerful predictor of intentions to exercise.

Fruin *et al.* (1991) presented high school students with information about the role of exercise in preventing cardiovascular disease. In the information, three components specified by protection motivation theory (response efficacy, response costs and self-efficacy) were manipulated in a factorial design with two levels (high versus low) for each variable. Manipulation checks found significant differences between the high and low conditions for each message variable. High self-efficacy information resulted in stronger endorsement of the behavioural intention to exercise. In this study information in the messages about response efficacy and response costs did not significantly influence the intention to exercise.

In another type of study, Wurtele (1988) provided information about osteoporosis to female students. In this study a factorial design was used to test the effectiveness of written communications varying in the described vulnerability to osteoporosis of female students and varying in the described effectiveness of increasing the amount of calcium in the diet to prevent osteoporosis. Manipulation checks revealed that the subjects exposed to the high-vulnerability essay reported stronger beliefs in their vulnerability to developing osteoporosis than did subjects in the low-vulnerability condition. Subjects in the high response efficacy condition reported significantly stronger beliefs in the effectiveness of a calcium-enriched diet for preventing osteoporosis than did the subjects in the low response efficacy condition. For intentions to increase the amount of calcium-rich food in the diet, vulnerability emerged as the best predictor, accounting for 23 per cent of the variance. Response efficacy entered as the second best predictor, accounting for an additional 5 per cent of the variance.

Beck and Lund (1981) exposed dental patients in a factorial design to persuasive communications designed to manipulate their beliefs about the seriousness of periodontal disease (high versus low) and their susceptibility to it (high versus low) in order to enhance patients' dental brushing and flossing behaviour. Dependent measures in this study were amount of fear arousal, perceived seriousness of periodontal disease, perceived vulnerability to periodontal disease, response efficacy of a number of dental hygiene behaviours, self-efficacy in performing a number of dental hygiene behaviours, intentions to engage in the recommended actions and the patient's dental hygiene behaviour. The last measure was taken later by an additional telephone interview. Manipulations checks revealed that both the severity manipulation and the vulnerability manipulation were successful in influencing respectively the perceived seriousness and the perceived vulnerability to periodontal disease. Regression analysis revealed that the only predictor of the intention to floss was the self-efficacy towards dental flossing. Additional regression analysis revealed that perceived seriousness of periodontal disease and self-efficacy of flossing were related to actual flossing behaviour.

3.3 Enhancing diagnostic health behaviours

Rippetoe and Rogers (1987) used written messages containing a high versus low threat essay (by varying the described severity of and vulnerability to breast cancer), a high versus low response efficacy essay and a high versus low self-efficacy essay. Manipulation checks revealed that the subjects who read the high-threat message perceived breast cancer as a more severe disease and perceived themselves as more vulnerable to breast cancer than did the subjects in the low-threat group. Stronger beliefs in the efficacy of breast self-examination were elicited in women exposed to the high response efficacy message when compared to those in the low response efficacy condition. Women who read the high self-efficacy message had stronger confidence in their ability to perform breast self-examination correctly than did women in the low self-efficacy condition. In this study the effects of the persuasive messages on both adaptive (e.g. intention to perform breast self-examination) and maladaptive (e.g. wishful thinking) coping reactions were studied. Subjects in the high-threat condition reported more adaptive and maladaptive coping compared to the subjects in the low-threat condition. Compared to the subjects in the low response efficacy group the subjects in the high response efficacy group reported more adaptive coping (intentions to perform breast self-examination) and less maladaptive coping (like fatalism) in response to the threat of breast cancer. Compared to the subjects in the low self-efficacy condition the subjects in the high self-efficacy condition reported more adaptive coping (intention to perform breast self-examination and rational problem-solving) and less maladaptive coping (feelings of hopelessness). Path analysis revealed that response efficacy was the major predictor of the intention to perform breast self-examination. Perceived severity of breast cancer and perceived self-efficacy in performing breast self-examination were also predictors of the intention to perform breast self examination.

Brouwers and Sorrentino (1993) provided students with information about a fictitious disease (Crevelling's disease) in order to enhance the use of a diagnostic test, the Crevelling's identification (CID) test. Students were presented with one of four versions of an information pamphlet varying on two dimensions: level of threat and level of effectiveness of the CID test. The high-threat essay described Crevelling's disease as an extremely debilitating illness which was most prevalent in unmarried students aged 15 to 24. The low-threat essay described Crevelling's disease as a disease with no long-term effects to which blue-collar workers aged 46 to 55 were most vulnerable. The high-efficacy essay stressed the effectiveness of the CID test and the ease with which one could do the test, while the low-efficacy essay stressed the inconsistent findings of the CID test and emphasized the difficulties associated with carrying out the procedure. Manipulation checks revealed that the essays were successful in manipulating perceived severity, perceived vulnerability and perceived response efficacy in the predicted direction. Results showed that highly threatening and highly efficacious information was effective in enhancing preventive behaviour, i.e. a request for a CID test kit. Unfortunately, in this study no data are provided on the relative role of the components of protection motivation theory in predicting the recommended preventive behaviour.

3.4 Prevention of disease

Van der Velde and van der Pligt (1991) tested the predictive value of the components of protection motivation theory with respect to AIDS-related behaviour. In their study, perceived severity and perceived vulnerability with respect to HIV infection, response efficacy of condom use and self-efficacy (the extent the subjects would be able to persist in using condoms) were measured in a sample of 231 people with multiple sex partners in the six months preceding the study. The study revealed that perceived response efficacy and perceived self-efficacy were significantly related to the intention to use condoms consistently.

Tanner *et al.* (1991) used protection motivation theory as a framework in the provision of information to students about sexually transmitted diseases. Subjects received one of the following versions of materials about responsible sexual behaviour: (a) high-threat information, (b) low-threat information, (c) high-threat information followed by coping response information, (d) low-threat information followed by coping response information, (e) coping response information, (f) a control group who received no information. The study revealed that in comparison with the coping response only information condition, the high-threat/coping response information condition was more effective in generating intention to use condoms. The authors conclude from this finding that this study provides support for an ordered protection motivation model, in which threat appraisal occurs prior to coping appraisal. The authors provided no information about the relative effectiveness of PMT components in predicting the recommended preventive behaviour.

4 Developments

To date, with regard to health-related behaviours, the main fields of application of protection motivation theory are reducing alcohol use, enhancing healthy lifestyles, enhancing diagnostic health behaviours and prevention of disease. With respect to reducing alcohol use, to date in only one study (Stainback and Rogers 1983) were the effects of persuasive messages studied. In these messages, however, only two components of PMT (the severity of the consequences of drinking and the probability that these consequences will occur) were varied. Only short-lived intentions to remain abstinent were produced in the high-fear group. The study by Runge et al. (1993), however, indicated that hospitalized individuals with alcohol abuse problems reported a lower response efficacy for moderate drinking than did their community counterparts. Future research could produce more effective messages by including more components of PMT in messages aimed at reducing alcohol use.

With respect to enhancing healthy lifestyles various studies aimed at promoting exercise behaviour indicated that messages containing information to enhance self-efficacy (Stanley and Maddux 1986; Wurtele and Maddux 1987; Fruin et al. 1991) or response efficacy (Stanley and Maddux 1986) were effective in promoting exercise behaviour. To date studies have mainly been performed using students as experimental subjects. Future development could be aimed at generalizing the results obtained with students to specific at-risk groups (e.g. subjects at risk of heart disease) or to groups with specific difficulties (e.g. cardiovascular patients).

With respect to enhancing diagnostic health behaviours, results showed that highly threatening and highly efficacious information was effective in enhancing preventive behaviour (Rippetoe and Rogers 1987; Brouwers and Sorrentino 1993). To date, however, these results were obtained in a specific group (students) in one study (Brouwers and Sorrentino 1993) using a fictitious disease. Future research should be aimed at other subjects and should try to apply protection motivation theory to enhance diagnostic health behaviours in specific risk groups.

In general it can be stated that future research should be aimed at the application of PMT to the enhancing of health behaviours in specific groups at risk. An example of the direction future research may take is provided by the study of van der Velde and van der Pligt (1991), who tested the predictive value of components of PMT with respect to AIDS-related behaviour in people with multiple sex partners. Adding persuasive messages designed according to PMT to these kind of applied field studies will further promote the development of PMT.

5 Operationalization of the model

5.1 Operationalization of messages

In one of the earliest analyses of the relation between fear arousal and persuasion (Hovland et al. 1953), fear appeals were characterized as communications describing the unfavourable consequences that might result from failure to adopt the recommendations in the message. This broad definition has led to various operationalizations of fear appeals. In studies using PMT as a framework for the design of the persuasive messages the components of the threat appraisal process (severity and vulnerability) have been operationalized in various ways. Some research has tried to operationalize the severity of the risk in the message, by arguing, for example, that excessive drinking produces either severe injury or minor irritation to the internal organs (Stainback and Rogers 1983). A typical example of various operationalizations of the severity of the threat in the message is offered by Rippetoe and Rogers (1987). In their study, high-threat and low-threat essays were compared. The high-threat essay described 'breast cancer in graphic detail, contained vivid descriptions of radical chemotherapy side effects and a radical mastectomy and emphasized college-age women's vulnerability to breast cancer because of stress and diets with increased fat. This essay was accompanied by graphic colour photographs of two young women with extremely advanced breast cancer' (Rippetoe and Rogers 1987: 599). The low-threat essay 'described breast cancer as a less severe disease with few physical or emotional consequences. It also emphasized the rarity of the disease among college-age women and college-age women's decreased vulnerability to the illness. This essay was accompanied by black and white photographs of the normal, healthy breasts of a young woman' (p. 599).

Response efficacy has been operationalized by, for example, essays arguing that there is no effective method to treat a disease or that a simple medical treatment cures it. For example, Brouwers and Sorrentino (1993) used persuasive messages based on PMT. In their study a pamphlet describing a fabricated medical condition (Crevelling's disease) and its associated adaptive diagnostic response (the Crevelling's identification test, a urine analysis test that can be done in the home after 12 hours of fasting) were used. The high response efficacy essay 'stressed the effectiveness of the Crevelling's Identification Test and its ability to detect the beginning signs of Crevelling's disease infection accurately.' The low response efficacy essay stressed 'the inconsistent and unreliable findings of the Crevelling's Identification Test' (Brouwers and Sorrentino 1993). In another study (Rippetoe and Rogers 1987: 599) the high response efficacy essay 'stressed the importance of breast self-examination and its efficacy in detecting breast cancer early, thus increasing life expectancy.' The low response efficacy essay argued that 'breast self-examination was not effective in detecting breast cancer early enough to increase life expectancy.'

The last component of persuasive messages based on PMT relates to the self-efficacy that is needed to perform the recommended action successfully. It must be argued in the message that the individual has the ability to complete successfully the recommended action. For example, in a high self-efficacy essay, Rippetoe and Rogers (1987) provided information that emphasized a woman's ability to perform breast self-examination correctly and to incorporate it in her health routine. The low self-efficacy essay focused on the difficulty of doing a good breast self-examination and the difficulty of actually detecting a lump. Brouwers and Sorrentino (1993) stressed in the high self-efficacy essay the ability and ease with which one could successfully do the test. The low self-efficacy essay emphasized the difficulties associated with carrying out the procedure, such as time calibration of each step and problems reading instruments involved in the process.

5.2 Operationalizations of measures of social cognitions

PMT (Rogers 1983) assumes that a fear appeal initiates a corresponding cognitive mediating process. In order to identify the corresponding cognitive mediating process several measures have been used. Although the exact content of the questions aimed at measuring the cognitive mediating process is, of course, dependent upon the content of the message, a general outline and some examples of questions that can be used are formulated below. Usually items are formulated in order to measure the subjects' beliefs in: (a) the severity of the threat, (b) their vulnerability to the threat, (c) the response efficacy, (d) their self-efficacy in performing the advised behaviour and (e) the intention to perform the advised behaviour. The items can be worded to enable responses on five-point scales, enabling the subjects to specify the answer that best corresponds to their opinion.

Items referring to the *severity of the threat* are directly or indirectly aimed at assessing the respondents' belief in the severity of the disease. Sometimes questioning is rather direct (e.g. 'I believe Crevelling's disease is a very serious illness'; Brouwers and Sorrentino 1993). Sometimes more items are used and the psychometric properties of the scale used to assess the severity are determined (Boer *et al.* 1993). In this study perceived severity of breast cancer was assessed with three questions ('I think that breast cancer is a more serious disease than other diseases that I know', 'Despite the advances of medical science breast cancer remains as serious as it was in the former days', 'I think breast cancer is a serious disease'). Questions could be answered on a three point scale with the response alternatives 'yes', 'don't know' and 'no'. The internal consistency of the scale was, however, rather low (Cronbach's alpha = 0.35).

In assessing the *vulnerability* to the threat one may emphasize either the vulnerability (e.g. 'Due to my present lifestyle and age, I feel personally vulnerable to contracting Crevelling's disease'; Brouwers and Sorrentino 1993) or one may emphasize the chance of contracting the disease (Boer *et al.* 1993). In this study perceived susceptibility to breast cancer was assessed with two questions ('It is rather probable that I will ever get breast cancer' and 'The chance that someone of my age in comparable conditions gets breast cancer is rather large'). Questions could be answered on a three-point scale, with the response alternatives 'yes', 'don't know' and 'no'. Both questions correlated reasonably ($r = 0.35$, $p < 0.0001$).

Response efficacy of the recommended behaviour can also be assessed with one item ('The Crevelling's Identification Test is a very accurate and informative procedure that will identify whether or not Crevelling's disease is present'; Brouwers and Sorrentino 1993), but other researchers prefer to use a formulation that is more in line with the traditional way consequences of behaviour are measured (see Fishbein and Ajzen 1975). In these studies consequences are linked to the recommended behaviour and it is assessed whether the subject thinks the consequences are the likely outcome of the recommended behaviour. In the Boer *et al.* (1993) study response efficacy of mammographic screening was assessed with four questions ('Participation in the mass screening on breast cancer leads to ... (1) certainty about my health status, (2) reassurance, (3) early detection if something is wrong, (4) the detection of small abnormalities'). Questions could be answered on a three-point scale with the response alternatives 'yes', 'don't know' and 'no'. The four items formed a reliable scale (Cronbach's alpha = 0.67).

Self-efficacy refers to the belief of the subject that the recommended behaviour can be executed successfully. In this respect one can use single-item measures or multiple-item measures with known psychometric properties. A representative single-item measure comes from the study of Brouwers and Sorrentino (1993), who assessed self-efficacy by asking the subject to indicate agreement or disagreement with the statement: 'I feel confident in my ability to accurately do the Crevelling's Identification Test at home.' A representative sample of items that might be used in a multiple-item measure comes from the Boer *et al.* (1993) study. They assessed women's self-efficacy with respect to participating in breast cancer screening by asking their agreement with seven questions ('It is difficult for me to participate ... (1) because I am nervous for the examination, (2) because of my bad health status, (3) because I fear the examination, (4) because I am afraid of the X-rays that are used, (5) because the examination is carried out during working hours, (6) because of the time it takes, (7) because of the transport to the site of the examination'). Questions could be answered on a three-point scale with the response alternatives 'yes', 'don't know' and 'no'. The items formed a reliable scale (Cronbach's alpha = 0.7()).

Protection motivation is usually indicated by the intention to perform the desired behaviour. An example is provided by a study by Boer *et al.* (1993). In this study the intention to participate in breast cancer screening was assessed with one question ('Do you intend to participate in the mass screening for breast cancer?'). The question could be answered on a six-point scale with the extremes 'definitely yes' and 'definitely no'.

It must be noted that the above descriptions of items are of course indicative. Depending on the topic, tailor-made questions have to be asked. This means that, *a priori*, no guarantee can be given about the psychometric properties of the scales that are used in the study. For this reason it is wise to pretest the formulated questions on a small group of subjects, before starting with the main research.

6 Application of the model

Based on the promising results of experimental projects (De Waard *et al.* 1984; Verbeek *et al.* 1984), mass screening with mammography was introduced in the Netherlands in 1989 to promote the early detection of breast cancer in women aged 50 to 70 years. In the current national screening programme women will be screened with mammography every two years. The expected effect of regular screening on later breast cancer mortality can only be accomplished if an appropriate percentage of the women from the target group use and keep using screening services.

Health education on mass screening with mammography might be an important instrument in attaining the desired level of participation. An integrative theory on the role of various cognitive factors in preventive health behaviour is provided by PMT. Health education aimed at influencing perceived vulnerability, response efficacy and self-efficacy expectancy may be effective in achieving and maintaining participation in the breast screening programme. In some studies perceived vulnerability to breast cancer was a significant predictor of participation in breast cancer screening (Calnan 1984; Lerman *et al.* 1990; Fulton *et al.* 1991). In other studies, response efficacy with regard to mammography was a major influence for the majority of women who participated in the mammogram programme (Rutledge *et al.* 1988; Fulton *et al.* 1991). Rutledge *et al.* (1988) made a qualitative analysis of data from small focus groups of women invited to participate in a breast screening programme to assess whether or not providing factual information would increase participation. They suggested that emotional fears having to do with impending expectations of ill health were the basis of non-participation. Providing positive reassurance to dispel those fears might improve acceptance (Leather and Roberts 1985). Based on the available evidence it was suggested that educational efforts on breast cancer screening would perhaps be more effective if directed at informing women that mammography can detect breast cancer in the absence of breast symptoms rather than increasing a woman's perception of her vulnerability by emphasizing the prevalence of breast cancer and its risk factors (see also Vernon *et al.* 1990). This suggestion is supported by empirical evidence on the relative importance of cognitive factors in preventive behaviour related to cancer (Seydel *et al.* 1990). A study was conducted to test the effects of health education based on protection motivation theory about breast cancer screening by mammography.

6.1 Materials and methods

Design
In a quasi-experiment, with an experimental group and a control group, it was tested whether health education on mass screening for breast cancer leads to improved information acquisition and subsequent changes in expectancies.

Subjects

The experimental group consisted of women from the city of Arnhem (the Netherlands) who were invited by letter by the East Netherlands Foundation for Cancer Screening to be screened with mammography. In the experimental group 386 women were invited to participate in the experiment and eventually 68 per cent filled in a questionnaire (*n* = 261).

The control group consisted of women from the city of Enschede (the Netherlands), where at the time of data collection no mass screening for breast cancer had been performed. The 500 women from the control group were randomly selected by municipal services from the municipal administration of the city of Enschede. In the selection process it was ensured that the women were within the same age range as the women from the experimental group (50 to 70 years). Of the women from the control group, 60 per cent filled in the questionnaire (*n* = 299).

Materials

The women in the experimental group received a leaflet titled 'Breast examination', which was sent with the invitation for the breast screening. The leaflet contained information on issues that, according to protection-motivation theory (Rogers 1983), determine protective health behaviour. The leaflet described the relatively high vulnerability of older women to breast cancer and the high response efficacy of mammographic screening as a means of cancer control, and tried to induce feelings of high self-efficacy with regard to participation by explaining that a mammographic breast examination is an easy procedure with only little discomfort.

Procedure

The women from the experimental group received a questionnaire three days after the receipt of the invitation and the leaflet 'Breast examination'. The day before the possible participation in the breast screening the questionnaires were collected. The women in the control group were sent a questionnaire by post, which could be returned in a postage-paid envelope.

Measures

In the questionnaire we measured: (a) knowledge of breast cancer and mass screening for breast cancer based on information from the leaflet 'Breast examination'; (b) general knowledge of breast cancer and breast self-examination; (c) perceived vulnerability to breast cancer; (d) perceived seriousness of breast cancer; (e) response efficacy of mammographic screening; (f) self-efficacy with respect to participation in the screening; (g) intention to participate in the screening; (h) fear of breast cancer; (i) demographic variables.

Questions on knowledge of breast cancer and mass screening were derived from the contents of the leaflet 'Breast examination'. Questions referred to the objective vulnerability to breast cancer, the benefits of early detection and the performance of a mammographic breast examination. Subjects could indicate the correctness of items like 'In the Netherlands breast cancer is the most frequent form of cancer in women' and 'Mass screening for breast cancer is repeated every two years'. Questions could be answered on a three-point scale, with the response alternatives 'correct', 'don't know' and 'not correct'. The eight items formed a reliable scale (Cronbach's alpha = 0.84).

Questions used in the assessment of general knowledge of breast cancer and breast self-examination only referred to issues not discussed in the leaflet. Subjects could indicate the correctness of items like 'Sudden pressure (e.g. a punch on the breast) can cause breast cancer' and 'Breast feeding enhances the risk of breast cancer'. Questions could be answered on a three-point scale with the response alternatives 'correct', 'don't know' and 'not correct'. The five items formed a reliable scale (Cronbach's alpha = 0.71).

Perceived vulnerability to breast cancer was assessed with two questions: 'It is rather probable that I will ever get breast cancer', 'The chance that someone of my age in comparable conditions gets breast cancer is rather large'. Questions could be answered on a three-point scale, with the response alternatives 'yes', 'don't know' and 'no'. Both questions correlated reasonably ($r = 0.35$, $p < 0.0001$).

Perceived severity of breast cancer was assessed with three questions ('I think that breast cancer is a more serious disease than other diseases that I know', 'Despite the advances of medical science breast cancer remains as serious as it was in former days', 'I think breast cancer is a serious disease'). Questions could be answered on a three-point scale, with the response alternatives 'yes', 'don't know' and 'no'. The internal consistency of the scale was rather low (Cronbach's alpha = 0.35).

Response efficacy of mammographic screening was assessed with four questions: 'Participation in the mass screening on breast cancer leads to: (a) certainty about my health status, (b) reassurance, (c) early detection if something is wrong, (d) the detection of small abnormalities.' Questions could be answered on a three-point scale, with the response alternatives 'yes', 'don't know' and 'no'. The four items formed a reliable scale (Cronbach's alpha = 0.67).

Self-efficacy expectation with regard to participation was assessed with seven questions: 'It is difficult for me to participate: (a) because I am nervous about the examination, (b) because of my bad health status, (c) because I fear the examination, (d) because I am afraid of the X-rays that are used, (e) because the examination is carried out during working hours, (f) because of the time it takes, (g) because of the transport to the site of the examination.' Questions could be answered on a three-point scale, with the response alternatives 'yes', 'don't know' and 'no'. The seven items formed a reliable scale (Cronbach's alpha = 0.70).

Intention to participate was assessed with one question ('Do you intend to participate in the mass screening for breast cancer?'). The question could be answered on a six-point scale, with the extremes 'definitely yes' and 'definitely no'.

Fear of breast cancer was assessed with an adapted version of the fear-of-cancer questionnaire (Kuttschreuter *et al.* 1984). In the adapted version the subject indicates the extent to which negative emotions would be aroused when confronted with the following situations: (a) a television programme on breast cancer, (b) a poster on breast self-examination, (c) an article in a newspaper on breast cancer, (d) an invitation for mass screening on breast cancer and (e) the experience of someone in one's neighbourhood having breast cancer. The subjects could indicate whether confrontation with the situations made them feel tense, nervous, restless or fearful. The items could be answered on a four-point scale, with the extremes 'not' and 'very much'. The 22 items formed a reliable scale (Cronbach's alpha = 0.95).

Demographic variables included characteristics such as age and level of education.

6.2 Results

Equality of groups

The women from the experimental group (mean = 57.1 years) were on average younger than the women from the control group (mean = 59.2 years; t = 4.2, p < 0.0001). The women from the experimental group also had a higher level of education than the women from the control group (χ^2 = 21.6, d.f. = 2, p < 0.0001). Finally, the women from the experimental group answered more questions correctly regarding general knowledge on breast cancer and breast self-examination ($F(1,518)$ = 21.8, p < 0.0001). Because of these differences between the experimental group and the control group the results presented are based on analysis of variance with age, level of education and general knowledge of breast cancer and breast self-examination used as covariates.

Health education

Table 4.2 shows that the applied health education leaflet had a clear effect on the level of knowledge with regard to breast cancer and mammographic screening. However, perceived severity of breast cancer and perceived vulnerability to breast cancer were not influenced by the health education intervention. The health education leaflet led to a significantly higher response efficacy, self-efficacy expectation and intention to participate in the experimental compared to the control condition. However, in each of these cases the differences were small.

Fear of breast cancer

The possible mediating effect of level of fear of breast cancer and the applied health education leaflet was investigated by analysing the effects of the health education leaflet separately for two levels of fear of breast cancer. The median score for the total group of subjects (3.727) was used as the criterion. The group with a relatively low level of fear of breast

Table 4.2 The effects of health education on knowledge about breast cancer screening and on variables derived from protection motivation theory

	Experimental group $n = 225$	*Control group* $n = 235$	*F(1,460)*
Knowledge	6.1	2.9	260.0***
Severity	2.3	2.4	< 1
Vulnerability	2.0	2.0	< 1
Response efficacy	2.9	2.8	4.7*
Self-efficacy expectation	2.9	2.7	15.0***
Intention to participate	4.9	4.6	27.6***

Note: In the analysis age, level of education and general knowledge on breast cancer were used as covariates.
*** $p < 0.001$; ** $p < 0.01$; * $p < 0.05$.

Table 4.3 The main effects of level of fear of breast cancer (FB) and the interaction effect between level of fear of breast cancer and health education (HE)

	Experimental group		*Control group*		*Main effect FB*	*Interaction FB × HE*
	Low FB $n = 93$	*High FB* $n = 71$	*Low FB* $n = 81$	*High FB* $n = 93$	*F(1,328)*	*F(1,328)*
Knowledge	6.3	6.3	3.3	3.0	< 1	< 1
Severity	2.2	2.3	2.2	2.4	6.6**	< 1
Vulnerability	1.9	2.0	1.9	2.1	6.8**	3.7
Response-efficacy	2.9	2.9	2.8	2.8	< 1	< 1
Self-efficacy expectation	2.9	2.8	2.9	2.7	11.1***	< 1
Intention to participate	4.9	4.9	4.6	4.7	< 1	< 1

Note: In the analysis age, level of education and general knowledge on breast cancer were used as covariates.
*** $p < 0.001$; ** $p < 0.01$; * $p < 0.05$.

cancer consisted of women with a score lower than or equal to the median score ($n = 181$) and the group with a relatively high level of fear of breast cancer consisted of women with a score higher than the median score ($n = 163$).

Table 4.3 shows that level of fear of breast cancer has a significant effect on the perceived severity of breast cancer, with the high fear of breast cancer group perceiving breast cancer as a more severe disease than the low fear of breast cancer group. Level of fear of breast cancer has a significant effect on the perceived vulnerability to breast cancer, with the high fear of breast cancer group feeling more vulnerable to breast cancer than the low fear of breast cancer group. Level of fear of breast cancer has an effect on the perceived self-efficacy with regard to participation, with the high fear of breast cancer group feeling less able to participate than the low fear of breast cancer group. Level of fear of breast cancer does not significantly interact with health education, either with regard to the amount of knowledge acquisition, or with regard to the variables derived from PMT.

Predicting intention to participate in breast cancer screening
Within-subjects regression analysis was used to determine the relation between the components of the theory and level of protection motivation. Using measures of existing cognitions rather than manipulated independent variables designed to influence those cognitions makes it possible to test the predicted interactions directly. By entering interaction terms in the regression analyses it is possible to determine whether a linear additive model is sufficient or whether a combination between an additive model and a multiplicative model is necessary to predict individual differences in level of protection motivation.

Table 4.4 shows the results of hierarchical multiple regression analyses to predict the intention to participate in breast cancer screening, with the main and interaction effects of the variables derived from protection motivation theory, knowledge of breast cancer screening as learned from the information leaflet and level of fear of breast cancer. Intention to participate in breast cancer screening was first predicted by the main effects

Table 4.4 Results of hierarchical multiple regression analyses to predict participation-intention from main and interaction effects of protection motivation variables, knowledge and fear of breast cancer

	Controls		Experimental	
	Cum. R	*Cum.* R^2	*Cum.* R	*Cum.* R^2
Severity	0.01	0.00	0.01	0.00
Vulnerability	0.02	0.00	0.05	0.00
Response efficacy	0.47	0.22	0.09	0.01
Self-efficacy expectation	0.60	0.36	0.25	0.06
Vulnerability × response efficacy	0.60	0.36	0.25	0.06
Vulnerability × self-efficacy exp.	0.60	0.36	0.38	0.15
Response eff. × self-efficacy exp.	0.60	0.36	0.41	0.17
Knowledge information leaflet	0.61	0.37	0.42	0.18
Fear of breast cancer	0.62	0.39[a]	0.44	0.20[b]

Note: [a] $F(9,201) = 14,4$, $p < 0.001$.
   [b] $F(9,192) = 6,7$, $p < 0.001$.

and then the other variables were added to the regression analysis in the indicated order.

In this study the women from the control group had not yet received health education about breast cancer screening; nor was breast cancer screening currently performed in that region. In these women, 39 per cent of the variance in the intention to participate in breast cancer screening could be predicted from the regression analyses. With respect to the role of the components of PMT in the prediction of the intention to participate, the following results were obtained. Vulnerability to breast cancer did not predict the intention to participate, perceived response efficacy explained 22 per cent of the variance and perceived self-efficacy explained an additional 14 per cent of the variance. The interaction between the components of protection motivation theory (vulnerability, response efficacy and self-efficacy) did not explain additional variance in the intention to participate. Variations in level of knowledge and fear of breast cancer explained the intention to participate in breast cancer screening only to a very limited extent.

The women in the experimental group had received health education about breast cancer screening and were invited to participate in the breast cancer screening. In these women in total 20 per cent of the variance in the intention to participate in the breast cancer screening could be predicted from the regression analyses. Vulnerability did not predict the intention to participate, the perceived response efficacy explained 1 per cent and perceived self-efficacy explained 5 per cent of the variance. The interaction between vulnerability and self-efficacy explained 9 per cent and the interaction between response-efficacy and self-efficacy explained 2 per cent; variations in level of knowledge explained 1 per cent and fear of breast cancer explained 2 per cent.

When the results of the regression analysis in the control group are compared with the results of the regression analysis on the data of the experimental group, it can be assumed that the women in both groups followed different decision rules in evaluating possible participation in breast cancer screening. In the women in the control group (who did not receive any health education and were not at that moment invited to participate), perceived response efficacy and perceived self-efficacy independently had a positive influence on the intention to participate. In the women in the experimental group (who received health education and were invited to participate in breast cancer screening), the decision-making process had concrete consequences. Under these circumstances women who judged themselves less vulnerable to breast cancer and who felt it to be less efficacious for them to participate were less inclined to participate. This means that when the behavioural intention has to be put into practice in the near future perceived self-efficacy plays a more prominent role as a determinant of behavioural intention. Under these circumstances response efficacy plays a less dominant role. In this study no separate analysis could be made of the role of the components in actual participation in the experimental group. The reason for this is that of the women who participated in this study 97 per cent participated in the screening. This means that the participation pattern showed too little variance to make a useful analysis of the role of the cognitive components in participation in breast cancer screening.

Predicting participation in the next screening round
Because in the first part of this study no useful analysis could be made of the role of the components of protection motivation theory in predicting participation in the first screening round, an extension was added to the study. The goal of the extension was to study the role of the components of PMT in predicting participation in the second screening round (two years later). In this part of the study an analysis was made of the ability of the components of PMT to predict health behaviours over longer periods of time.

Of the 372 women from the experimental group who participated in the first screening round in March 1989, 20 women were not invited to participate in the second screening round in the spring of 1991, because they had grown older than 70. In total, 14 women were not invited to participate in the second screening round, because they were missing from the database, which was provided by the municipal administration to the East Netherlands Breast Cancer Screening Authority. Of the 338 women who were invited to participate in the second screening round, 263 women (78 per cent) participated, while 75 women (22 per cent) did not.

Table 4.5 shows the results of hierarchical multiple regression analyses to predict participation status in the second screening round (two years

Table 4.5 Results of hierarchical multiple regression analyses to predict participation in the next screening round from main and interaction-effects of protection motivation variables, knowledge and fear of breast cancer prior to first screening round

	Cum. R	Cum. R^2
Severity	0.01	0.00
Vulnerability	0.08	0.01
Response efficacy	0.12	0.02
Self-efficacy expectation	0.13	0.02
Intention (protection motivation)	0.16	0.03
Vulnerability × response efficacy	0.16	0.03
Vulnerability × self-efficacy expectation	0.16	0.03
Response efficacy × self-efficacy expectation	0.16	0.03
Knowledge information leaflet	0.18	0.03
Fear of breast cancer	0.23	0.05[a]

Note: [a] $F(10,172) < 1.0$, n.s.

later) from main and interaction effects of PMT variables, knowledge about breast cancer screening and fear of breast cancer prior to the first screening round.

Results indicate that participation status in the second screening round could not be predicted from the variables derived from PMT (total explained variance is 3 per cent). Fear of breast cancer contributes most to predicting participation status in the second screening round. Additional analysis indicated that the level of fear for breast cancer was higher among the participants than among the non-participants in the second screening round. This finding supports the idea that a minimal amount of fear or worry promotes compliance in breast cancer screening.

6.3 Discussion

Early detection of breast cancer by means of mammographic screening can, if a desired minimal participation level is reached, lead to a reduction in cancer mortality in the target population (women between 50 and 70 years of age). Effective health education may help to achieve (and maintain) the desired minimal rate of participation. In a quasi-experiment we investigated the effects of health education on knowledge acquisition about mass screening on breast cancer and on expectancies, which according to PMT (Rogers 1983) determine self-protective health behaviour. Protection motivation theory stresses that not only risk appraisal but also response efficacy and self-efficacy expectancy play an important role in the development of protective behaviour.

The applied health education leaflet had a marked effect on the level of knowledge about breast cancer and breast cancer screening. After the health education leaflet the experimental group had a significantly higher response-efficacy with regard to mammographic screening, a significantly higher self-efficacy expectation with regard to participation and a significantly higher intention to participate in the screening. The perceived severity of breast cancer and the perceived vulnerability to breast cancer were not influenced by the applied health education leaflet. This finding gives empirical support to the suggestion of Vernon et al. (1990) that educational efforts would be more effective if directed at informing women that mammography can detect breast cancer in the absence of breast symptoms (benefits of early detection) than at increasing a woman's perception of her vulnerability.

In this study it was found that in the subjects in the control condition (who did not receive health information about breast cancer screening), response efficacy and self-efficacy were major predictors of the intention to participate in breast cancer screening. In the subjects in the experimental condition (who were informed about breast cancer screening and invited to participate in a breast examination) the interaction between perceived vulnerability and self-efficacy was the major predictor of the intention to participate. The results indicate that the components of PMT that determine the intention to participate may be dependent upon a phase in the decision-making process.

7 Future directions

The results of research into the effects of health education using PMT as a framework are rather ambiguous. There are some strengths, but also some weaknesses which have to be pointed to. PMT can be seen as a hybrid theory (see Prentice-Dunn and Rogers 1986), in which three components originate from the health belief model (Becker 1974; see Sheeran and Abraham, Chapter 2 in this volume): vulnerability, severity and response efficacy. The fourth component, self-efficacy, originates from social learning theory (Bandura 1977; see Schwarzer and Fuchs, Chapter 6 in this volume).

In evaluating PMT as a social cognition model for preventive health behaviour several criteria can be used. The first criterion refers to the percentage of the variance of the preventive behaviour that can be explained by using the components of PMT as predictors. Applying PMT to the prediction of breast cancer screening in the control group (which received no health education), 36 per cent of the variance in the intention to participate could be explained using the components from PMT. In the women who had received health education about breast cancer screening, 17 per cent of the variance in the intention to participate could be explained using the components from PMT. Based on the multiple correlations that have been found in various studies, it can be stated that PMT can be used as a fruitful model for the prediction of intention to engage in preventive health behaviour.

With respect to the role of the various components in the prediction of preventive health behaviour, the picture emerges that only in those cases where the subjects learn about a new, previously unknown, threat does threat appraisal play a role in the adoption of preventive health behaviours (Wurtele and Maddux 1987; Wurtele 1988; Brouwer and Sorrentino 1993). With respect to the role of response efficacy, various studies provide positive evidence that it plays a role in the adoption of preventive health behaviours (Stanley and Maddux 1986; Rippetoe and Rogers 1987; Wurtele 1988; van der Velde and van de Pligt 1991). Most positive evidence has been found for the role of self-efficacy in the adoption of preventive health behaviours. In several studies it has been found that variations in perceived self-efficacy are important in predicting preventive health behaviour (Beck and Lund 1981; Stanley and Maddux 1986; Rippetoe and Rogers 1987; Fruin *et al.* 1991; van der Velde and van der Pligt 1991).

An important theme for future research is the dependency of the components of PMT in predicting health behaviour on the phase of decision-making within the individual (see also Schwarzer and Fuchs, Chapter 6 in this volume). The 'health action process approach' formulated by Schwarzer (1992) might be a useful approach in this respect (see also Rakowski *et al.*

1992, 1993). Another important theme for future research is the stability of measures of social cognitions over longer periods of time. Longitudinal research in specific risk groups using within-subjects research designs seems to be a useful approach to promote the further development of PMT.

Acknowledgements

The empirical research reported in this chapter was supported by the Dutch Cancer Society. This chapter is dedicated to the remembrance of the father of the first author, Evert Boer, who died on 16 November 1994 in the period of revision of the final manuscript.

References

Bandura, A. (1977) Self-efficacy: toward a unifying theory of behavioral change, *Psychological Review*, **84**, 191–215.

Bandura, A. (1986) *Social Foundations of Thought and Action: a Social Cognitive Theory*. Englewood Cliffs, NJ: Prentice-Hall.

Beck, K.H. and Lund, A.K. (1981) The effects of health threat seriousness and personal efficacy upon intentions and behaviour, *Journal of Applied Social Psychology*, **11**, 401–15.

Becker, M.H. (ed.) (1974) The Health Belief Model and personal health behaviour, *Health Education Monograph*, **2**, (special issue).

Boer, H., Seydel, E.R. and Stalpers, R. (1993) Prospective study of factors associated with repeat participation in breast cancer screening. In H. Schröder, K. Reschke, M. Johnston and S. Maes (eds) *Health Psychology: Potential in Diversity*. Regensburg: Roderer Verlag, 230–41.

Boer, H., Seydel, E.R. and Taal, E. (1994) Knowledge gap effects in health education on mass screening with mammography. In J.-P. Dauwalder (ed.) *Psychology and Promotion of Health*. Seattle: Hogrefe and Huber, 178–86.

Brouwers, M.C. and Sorrentino, R.M. (1993) Uncertainty orientation and protection motivation theory: the role of individual differences in health compliance, *Journal of Personality and Social Psychology*, **65**, 102–12.

Calnan, M. (1984) The health belief model and participation in programmes for the early detection of breast cancer: a comparative analysis, *Social Science and Medicine*, **19**, 823–30.

De Warrd, F., Collette, H.J.A., Rombach, J.J., Baanders-van Halewijn, E.A. and Honing, C. (1984) The DOM project for the early detection of breast cancer, Utrecht, The Netherlands, *Journal of Chronic Diseases*, **37**, 1–44.

Fishbein, M. and Ajzen, I. (1975) *Belief, Attitude, Intention and Behavior: an Introduction to Theory and Research*. Reading, MA: Addison Wesley.

Fruin, D.J., Pratt, C. and Owen, N. (1991) Protection motivation theory and adolescents' perceptions of exercise, *Journal of Applied Social Psychology*, **22**, 55–69.

Fulton, J.P., Buechner, J.S., Scott, H., DeBuono, B.A., Feldman, J.P., Smith, R.A. and Kovenock, D. (1991) A study guided by the health belief model of the predictors of breast cancer screening of women ages 40 and older, *Public Health Reports*, **106**, 410–20.

Hass, J.W., Bagley, G.S. and Rogers, R.W. (1975) Coping with the energy crisis: effects of fear appeals upon attitudes toward energy consumption, *Journal of Applied Psychology*, 60, 754–6.

Hovland, C.I., Janis, I.L. and Kelley, G.H. (1953) *Communication and Persuasion*. New Haven, CT: Yale University Press.

Janis, I.L. (1967) Effects of fear arousal on attitude change: recent developments in theory and experimental research. In L. Berkowitz (ed.) *Advances in Experimental Social Psychology*, Vol. 3. New York: Academic Press, 166–224.

Janis, I.L. and Feshbach, S. (1953) Effects of fear-arousing communications, *Journal of Abnormal and Social Psychology*, 48, 78–92.

Kantola, S.J., Syme, G.J. and Nesdale, A.R. (1983) The effects of appraised severity and efficacy in promoting water conservation: an informational analysis, *Journal of Applied Social Psychology*, 13, 164–82.

Kuttschreuter, M., Gutteling, J.M., Seydel, E.R. and Wiegman, O. (1984) Angst voor kanker (fear of cancer), *Gezondheid en Samenleving*, 5, 281–5.

Lazarus, R.S. (1966) *Psychological Stress and the Coping Process*. New York: McGraw-Hill.

Leather, D.S. and Roberts, M.M. (1985) Older women's attitudes towards breast disease, self examination, and screening facilities: implications for communication, *British Medical Journal*, 290, 668–70.

Lerman, C., Rimer, B., Trock, B., Balshem, A. and Engstrom, P.F. (1990) Factors associated with repeat adherence to breast cancer screening, *Preventive Medicine*, 19, 279–90.

Leventhal, H. (1970) Findings and theory in the study of fear communications. In L. Berkowitz (ed.) *Advances in Experimental Social Psychology*, Vol. 5. New York: Academic Press, 119–86.

Maddux, J.E., Norton, L.W. and Stoltenberg, C.D. (1986) Self-efficacy expectancy, outcome expectancy and outcome value: relative effects on behavioural intentions, *Journal of Personality and Social Psychology*, 51, 783–9.

Maddux, J.E. and Rogers, R.W. (1983) Protection motivation and self-efficacy: a revised theory of fear-appeals and attitude change, *Journal of Experimental Social Psychology*, 19, 469–79.

Mewborn, C.R. and Rogers, R.W. (1979) Effects of threatening and reassuring components of fear appeals on physiological and verbal measures of emotion and attitudes, *Journal of Experimental Social Psychology*, 15, 242–53.

Mulilis, J.P. and Lippa, R. (1990) Behavioural change in earthquake preparedness due to negative threat appeals: a test of protection motivation theory, *Journal of Applied Social Psychology*, 2, 619–38.

Prentice-Dunn, S. and Rogers, R.W. (1986) Protection motivation theory and preventive health: beyond the health belief model, *Health Education Research*, 1, 153–61.

Rakowski, W., Dube, C.E., Marcus, B.H., Prochaska, J.O., Velicer, W.F. and Abrams, D.B. (1992) Assessing elements of women's decisions about mammography, *Health Psychology*, 11, 111–18.

Rakowski, W., Fulton, J.P. and Feldman, J.P. (1993) Women's decision making about mammography: a replication of the relationship between stages of adoption and decisional balance, *Health Psychology*, 12, 209–14.

Rippetoe, P.A. and Rogers, R.W. (1987) Effects of components of protection motivation theory on adaptive and maladaptive coping with a health threat, *Journal of Personality and Social Psychology*, 52, 596–604.

Rogers, R.W. (1975) A protection motivation theory of fear appeals and attitude change, *Journal of Psychology*, **91**, 93–114.

Rogers, R.W. (1983) Cognitive and physiological processes in fear appeals and attitude change: a revised theory of protection motivation. In J.T. Cacioppo and R.E. Petty (eds) *Social Psychophysiology: a Source Book*. New York: Guilford Press, 153–76.

Runge, C., Prentice-Dunn, S. and Scogin, F. (1993) Protection Motivation Theory and alcohol use attitudes among older adults, *Psychological Reports*, **73**, 96–8.

Rutledge, D.N., Hartman, W.H., Kinman, P. and Winfield, H. (1988) Exploration of factors affecting mammography behaviours, *Preventive Medicine*, **17**, 412–22.

Schwarzer, R. (1992) Self-efficacy in the adoption and maintenance of health behaviours: theoretical approaches and a new model. In R. Schwarzer (ed.) *Self-efficacy: Thought Control of Action*. Washington, DC: Hemisphere, 217–43.

Seydel, E., Taal, E. and Wiegman, O. (1990) Risk-appraisal, outcome and self-efficacy expectancies: cognitive factors in preventive behaviour related to cancer, *Psychology and Health*, **4**, 99–109.

Stainback, R.D. and Rogers, R.W. (1983) Identifying effective components of alcohol abuse prevention programs: effects of fear appeals, message style and source expertise, *International Journal of Addictions*, **18**, 393–405.

Stanley, M.A. and Maddux, J.E. (1986) Cognitive processes in health enhancement: investigation of a combined protection motivation and self-efficacy model, *Basic and Applied Social Psychology*, **7**, 101–13.

Sutton, S.R. (1982) Fear-arousing communications: a critical examination of theory and research. In J.R. Eiser (ed.) *Social Psychology and Behavioural Medicine*. London: Wiley, 303–37.

Tanner, J.F., Hunt, J.B. and Eppright, D.R. (1991) The Protection Motivation Model: a normative model of fear appeals, *Journal of Marketing*, **55**, 36–45.

Van der Velde, F.W. and van der Pligt, J. (1991) AIDS-related health behaviour: coping, protection motivation and previous behaviour, *Journal of Behavioural Medicine*, **14**, 429–51.

Verbeek, A.L.M., Hendriks, J.H.C.L. and Holland, R. (1984) Reduction of breast cancer mortality through mass screening with modern mammography: first results of the Nijmegen project, 1975–1981, *Lancet*, **i**, 1222–4.

Vernon, S.W., LaVille, E.A. and Jackson, G.L. (1990) Participation in breast screening programs: a review, *Social Science and Medicine*, **30**, 1107–18.

Wiegman, O., Taal E., Van den Bogaard, J. and Gutteling, J.M. (1992) Protection motivation theory variables as predictors of behavioural intentions in three domains of risk management. In J.A.M. Winnubst and S. Maes (eds) *Lifestyles, Stress and Health: New Developments in Health Psychology*. Leyden: DSWO Press, 55–70.

Wolf, S., Gregory, W.L. and Stephan, W.G. (1986) Protection motivation theory: predictions of intentions to engage in anti-nuclear war behaviours, *Journal of Applied Social Psychology*, **16**, 310–21.

Wurtele, S.K. (1988) Increasing women's calcium intake: the role of health beliefs, intentions and health value, *Journal of Applied Social Psychology*, **18**, 627–39.

Wurtele, S.K. and Maddux, J.E. (1987) Relative contributions of protection motivation theory components in predicting exercise intentions and behavior, *Health Psychology*, **6**, 453–66.

5 MARK CONNER AND
PAUL SPARKS

THE THEORY OF PLANNED
BEHAVIOUR AND
HEALTH BEHAVIOURS

1 General background

The theory of planned behaviour (TPB: Ajzen 1985, 1988, 1991) is an extension of the earlier theory of reasoned action (TRA: Fishbein and Ajzen 1975; Ajzen and Fishbein 1980) that continues to attract a great deal of attention in psychology (Sheppard *et al.* 1988; Tesser and Shaffer 1990; Olson and Zanna 1993). Both models can be considered to be deliberative processing models in that they appear to imply that individuals make behavioural decisions based upon a careful consideration of available information. The TRA itself had its origins in Fishbein's early work on the psychological processes by which attitudes might cause behaviour (Fishbein 1967a) and in an analysis of the failure to predict behaviour from knowledge of individuals' attitudes. The former work used an expectancy-value framework (Peak 1955) to explain the relationship between beliefs and attitudes, and interposed a new variable, behavioural intentions, between attitudes and behaviour; the latter work generated a powerful explanation of when strong attitude–behaviour relationships might be expected (the principle of compatibility). These are both explained in detail below, beginning with the principle of compatibility and followed by the full details of the TRA/TPB in the subsequent section.

Based upon an analysis of previous studies of the relationship between attitudes and behaviour, Fishbein and Ajzen (1975) and Ajzen and Fishbein (1977) developed the principle of compatibility (Ajzen 1988).[1] This principle is based upon the assertion that each attitude and behaviour has the four elements of action, target, context and time, and states that correspondence between attitudes and behaviour will be greatest when both are measured at the same level with respect to each of these elements. Hence, any particular behaviour consists of (a) an action (or behaviour), (b) performed on or toward a target, (c) in a context, (d) at a time or occasion. For example, a person concerned about oral hygiene (a) brushes (b) her teeth (c) in the bathroom (d) every morning after breakfast. This example illustrates how a behaviour can be aggregated over a range of occasions. Each element can be specified at any level, from the very general to the very specific. Indeed, commonly in the study of health behaviours it is the repeat performance of a single behaviour (e.g. teeth brushing) or even a general class of behaviours (e.g. healthy eating) that we are interested in predicting (Ajzen 1988).

Attitudes may also be defined with reference to each of these four elements at any level of specificity, although attitudes may commonly only specify a target or an action, as in studies of attitudes towards healthy food or healthy eating. In emphasizing that attitudes and behaviour will be most strongly related when both are assessed at the same level of specificity with regard to these four elements, Fishbein and Ajzen highlighted the proposal that general attitudes should predict general classes of behaviours. More importantly for our present purposes, they also demonstrated the need to study specific attitudes when attempting to predict specific behavioural acts. In addition, the claimed causal role for such specific attitudes in their relationship to target behaviours formed one important basis of the TRA and TPB. Considerations of compatibility will be particularly important when developing appropriate measures for components of the TRA/TPB.

2 Description of the model

The TRA suggests that the proximal determinant (or cause) of volitional behaviour is one's intention to engage in that behaviour. Intentions represent a person's motivation in the sense of her or his conscious plan or decision to exert effort to perform the behaviour. Attitudes towards a specific behaviour exert their impact upon performance of that behaviour via their impact upon intentions. Thus, in the TRA, the issue of how the unobservable cognitive construct of an attitude is transformed into observable action is clarified by interposing another psychological event: the formation of an intention between the attitude and the behaviour. In suggesting that behaviour is under the control of intention the TRA restricts itself to volitional behaviours. Those behaviours which require skills, resources or opportunities that are not freely available are not considered to be within the domain of applicability of the TRA or, rather, are likely to be poorly predicted by the TRA components (Fishbein 1993).

The TPB was developed as a deliberate attempt to broaden the applicability of the TRA to include such non-volitional behaviours by incorporating explicit considerations of perceptions of control over performance of the behaviour as an additional predictor of behaviour. Ajzen (1988, 1991) argues that it is only in the case of volitional behaviours that the

TRA will provide adequate predictions. However, considerations of perceptions of control are important because they extend the applicability of the theory beyond easily performed, volitional behaviours to those complex goals and behaviours which are dependent upon performance of a complex series of other behaviours, but which are often of considerable importance in terms of health outcomes (e.g. healthy eating).

Hence, the TPB depicts behaviour as a linear regression function of behavioural intentions and perceived behavioural control:

$$B = w_1BI + w_2PBC \qquad\qquad (1)$$

where B is behaviour, BI is behavioural intention, PBC is perceived behavioural control and w_1 and w_2 are regression weights.

The link between intentions and behaviour reflects the fact that people tend to engage in behaviours they intend to perform. However, the link between behaviour and PBC is more complex. This relationship suggests that we are more likely to engage in (attractive/desirable) behaviours we have control over (and suggests that we are prevented from carrying out behaviours over which we have no control). Ajzen (1988) is explicit in stating that it is actual control which is important here, in that people will tend to perform (and exert extra effort to perform) desirable behaviours they have control over, and not perform behaviours they have little or no control over. Hence, measures of actual control would be desirable here. However, because such measures are difficult to obtain, perceptions of control (PBC) are used as proxy measures for actual control. PBC will predict behaviour directly to the extent that the measure matches actual control (Ajzen 1988).

2.1 Determinants of intentions

In the TRA attitudes are one predictor of behavioural intentions. Attitudes are the overall evaluations of the behaviour by the individual. Applying the principle of compatibility, the relevant attitudes are those towards performance of the behaviour, assessed at a similar level of specificity to that used in the assessment of behaviour. The TRA also specifies subjective norms as the other determinant of intentions. Subjective norms consist of a person's beliefs about whether significant others think he or she should engage in the behaviour. Significant others are individuals whose preferences about a person's behaviour in this domain are important to him or her. Subjective norms are assumed to assess the social pressures individuals feel to perform or not perform a particular behaviour.

The TPB incorporates a third predictor of intentions, perceived behavioural control, which is the individual's perception of the extent to which performance of the behaviour is easy or difficult. The concept is similar to Bandura's (1982) concept of self-efficacy (see Schwarzer and Fuchs, Chapter 6 in this volume). Control is seen as a continuum with easily executed behaviours at one end (e.g. eating a readily available liked food) and behavioural goals demanding resources, opportunities and specialized skills (e.g. becoming a world-class chess player) at the other end. Hence, behavioural intention is a linear regression function of attitudes, subjective norms and perceived behavioural control:

$$BI = w_3 A_B + w_4 SN + w_5 PBC \tag{2}$$

where BI is behavioural intention, A_B is attitude toward the behaviour, SN is subjective norm, PBC is perceived behavioural control, and w_3 to w_5 are empirical weights indicating the relative importance of the determinants of intentions. The equation indicates that intentions are a function of one's evaluation of personally engaging in the behaviour, one's perception that significant others think you should or should not perform the behaviour, and perceptions of one's control over performance of the behaviour. Without the PBC component the equation represents the TRA. The PBC component has links with both the intentions and behaviour components.

2.2 Determinants of attitudes

Just as intentions are held to have determinants, so the attitude, subjective norm and perceived behavioural control components are also held to have determinants. The attitude component is a function of a person's salient behavioural beliefs, which represent perceived consequences of the behaviour. Following expectancy-value conceptualizations (Peak 1955), the model quantifies consequences as being composed of the multiplicative combination of the perceived likelihood that performance of the behaviour will lead to a particular outcome and the evaluation of that outcome. These expectancy-value products are then summed over the various salient consequences:

$$A_B = \sum_{i=1}^{i=l} b_i \cdot e_i \tag{3}$$

where b_i is the behavioural belief that performing the behaviour, B, leads to some consequence i (subjective probability that the behaviour has the consequence i), e_i is the evaluation of consequence i, and l is the number of salient consequences. It is worth noting that it is not claimed that an individual performs such calculations each time he or she is faced with a decision about whether to perform a behaviour, but rather that the results of such considerations are maintained in memory and retrieved and used when necessary (Eagly and Chaiken 1993). However, it is also possible for the individual to retrieve the relevant individual beliefs and evaluations when necessary. Fishbein (1993) claims that equation (3) is not a model of a process but is a computational representation aimed to capture the output of a process that occurs automatically as a function of learning.

This part of the model, the relationship between attitudes and beliefs, has its origins in Fishbein's (1967a, b) summative model of attitudes. It is assumed that a person may possess a large number of beliefs about a particular behaviour, but that at any one time only some of these are likely to be salient. It is the salient beliefs which are assumed to determine a person's attitude. This link between attitudes and behavioural beliefs is generally strong; van den Putte (1993) reports a mean correlation of 0.53 across the 113 studies he reviewed. A number of authors have also suggested that the prediction of attitudes might be improved by adding a measure of importance or relevance of the attribute to the attitude towards the object. However, most evidence collected to date suggests that this additional variable does not further improve the predictability of attitudes (e.g. Holbrook and Hulbert 1975). This may be because salient attributes are all of equal importance to the individual, or because outcome evaluation encompasses this importance issue and so the rating of importance adds no new information. Moreover, the difficulty of measuring attitude importance should not be underestimated (Jaccard *et al.* 1986; Krosnick *et al.* 1994).

2.3 Determinants of subjective norms

Subjective norm is a function of normative beliefs, which represent perceptions of specific significant others' preferences about whether one should or should not engage in a behaviour. This is quantified in the model as the subjective likelihood that specific salient groups or individuals (referents) think the person should or should not perform the behaviour, multiplied by the person's motivation to comply with that referent's expectation. Motivation to comply is the extent to which the person wishes to comply with the specific wishes of the referent on this issue. These products are then summed across salient referents:

$$SN = \sum_{j=1}^{j=m} nb_j \cdot mc_j \tag{4}$$

where SN is the subjective norm, nb_j is the normative belief (i.e. a subjective probability) that some referent j thinks one should perform the behaviour, mc_j is the motivation to comply with referent j, and m is the number of salient referents. It should be noted that the distinction between behavioural beliefs and normative beliefs is somewhat arbitrary (Miniard and Cohen 1981) and there is often found to be considerable correlation between the two (O'Keefe 1990). However, there is some merit in maintaining a distinction between the determinants of behaviour that are attributes of the person and those that are attributes of the social environment (see Eagly and Chaiken 1993: 171).

The expectancy-value nature of equation (4) has been noted by a number of authors (e.g. Eagly and Chaiken 1993) and is generally taken to be supported by correlations between normative beliefs and subjective norms in the range 0.50 to 0.70 (van den Putte (1993) reports a mean value of

0.53 across the 113 studies he reviewed). However, more controversy has surrounded the wording of these items. Cialdini *et al.* (1991) call the normative beliefs used in the TRA/TPB injunctive social norms, as they concern others' social approval, and distinguish them from descriptive social norms which describe perceptions of what others do. The relative predictive power of these normative items is an issue of some debate (e.g. Lewis *et al.* 1989), although Fishbein (1993) suggests that both can be considered indicators of the same underlying concept, social pressure. Others have debated the most appropriate level of specificity to use in the wording of motivation to comply item (e.g. O'Keefe 1990).

2.4 Determinants of perceived behavioural control

Judgements of perceived behavioural control are influenced by beliefs concerning whether one has access to the necessary resources and opportunities to perform the behaviour successfully, weighted by the perceived power of each factor (Ajzen 1988, 1991). The perceptions of factors likely to facilitate or inhibit the performance of the behaviour are referred to as control beliefs. These factors include both internal control factors (information, personal deficiencies, skills, abilities, emotions) and external control factors (opportunities, dependence on others, barriers). People who perceive they have access to the necessary resources and perceive that there are the opportunities (or lack of obstacles) to perform the behaviour are likely to perceive a high degree of behavioural control (Ajzen 1991). There has been some variation in how control beliefs are operationalized. Ajzen and Madden (1986) assessed *PBC* to be based upon the sum of frequency of occurrence of various facilitators and inhibitors. Ajzen (1991) has suggested that each control factor is weighted by its perceived power to facilitate or inhibit performance of the behaviour. The model quantifies these beliefs by multiplying the frequency or likelihood of occurrence of the factor by the subjective perception of the power of the factor to facilitate or inhibit the performance of the behaviour:

$$PBC = \sum_{k=1}^{k=n} c_k \cdot p_k \tag{5}$$

where PBC is perceived behavioural control, c_k is the perceived frequency or likelihood of occurrence of factor k, p_k is the perceived facilitating or inhibiting power of the factor k, and n is the number of control factors.

Relatively few studies have examined this relationship. At the time of writing we found only a handful of studies which reported this relationship clearly (Ajzen and Driver 1991; Kimiecik 1992; Godin *et al.* 1993; Conner and Sherlock 1993; Norman and Smith 1995), and the mean correlation was 0.41. Ajzen (1991) reports a correlation of 0.50 for this relationship, based on data in Ajzen and Driver (1991). Valois *et al.* (1993)

specifically investigated equation (5) and its relationship to *PBC* and *BI*. They were generally supportive of the multiplicative composite. However, further research may be required to clarify the best way to assess the determinants of *PBC*.

2.5 Commentary

The causal model which the TPB represents is illustrated in Figure 5.1. Behaviour is determined by intention to engage in the behaviour and perceptions of control over performance of the behaviour. Intention is determined by attitude towards the behaviour, subjective norms and perceived behavioural control. Attitude is determined by perceptions of the likelihood of salient outcomes and their evaluation. Subjective norm is determined by normative beliefs and motivation to comply with salient referents. PBC is determined by the perceived presence or absence of requisite resources and opportunities and the perceived power of these factors to facilitate or inhibit performance of the behaviour.

The model is held to be a complete theory of behaviour in that any other influences on behaviour are held to have their impact upon behaviour via influencing components of the TPB. However, it is perhaps more correctly regarded as a theory of the proximal determinants of behaviour. Indeed, Ajzen (1991) describes the model as open to further elaboration if further important proximal determinants are identified. The model does give a clear description of the processes by which attitudes and beliefs determine behaviour. It has been criticized as being too elaborate (Fischhoff *et al.* 1982; Fazio 1986) to be regarded as a realistic description of individual decision-making processes. However, the TRA and TPB are models of the processes by which individuals form attitudes and intentions, which may be subsequently stored in memory and retrieved when the individual faces a behavioural decision. Research supporting the application of the TRA to a range of behaviours is extensive, while that on the TPB is growing and is considered below.

3 Summary of research

The TRA/TPB has been applied to the prediction of a number of different behaviours, including health-relevant behaviours, with varying degrees of success. Excellent reviews of the large number of studies using the TRA can be found in Sheppard *et al.* (1988) and van den Putte (1993). Ajzen (1991) provides the most comprehensive review to date of research using the TPB. Here we concentrate on reviewing published studies using the TPB, focusing on those which have been used to predict health behaviours and referring to studies using the TRA where appropriate. Specific discussions of applications to the study of a number of health behaviours are followed by a general overview of results using the TPB.

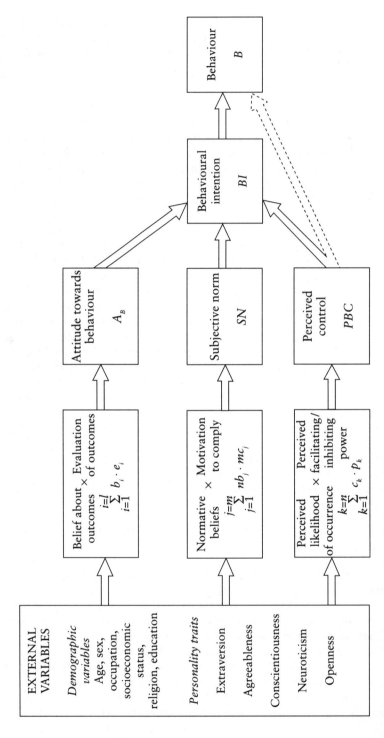

Figure 5.1 The theory of planned behaviour (TPB).

3.1 Smoking

A number of studies have employed the TRA to investigate smoking initiation (Sherman *et al.* 1982; Sutton 1989), frequency of smoking (Chassin *et al.* 1981; Fishbein 1982; Budd 1986; Grube *et al.* 1986) and cessation (De Vries and Kok 1986; Marin *et al.* 1990). Only a couple of studies have currently employed the TPB in relation to smoking (Babrow *et al.* 1990; Godin *et al.* 1992). For example, Godin *et al.* (1992) looked at the prediction of the frequency of smoking in the general public over a six-month period. The prediction of intentions was significantly improved by the addition of the *PBC* component (27 versus 15 per cent of variability accounted for), and actual smoking behaviour appeared to be primarily related to *PBC*.

3.2 Alcohol consumption

Frequency of drinking has been explored using the TRA by a number of studies, in samples both with (Fishbein *et al.* 1980; Budd and Spencer 1984) and without (Schlegel *et al.* 1977; London 1982) drinking problems. A single study using TPB on drinking behaviour (Schlegel *et al.* 1992) has been published. This study found that *PBC* contributed to the predictions of intentions, but not frequency of getting drunk in non-problem drinkers. In problem drinkers the *PBC* also contributed to predictions of frequency of getting drunk. The authors interpreted the findings as supporting the need to incorporate measures of *PBC* for non-volitional behaviours.

3.3 Sexual behaviours

The TRA has been extensively applied in relation to oral contraceptive use (Davidson and Jaccard 1979; Werner and Middlestadt 1979; Doll and Orth 1993) and other forms of contraception (McCarty 1981; Pagel and Davidson 1984), and more specifically condom use in relation to the threat of AIDS in heterosexual (Chan and Fishbein 1993; Terry *et al.* 1993a) and homosexual samples (Fishbein *et al.* 1992).

Several studies have also applied the TPB, particularly in relation to condom use (Boldero *et al.* 1992; Wilson *et al.* 1992; Terry *et al.* 1993a, b; Conner and Graham 1994; van der Pligt and De Vries 1995). Nucifora *et al.* (1993) examined undergraduates' use of condoms using the TPB. *PBC* was found to make a small but significant contribution to the predictions of intentions to use condoms and actual condom use. However, intentions appeared to be principally determined by attitudes and subjective norms, while behaviour was mainly influenced by intentions.

3.4 Health screening attendance

Health screening attendance has not been investigated using the TRA, although the TPB has been applied in a couple of studies (De Vellis *et al.*

1990; Norman and Conner 1993). Norman and Conner found that *PBC* did not significantly contribute to the predictions of either intentions or behaviour, although the level of prediction of behaviour from intentions was also low.

3.5 Exercise

Participation in a range of exercise behaviours has been studied using the TRA (Sejwacz *et al.* 1980; Theodorakis *et al.* 1991). With the TPB a number of studies have investigated exercise in various samples (Godin and Shepherd 1987; Dzewaltowski *et al.* 1990; Kimiecik 1992; Theodorakis 1992, 1994; Godin *et al.* 1993; Yordy and Lent 1993; Norman and Smith 1995), including pregnant women (Godin *et al.* 1989). Dzewaltowski *et al.* (1990) reported the application of the TPB to exercise participation. Intentions were based both upon attitudes and *PBC*, but not subjective norms, while actual behaviour seemed to be principally determined by intentions.

3.6 Food choice

Food choice, whether or not related to health outcomes, has been a focus of TRA studies by a number of authors. For example, Manstead *et al.* (1983, 1984) investigated infant feeding, while Brinberg and Durand (1983) looked at visiting fast food restaurants. The TPB has also been applied to food choices by a number of authors (Beale and Manstead 1991; Sparks *et al.* 1992; Sparks and Shepherd 1992; Towler and Shepherd 1992; Lloyd *et al.* 1993). Towler and Shepherd looked at chip consumption. Intentions were found to be principally based upon attitudes, with *PBC* not adding any further predictive power. This was similarly the case for actual consumption, with intentions being the sole predictor. However, these results should be interpreted with caution as the data were cross-sectional and the measure of control used an atypical single item measure ('If you were to try, what is the likelihood that you will reduce the total intake of chips in your diet?', likely–unlikely).

3.7 Breast/testicle self-examination

Both breast (Lauver and Chang 1991) and testicle (Brubaker and Fowler 1990; Brubaker and Wickersham, 1990) self-examination have been studied using the TRA. A couple of studies have used the TPB to predict breast/testicle self-examination (Young *et al.* 1991; McCaul *et al.* 1993). McCaul *et al.* showed the TRA components to predict breast/testicle self-examination intentions and behaviours, with *PBC* adding significantly to predictions of intentions but not behaviour.

3.8 Other behaviours

While the TRA has been applied to a very long list of other behaviours, the TPB has to date been used in a more limited number of circumstances despite its claimed wider applicability. These include leisure activities (Ajzen and Driver 1992), studying (Lay and Burns 1991), class attendance (Prislin and Kovrlija 1992; Prislin 1993; Valois *et al.* 1993), getting an A on a course (Ajzen and Madden 1986), course enrolment (Crawley and Black 1992; Crawley and Koballa 1992), teaching methods (Crawley 1990), transport choice (Bamberg and Schmidt 1993), cheating, lying and shoplifting (Beck and Ajzen 1991), kidney donation (Borgida *et al.* 1992), drug use (Conner and Sherlock 1993) and drug compliance (Hounsa *et al.* 1993), patient education (Kinket *et al.* 1992), pain assessment (Nash *et al.* 1993), weight loss (Schifter and Ajzen 1985; Netemeyer *et al.* 1991), playing computer games (Doll *et al.* 1991; Doll and Ajzen 1992), stocks and shares buying (East 1993), voting (Netemeyer and Burton 1990; Netemeyer *et al.* 1991), driving behaviours (Parker *et al.* 1992a, b, 1995), reporting a colleague for unethical behaviour (Randall and Gibson 1991), visiting public houses (Traen and Nordlund 1993) and job search (Van-Ryn and Vinokur 1992).

3.9 Overview

The published studies applying the TRA have been reviewed by Sheppard *et al.* (1988) and van den Putte (1993), with Ajzen (1991) reviewing 16 studies using the TPB. The findings are generally supportive of the TRA/TPB. For example, the multiple correlation of intentions with attitudes and subjective norms is between 0.66 (Sheppard *et al.* 1988, from 87 studies) and 0.68 (van den Putte 1993, from 113 studies). Ajzen (1991) reports the multiple correlation between intentions and A, SN and PBC to be 0.71 across the 16 studies he reviewed. Van den Putte (1993) computes a value of $R = 0.64$, but notes the large variation in results between behaviours. The mean correlation between intentions and behaviour is reported to be 0.45 by Randall and Wolff (1994), 0.53 by Sheppard *et al.* and 0.62 by van den Putte. Ajzen reports the mean R between BI, PBC and behaviour to be 0.51, while van den Putte computes a value of 0.46. However, such values are not directly comparable because of considerable variation between behaviours. Ajzen (1991) and Madden *et al.* (1992) do, however, report empirical evidence that PBC significantly improves predictions of both intentions and behaviour.

4 Developments

Two areas of development in the use of the TRA/TPB will be commented upon here. The first is the extra complexity required in the application of these models to the prediction of choices between behaviours and to the prediction of goals. The second development concerns further variables which represent possible candidates for additions to the model.

4.1 Behavioural choices and goals

Where a behaviour represents a choice between two or more alternatives it has been recommended that the TRA/TPB components be assessed in relation to each alternative (Ajzen and Fishbein 1980). For example, an individual may have similarly valenced attitudes towards smoking and not smoking, but smoke because his or her attitudes towards smoking are less negative. If the components of the model are assessed in relation to each alternative, then the difference scores may provide better predictions of behaviour (Sheppard *et al.* 1988; Fishbein *et al.* 1986; van den Putte 1993). Davidson and Morrison (1982) demonstrated the importance of considering multiple alternatives in considering contraceptive choices. Courneya (1994) makes the important point that in studying frequently repeated behaviours (e.g. exercise, eating), different frequencies of performance of the behaviour may represent distinct alternatives and good predictions may require application of the TRA/TPB to each of the alternatives of interest.

In predicting the achievement of goals (e.g. weight loss) there are additional problems in applying the TRA (Sheppard *et al.* 1988). For example, intentions to lose weight only correlate weakly with actual weight loss (Sejwacz *et al.* 1980). However, weight loss is somewhat better predicted by application of the TRA to the component behaviours necessary for weight loss (e.g. avoiding high calorie foods, exercise) (Sejwacz *et al.* 1980). In contrast, the TPB should be directly applicable to the prediction of goals such as weight loss (and predictive of success to the extent that *PBC* matches actual control), and Schifter and Ajzen (1985) specifically applied the TPB to this goal. However, the extent to which *BI* and *PBC* alone are sufficient to predict the attainment of distant goals remains to be demonstrated, and other variables may need to be considered (see Schwarzer 1992; Schwarzer and Fuchs, Chapter 6 in this volume). For example, the TPB tells us little about the processes by which individuals form and act upon plans to achieve particular goals (Eagly and Chaiken 1993). In addition, it remains to be demonstrated that *PBC* and *BI* towards a goal such as weight loss are more predictive of weight loss than consideration of *BI* (and even *PBC*) towards each component behaviour relevant to achieving that goal (Fishbein 1993).

4.2 Additional predictors

A number of potential candidate variables for addition to the TRA/TPB have been suggested. In each case both theoretical and empirical justifications are necessary (Fishbein 1993). A number of studies have suggested direct impact of past behaviour on current behaviour unmediated by components of the TRA/TPB (e.g. Bentler and Speckhart 1979, 1981; Bagozzi 1981) and the available evidence is supportive of such a relationship (see Eagly and Chaiken 1993, for a discussion). However, while such studies have been used to support the contention that past behaviour is an important predictor of many behaviours, the intellectual cul-de-sac this represents for those interested in changing behaviours (Abraham and Sheeran 1994) is worth noting (see Norman and Conner, Chapter 7 in this volume).

Moral norms (personal beliefs about right and wrong) have been found to be significant, independent predictors of intentions and behaviour for particular classes of behaviours (e.g. Beck and Ajzen 1991), while self-identity, for example as a 'green' consumer, has been found to be important in addition to components of the TPB in other studies (e.g. Sparks and Shepherd 1992). Finally, a number of studies have looked at affective outcomes (e.g. regret, pleasure) as distinct from cognitive outcomes as determinants of attitudes (Bagozzi 1989; Ajzen and Driver 1991; Richard *et al.* 1995) and in a number of cases it may be worth considering both forms of outcomes. The status of these three additional variables in the context of the TPB is likely to become clearer as they are employed more widely.

5 Operationalization of the model

This section describes the development of adequate measures of each of the differing components of the model, while the following section considers an application of the TPB to healthy food choice and dietary change. Extensive details of applying the TRA can be found in Ajzen and Fishbein (1980), while Ajzen (1991) provides the most extensive coverage of applying the TPB (see also Terry *et al.* 1993c).

Perhaps the first decision concerns the definition of the population of interest. This decision is likely to be based upon theoretical and pragmatic grounds. Within the selected population, it is important to ascertain if there are likely to be within-group differences that the research may wish to address. It may also be that additional work will be required to ensure that the different measures are applicable to each identified sub-group. Pilot work may be necessary to investigate such divisions in the population.

5.1 Behaviours

In considering the development of appropriate measures of each of the components of the TPB, it is common to begin with developing a clear conceptualization of the behaviour or goal we wish to predict. The principle of compatibility discussed earlier makes it clear that the measures of behaviours and attitudes need to be formulated at the same level of specificity with regard to action, target, context and time. Hence, we need to be clear about the level at which we wish to predict behaviour with regard to these four elements. Clear specification of the action, target, context and time frame for the behaviour will make clearer the specification of the TPB measures. For example, we may wish to predict eating (action) of fruit (target) as part of a midday meal (context) tomorrow (time frame). In such a case the TPB measures would be taken on one day and the measure of behaviour would need be taken the next day. Obviously aggregation of behaviours across time frames, contexts, targets and actions is possible. The minimum specification would require an action and time frame to be stated. Such clear specification allows easy application of the principle of compatibility with respect to the TPB measures. Assessment of such a behaviour might involve simple self-reports of whether the behaviour was performed in the specified context over the appropriate time period:

I ate fruit as part of my midday meal today.   Definitely did not   1 2 3 4 5 6 7   Definitely did

An alternative item might simply require the respondent to mark whether the behaviour was or was not performed:

I did/did not eat fruit as part of my midday meal today.

More complex goals (e.g. weight loss) may require specification of a series of simpler behaviours (e.g. exercise, avoiding fatty foods) and assessing the TPB components in relation to each of these. In all cases it is important to consider carefully the nature of the behaviour.

For assessing frequently repeated behaviours, Courneya (1994) points out that a range of alternative response formats are possible. For example, the above responses would be continuous, closed and dichotomous, closed respectively. Open response formats (e.g. 'How many times did you eat fruit as part of your lunch in the past month?____times') are also possible. Courneya also notes both the need to match the measures of behaviour to that used to assess intention and, in using continuous response formats, the need to obtain measures of each of the components of the TPB towards performing each of the behavioural options, because each may be considered a different behaviour by the respondent.

5.2 Behavioural intentions

Behavioural intention measures tend to use a number of standard wordings that use the same level of specificity with respect to action, target, context and time frame as used in the behaviour measure. Traditionally, this is defined as a subjective probability judgement of how the individual intends to behave. For example, a single item intention measure matched to the above behaviour might be worded:

I intend to eat fruit as part of my midday meal tomorrow.   Likely   1 2 3 4 5 6 7   Unlikely

However, from a psychometric point of view, multiple-item measures are more appropriate. Such measures commonly assess not only intentions which are commonly thought of as plans, but also desire and self-prediction concerning performance of the behaviour (Sheppard *et al.* 1988; Fishbein and Stasson 1990; Norman and Smith 1995), each of which are typically highly intercorrelated (e.g. Figure 5.2). We have found the group of six items shown in Figure 5.2 to be highly intercorrelated, as indicated by high internal reliability measures (alpha > 0.9) for a range of behaviours. Principal components analysis of such measures suggest one factor explaining at least 70 per cent of the variance. Reporting of internal reliability data is to be encouraged for this and all components of the TPB.

5.3 Attitudes

Attitudes are personal evaluations of the target behaviour and are typically measured by using items such as:

My eating fruit as part of my midday   Good 1 2 3 4 5 6 7 Bad
meal tomorrow would be: Harmful 1 2 3 4 5 6 7 Beneficial
                                               Pleasant 1 2 3 4 5 6 7 Unpleasant

Here respondents are required to evaluate the behaviour described at the appropriate level of specificity on a series of semantic differentials (taken from the evaluative dimension of Osgood *et al.* 1957). Typically, four to six such differentials are used and these tend to show high internal reliability (alpha > 0.9) (Figure 5.2).

5.4 Subjective norms

Subjective norms are operationalized as the person's subjective judgement concerning whether significant others would want him or her to perform the behaviour or not. These are traditionally measured by a single item such as:

Most people who are important to me think I:
Should 1 2 3 4 5 6 7 Should not
eat fruit as part of my midday meal tomorrow.

There are a number of well-known problems with the use of single items and a number of multiple item measures have been suggested (Figure 5.2), although there are few reliability data on such measures.

5.5 Perceived behavioural control

PBC represents the overall control the individual perceives him or herself to have over performance of the behaviour. It has commonly been measured by the following three items (Ajzen and Madden 1986):

How much control do you feel you have over eating fruit
as part of your midday meal tomorrow?   No control 1 2 3 4 5 6 7 Complete control

For me to eat fruit as part of my midday
meal tomorrow is . . .   Difficult 1 2 3 4 5 6 7 Easy

If I wanted to I could easily eat fruit as
part of my midday meal tomorrow.   Likely 1 2 3 4 5 6 7 Unlikely

Figure 5.2 Measuring components of the theory of planned behaviour: example item wordings and response formats.

Behavioural intentions

(a) Intention

I intend to eat fruit as part of my midday meal tomorrow.   Definitely do not 1 2 3 4 5 6 7 Definitely do

I plan to eat fruit as part of my midday meal tomorrow.   Definitely do not 1 2 3 4 5 6 7 Definitely do

(b) Desire

I would like to eat fruit as part of my midday meal tomorrow.   Definitely yes 1 2 3 4 5 6 7 Definitely no

I want to eat fruit as part of my midday meal tomorrow.   Strongly disagree 1 2 3 4 5 6 7 Strongly agree

(c) Expectation

I expect to eat fruit as part of my midday meal tomorrow.   Unlikely 1 2 3 4 5 6 7 Likely

How likely is it that you will eat fruit as part of your midday meal tomorrow.   Unlikely 1 2 3 4 5 6 7 Likely

Attitudes

My eating fruit as part of my midday meal tomorrow would be:

(a) Bad	1	2	3	4	5	6	7	Good
(b) Harmful	1	2	3	4	5	6	7	Beneficial
(c) Unpleasant	1	2	3	4	5	6	7	Pleasant
(d) Unenjoyable	1	2	3	4	5	6	7	Enjoyable
(e) Foolish	1	2	3	4	5	6	7	Wise

Behavioural beliefs

Eating fruit as part of my midday meal tomorrow would make me healthier.   Unlikely 1 2 3 4 5 6 7 Likely

Outcome evaluations

Being healthier would be . . .   Bad 1 2 3 4 5 6 7 Good

Subjective norms

People who are important to me think I:

Should 1 2 3 4 5 6 7 Should not

eat fruit as part of my midday meal tomorrow.

People who are important to me would:
  Approve 1 2 3 4 5 6 7 **Disapprove**
      of my eating fruit as part of my midday meal tomorrow.

People who are important to
  me want me to eat fruit
  as part of my midday
  meal tomorrow.   **Likely** 1 2 3 4 5 6 7 **Unlikely**

I feel under social
  pressure to eat fruit as
  part of my midday
  meal tomorrow.   **Strongly disagree** 1 2 3 4 5 6 7 **Strongly agree**

Normative beliefs
      My friends think I:
      Should 1 2 3 4 5 6 7 **Should not**
          eat fruit as part of my midday meal tomorrow.

Motivation to comply
With regard to your diet
  how much do you
  want to do what your
  friends think you
  should.   **Not at all** 1 2 3 4 5 6 7 **Very much**

Perceived behavioural control
Whether I do or do not
  eat fruit as part of my
  midday meal tomorrow
  is entirely up to me. **Strongly disagree** 1 2 3 4 5 6 7 **Strongly agree**

How much control do
  you feel you have over
  eating fruit as part of
  your midday meal
  tomorrow?   **No control** 1 2 3 4 5 6 7 **Complete control**

I would like to eat fruit
  as part of my midday
  meal tomorrow but I
  don't really know if I
  can.   **Strongly disagree** 1 2 3 4 5 6 7 **Strongly agree**

I am confident that I
  could eat fruit as
  part of my midday
  meal tomorrow if I
  wanted to.   **Strongly disagree** 1 2 3 4 5 6 7 **Strongly agree**

For me to eat fruit as
  part of my midday
  meal tomorrow is . . .   Difficult 1 2 3 4 5 6 7 Easy

Control beliefs
When eating out, there
  is a limited choice of
  fruit available . . .   Likely 1 2 3 4 5 6 7 Unlikely

Power
The limited choice of
  fruit when eating out
  makes my eating fruit
  as part of my midday
  meal tomorrow . . .   Less likely 1 2 3 4 5 6 7 More likely

---

However, the internal reliability of these items has frequently been found to be low (e.g. Beale and Manstead 1991; Sparks 1994). For example, in the Beale and Manstead (1991) study, the authors measured *PBC* by way of three items: (a) 'If I wanted to, it would be easy for me not to let my baby eat or drink anything which contains sugar between meals' (seven-point response scale ranging from likely to unlikely); (b) 'My not letting my baby eat or drink anything which contains sugar between meals is . . .' (easy–difficult); and (c) 'There is very little that I can do to make sure that my baby does not eat or drink anything which contains sugar between meals' (agree–disagree). They found it necessary to delete the last of the three items in order to improve alpha from 0.40 to 0.56. Sparks *et al.* (1992) also reported low coefficients in a study of attitudes towards biscuit and wholemeal bread consumption (alpha = 0.49), as did Sparks and Shepherd (in preparation) in a study of attitudes towards dietary change (alpha = 0.48). In a different health domain, Chan and Fishbein (1993) have also reported similar problems of inter-item reliability in a study of women's intentions to tell their partners to use condoms. Figure 5.2 contains a number of alternatives which we have found to have higher internal reliability than those reported in the above studies.

This problem of the adequate measurement of *PBC* requires greater attention than it has been given to date. Consider the sorts of item that are currently used to assess the construct (see above): part of the problem with inter-item reliability may be differences in the way that lay people conceptualize the notion of 'control' and how they conceptualize the notion of 'difficulty' (Chan and Fishbein 1993; Sparks 1994). People may consider the performance of a behaviour to be 'under their control' yet at the same time consider it to be difficult to carry out. The mix of unipolar and bipolar scales among *PBC* items may contribute to this problem, which may also be exacerbated by question order context effects when items are either randomly or systematically ordered in questionnaires (e.g. Budd 1987; Schwarz and Sudman 1992; van den Putte 1993; Sheeran and Orbell

1995). There now exist a number of studies that have pointed to the importance of perceived behavioural control in predicting behavioural intentions and behaviour itself: this should not lead to complacency regarding conceptual issues which in turn have implications for construct measurement and consequently for the relevance of *PBC* for practical issues.

5.6 Behavioural beliefs

In the TRA/TPB the relevant behavioural beliefs are those salient to the individual. However, most applications of these models employ modal salient beliefs derived from pilot studies with a representative sample of individuals drawn from the population of interest (see Rutter and Bunce 1989, for an exception). The pilot studies typically consist of semi-structured interviews where respondents are asked to list the characteristics, qualities and attributes of the object or behaviour (Ajzen and Fishbein 1980: 64–71). For example, respondents are asked 'What do you see as the advantages and disadvantages of eating fruit as part of your midday meal?' The most frequently mentioned (modal) beliefs are then used in the final questionnaire, with commonly between six and 12 beliefs being employed.

Examples of belief strength and outcome evaluation items are given in Figure 5.2. Belief strength assesses the subjective probability that a particular outcome will be a consequence of performing the behaviour. Such items commonly use response formats such as 'likely–unlikely', 'probable–improbable' or 'true–false', which are scored in a bipolar fashion, i.e. –3 unlikely to +3 likely (see Ajzen and Fishbein 1980, for a justification). Outcome evaluations assess the overall evaluation of that outcome and are also treated as bipolar (–3 negative evaluation to +3 positive evaluation) and are responded to on 'good–bad' or 'pleasant–unpleasant' response formats (Ajzen and Fishbein 1980). Belief strength and evaluation are then multiplicatively combined and summed (equation 3) to give an indirect measure of attitude. The problem with such calculations on interval level data has been noted by a number of authors (e.g. Evans 1991), although no completely satisfactory solution has been found.

5.7 Normative beliefs

As for behavioural beliefs, most studies employ modal rather than individually salient referent groups as the basis of normative items and derive these from pilot studies with a representative sample of individuals from the population of interest. Ajzen and Fishbein (1980: 74–5) suggest that we ask about the groups or individuals who would approve or disapprove of you performing the behaviour or who come to mind when thinking about the target behaviour. For example, respondents might be asked, 'Are there any groups or individuals who come to mind when thinking about eating fruit as part of your midday meal?' The most frequently mentioned (modal) referents are then incorporated in the final questionnaire. Typically two to six referent groups are included. Figure 5.2 shows examples of normative belief and motivation to comply items. Normative beliefs are the person's perceptions of whether specific referents would want him or her to perform the behaviour under consideration. These items are typically responded to on a 'should–should not' or 'likely–unlikely' response format and scored in a bipolar fashion, i.e. −3 strong negative pressure to perform to +3 strong positive pressure to perform. Motivation to comply is operationalized as the person's willingness to comply with the expectations of the specific referents. Such items are typically responded to on 'not at all–strongly' or 'likely–unlikely' response formats and treated as unipolar scales, i.e. +1 low motivation to comply, +7 strong motivation to comply. This is because people are considered unlikely to be motivated to do the opposite of what they perceive significant others want them to do. The relevant normative beliefs and motivations to comply are then multiplicatively combined and summed (equation 4) to give an indirect measure of normative pressure.

5.8 Control beliefs

Finally for control beliefs, the few studies which have reported these items have also used modal control beliefs derived from pilot studies with samples representative of the target population, although presumably salient control factors are the most appropriate measures. Ajzen and Driver (1991) suggest that individuals are asked to list the factors and conditions that make it easy or difficult to perform the target behaviour and the most frequently mentioned (modal) items are used in the final questionnaire. For example, respondents might be asked, 'What factors might prevent you or help you eat fruit as part of your midday meal?' However, perhaps because they have so infrequently been used to date, there has been some variation in how control beliefs have been operationalized. Figure 5.2 gives examples of a control belief and power item. Control beliefs assess the presence or absence of facilitating or inhibiting factors and are commonly scored on 'never–frequently', 'false–true', 'available–unavailable' or 'likely-unlikely' response formats. Ajzen (1991) suggests that control is best treated as a bipolar scale (−3 inhibits to +3 facilitates), although a unipolar scoring appears more appropriate for certain response formats (e.g. +1 'never' to +7 'frequently'). Perceived power items assess the power of the item to facilitate or inhibit performance of the behaviour. Power items are also problematic: response formats include 'more likely–less likely', 'easier–more difficult' and 'not important–very important'. Ajzen (1991) reports mixed evidence concerning whether these should be scored as unipolar or bipolar, although the wording of the response format may suggest the most appropriate scoring to use. The relevant items are then multiplicatively combined and summed (equation 5) to give an indirect measure of perceived behavioural control. This offers a promising avenue for exploration, offering an opportunity to identify those factors that underpin people's perceptions of control. However, precisely how these control beliefs combine to influence *PBC* requires more attention since this research is currently at a very preliminary stage.

6 Application of the model: food choice

In this section we discuss the application of the theory of planned behaviour to a particular health issue – that of healthy food choices and dietary change. There is a large body of evidence that links the diets of many people in the Western world to particular serious diseases (Cannon 1992). Although this link is sometimes challenged, the weight of evidence seems to be firmly on the side of those who suggest, for example, a connection between fat consumption and heart disease. Whereas in the United States fat consumption declined between the mid-1960s and the mid-1980s (Stephen and Wald 1990), in the UK fat consumption levels (as a percentage of dietary energy) have remained very constant (at about 42 per cent of food energy) (Secretary of State for Health 1992). The available evidence suggests that the percentage of energy derived from fat is very similar for women and men. This is also a problem that cuts across social class lines (Gregory *et al.* 1990). Those involved in health research and health promotion are understandably keen to find out why consumption levels have remained so static and what barriers to change are likely to present themselves in the future. In this section, we look at the potential contribution of the TPB in addressing these issues.

By now a number of diverse studies have pointed to the influential role that *PBC* plays in people's dietary intentions and behaviour. In an early application of the TPB, Ajzen and Timko (1986) found that measures of perceived behavioural control over a variety of behaviours 'related to matters of health' (including eating three meals a day, avoiding drinks containing caffeine, avoiding high cholesterol foods, eating fresh fruit and vegetables, taking vitamin supplements) made a contribution, independent of attitudes, to the prediction of the behaviours in question. This extended model has also proved useful in predicting mothers' intentions to limit their infants' sugar consumption (Beale and Manstead 1991) and people's intentions to use skimmed milk (Raats *et al.* 1995), to consume biscuits (Sparks *et al.* 1992) and to eat organically produced vegetables (Sparks and Shepherd 1992). Predictions of intentions to make specific dietary changes also appear to benefit from an assessment of *PBC*: Sparks and Shepherd (in preparation) found, *inter alia*, that perceptions of control contributed to intentions to reduce consumption of meat, cheese, chocolate and biscuits[2] (see also Sparks *et al.* 1995). Of course, these latter examples make reference to reducing or increasing consumption of a food: this doesn't really involve a behaviour, *per se*, as much as a difference between behaviours at different (but unspecified) time points. We return to this issue later.

Not all food consumption behaviours are likely to be influenced by perceived control problems: the TPB, as we indicated earlier, is understood as applicable to behaviours characterized by 'incomplete volitional control'

(Ajzen 1988: 132). However, it is apparent that people often do experience difficulties in relation to diet and dietary change. It is worth bearing in mind in this regard that many of the difficulties faced are not difficulties with carrying out particular behaviours but difficulties experienced in refraining from certain behaviours: while some people (in the UK) may not be able to eat what they would prefer to eat because of, for example, constraints presented by low income and poor access to retail outlets, a different kind of control problem exists where people experience problems of resisting certain foods, of restraint, craving, 'addiction' and temptation.

So, in considering the role of *PBC* in the context of food choice, we have to consider not only the difficulties that people may have in acquiring or eating certain foods but also difficulties experienced in not eating (or overeating) certain foods. People in the Western world are concerned about eating too much food as well as about eating too little (see Goodman and Redclift 1991) and huge sums of money are spent each year on products to promote weight loss (for either health or body image reasons). While the application of the TPB is likely to help to predict intentions and behaviour in many food choice situations, the knowledge that people experience control problems needs to be supplemented by an understanding of what those control problems are, if the theory is to be of practical benefit for health promotion. In the Sparks *et al.* (1992) study alluded to above, there was some indication that problems of not being able to resist eating biscuits were important for predicting perceptions of control over their consumption, while perceptions of problems of lack of availability in the shops seemed to be important for the prediction of consumption of organic vegetables. Here, we have examples of the two different kinds of control problems to which we referred earlier: what Ajzen (1988: 128–31) would call internal control factors (in the case of the problem of restraint) and external control factors (in the case of availability). The relationship between perceived behavioural control and specific problems was assessed by multiple regression techniques (see Table 5.1). The percentage variance accounted for is very small – so clearly better methods are required if we are to come to a reasonable understanding of the control problems that people experience.

6.1 An example: dietary change

The notion of dietary change is usually associated with the changes that people make to their proportional intake of macronutrients such as fats and carbohydrates, or to their overall consumption levels more generally. Here, we illustrate the use of the TPB through the example of Conner *et al.*'s (1994) study of attitudes towards healthy eating. This was a questionnaire study in which respondents were selected from a number of general practices. Two hundred and forty-one people took part in the study, a number which reflected a response rate of approximately 50 per cent (respondents, therefore, should not be thought of as representing a random sample of the

Table 5.1 Regression of (a) perceived behavioural control on problems associated with biscuit consumption and (b) perceived behavioural control on problems associated with consumption of 'organic' vegetables (from Sparks *et al.* 1992)

	Beta
(a) Biscuits ($R = 0.46$)	
Problem of availability	−0.05
Problem of cost	−0.14
Problem of resisting	−0.44***
Problem of others' preferences	−0.08
(b) 'Organic' vegetables ($R = 0.22$)	
Problem of availability	−0.18*
Problem of family influence	−0.11
Problem of friends' influence	0.13
Problem of cost	−0.03

Note: * $p < 0.05$; *** $p < 0.001$.

population). The questionnaire included the following measures to assess central components of the TPB (applications of the TRA and TPB usually adopt their measures from those suggested in Ajzen and Fishbein (1980), Ajzen (1988) or research papers produced by these authors). All responses were made on seven-point scales.

Behaviour. This was assessed at the time of, and six months after, the TPB measures and consisted of a 33-item food frequency measure. From this measure the percentage of calories in the individual's diet derived from fat at each time point was calculated. The change in the percentage calories from fat was then calculated as one indicator of a healthy diet.

Behavioural intentions. Five measures were used, which included traditional intention measures and what we have characterized as desire and expectation measures (Figure 5.2, with end options given in parenthesis): (a) I intend to eat a healthier diet during the next six months (definitely do–definitely do not); (b) I will try to eat a healthier diet during the next six months (unlikely–likely); (c) I want to eat a healthier diet over the next six months (strongly agree–strongly disagree); (d) I expect to eat a healthier diet during the next six months (unlikely–likely); (e) how likely is it that you will eat a healthier diet during the next six months? (unlikely–likely). These items were then summed to give an overall intention score. Inter-item reliability (Cronbach's alpha) for these items was 0.95.

Attitude. The measure was taken as the sum of five semantic differential scales: my eating a healthier diet is . . . (bad–good, harmful–beneficial, unpleasant–pleasant, unenjoyable–enjoyable, foolish–wise). Cronbach's alpha for these items was 0.95.

Subjective norm. This question was asked in the following format: people who are important to me think I should eat a healthier diet (unlikely–likely).

Perceived behavioural control. This was measured using the following six items (with end options given in parenthesis): (a) I am confident that if I ate a healthier diet I could keep to it (strongly disagree–strongly agree); (b) whether I do or do not eat a healthier diet over the next six months is entirely up to me (strongly disagree–strongly agree); (c) how much control do you have over eating a healthier diet over the next six months? (no control–complete control); (d) I would like to eat a healthier diet but don't really know if I can (strongly disagree–strongly agree); (e) I am confident that I could eat a healthier diet if I wanted to (strongly disagree–strongly agree); (f) for me to eat a healthier diet in the next six months is . . . (difficult–easy). The alpha coefficient for these six items was 0.74, and the items were subsequently summed in order to form a measure of perceived behavioural control.

Behavioural beliefs. Seven beliefs were assessed (these had been elicited from another sample of subjects via a pretest questionnaire, following Ajzen and Fishbein 1980: Chapter 6). These were: (a) eating a healthier diet would make me physically fitter; (b) eating a healthier diet would make me healthier; (c) by eating a healthier diet I would lose weight; (d) eating a healthier diet would help me live longer; (e) eating a healthier diet would make me feel good about myself; (f) eating a healthier diet would take time (e.g. choosing healthier foods, preparing healthier foods); (g) A healthier diet would be expensive. The response scales were marked unlikely and likely at their end points and were scored from –3 to +3. The 'outcomes' identified in the behavioural belief questions were evaluated on a response scale labelled from bad to good (scored –3 to +3) in response to questions of the form: being physically fitter would be . . . (bad–good). Each behavioural belief was multiplied by the corresponding outcome evaluation and these products were summed. The alpha for this scale was 0.70.

Normative beliefs. Four beliefs were assessed (the referent groups were derived from pilot interviews). The referents were friends, health experts, family and workmates. The normative belief questions were all of the same format: my friends think I should eat a healthier diet (likely–unlikely). Corresponding to each normative belief was a motivation to comply question, assessed by statements worded in the form: with regard to eating, I want to do what friends think I should (strongly agree–strongly disagree). Each normative belief was multiplied by the corresponding motivation to comply and these products were summed. The alpha for this scale was 0.75.

Control beliefs. Eleven beliefs were assessed (the control factors were derived from pilot interviews). These were: (a) lack of support from people with whom I share food; (b) the limited choice of healthier food when eating out; (c) obscure and difficult to understand advice about healthier eating; (d) stressful situations; (e) having free time on my hands; (f) being anxious/upset; (g) seeing others eat unhealthy foods; (h) feeling depressed; (i) the poor taste of a healthier diet; (j) being in a hurry at meal times; (k) lack of easy access to places selling healthier foods (e.g. large supermarkets).

Table 5.2   Correlations among TPB components (from Conner *et al.* 1994). Note all correlations above 0.15 are significant.

	BI	ATT	SN	PBC	BE	NB	CB
Behaviour	0.01	0.05	0.01	0.17	0.04	0.03	0.01
Behavioural intentions (BI)		0.35	0.23	0.60	0.50	0.24	0.22
Attitudes (ATT)			0.07	0.37	0.24	0.08	0.12
Subjective norm (SN)				−0.02	0.39	0.60	0.14
Perceived control (PBC)					0.23	0.06	0.37
Beliefs × evaluation (BE)						0.42	0.21
Normative beliefs × motivation to comply (NB)							0.20
Control beliefs × power (CB)							

Note: all correlations above 0.15 are significant.

The power items were all of the same format: Lack of support from whom I share food makes my eating a healthier diet . . . (unlikely–likely; scored −3 to +3). Control belief items corresponded to each of the above power items (e.g. people with whom I eat food support me in eating a healthier diet, 'never–frequently'; scored 1 to 7). Each power item was multiplied by the corresponding control belief and these products were summed. The alpha for this scale was 0.77.

For the basic analysis, the correlations among the TPB components were calculated. These are reported in Table 5.2. The correlations are similar to those reported by van den Putte (1993), which we cited earlier. However, it is perhaps worth noting that, contrary to the TPB, the correlation between intentions and outcome beliefs (*b.e*) was significantly higher than the correlation between intentions and attitudes.

Next, multiple regressions of behavioural intentions on to attitudes, subjective norms and perceived behavioural control were computed. The final beta coefficients showed that all three variables exerted an independent predictive effect on behavioural intentions (see Table 5.3). The multiple correlation (R) between the three predictors and behavioural intention was 0.64. This means that 41 per cent (R^2) of the variance in intention scores could be 'explained' by these predictors.

The behaviour measure (change in percentage of calories derived from fat) was then regressed on to intentions and perceived behavioural control to assess their predictive effects. Each of these two predictors accounted for a small but significant proportion of the variance in behaviour (Table 5.4), with PBC being the more powerful predictor. However, the lack of a significant simple correlation between intentions and behaviour suggests that the multiple regression results should be interpreted with caution. The multiple correlation (R) between the two predictors and behaviour was 0.21. This indicates that 5 per cent (R^2) of the variance in changes in the behaviour score could be 'explained' by these predictors.

Table 5.3 Regressions of behavioural intentions to eat a healthier diet during the next six months on to attitudes, subjective norm and perceived behavioural control (from Conner *et al.* 1994)

	Beta	r	R^2
Attitudes	0.13*	0.35**	0.41**
Subjective norm	0.23**	0.23**	
Perceived behavioural control	0.53**	0.60**	

Note: * $p < 0.01$; ** $p < 0.001$.

Table 5.4 Regressions of change in percentage of calories derived from fat in the diet on to behavioural intentions to eat a healthier diet during the next six months and perceived behavioural control (from Conner *et al.* 1994)

	Beta	r	R^2
Behavioural intentions	0.16*	0.01	0.05*
Perceived behavioural control	0.27**	0.17**	

Note: * $p < 0.05$; ** $p < 0.001$.

6.2 Summary of study findings and implications

The above study demonstrates the application of the TPB to understanding healthy eating. In this study intentions were well predicted by the other components of the model. However, only a modest amount of the variability in behaviour could be explained. There may be a number of reasons for this low predictive power. First, it may be that intentions changed during the six-month period between the assessment of the TPB variables and the final measure of behaviour. This would act to reduce the level of correlation between the TPB components and the behaviour measure. Second, the behaviour measure used here only taps one aspect of healthy eating, whereas the TPB measures assessed views on healthy eating in general. As a consequence, the respondents in the study may have thought about healthy eating as increased consumption of fruit and vegetables, which need not necessarily have had a major impact upon amount of calories consumed as fat in the diet. This illustrates the fact that compatibility of measures may be a more difficult issue to resolve than our earlier discussion suggested, especially for 'general' behaviours where multiple behaviour measures may be more appropriate (see Ajzen and Timko 1986).

6.3 'Control' over dietary change

If we wish to use the TPB to assess attitudes towards dietary change, we have to recognize that change represents a difference (of consumption) between two time points. Consumption levels will be different for different people: thus closely specified behaviours are difficult to identify (at least for groups, rather than individuals). It is questionable therefore whether the TPB is strictly applicable to such issues, given that a single 'objectively defined' behaviour is not of primary interest here. However, if attitudes towards dietary changes are what are of interest, then it behoves us to investigate the theoretical and conceptual problems associated with addressing this issue via the TPB, and the empirical and methodological issues which it raises and demonstrates. We have already alluded to some research that indicates that the TPB may be useful in predicting intentions to make dietary changes (Sparks and Shepherd, in preparation). However, other research on a similar theme (Paisley 1994) found no such independent effect for *PBC*.

6.4 Control over food choice

While many of the applications of the TPB in the domain of food-related behaviours have focused on consumption behaviours that have direct implications for health, it is also of interest to examine attitudes towards behaviours involving the technologies and processes of food production, since these may also be perceived as potentially hazardous or beneficial to health.[3] For example, health concerns about pesticide residues have been with us for some time, whereas similar concerns about the application of genetic engineering techniques in food production are relatively recent. When we wish to address people's attitudes to these issues, we are often less concerned with specific behaviours than with more general attitudes, possibly attitudes towards 'targets' (see Eagly and Chaiken 1993: 202–15). Of course, people may oppose or support technologies in ways other than through the foods that they buy and eat: this may take any number of forms, from arguing and discussing their point of view in private and public discussions, through to 'ethical investments'. Perceived behavioural control may not really be an issue in such cases, although perceptions of control over the 'target' (the technology, or the use of the technology) may be. Such perceptions of control may be influential with respect to the attitudes that people adopt towards those technologies (we return to this point later).

6.5 Applying the model

Some of the considerations that have been discussed so far make it clear that, in applications of the TPB, concepts, methods and findings need to be carefully considered. Although a major attraction of the TRA and TPB has been the clarity with which measurement techniques have been described (Ajzen and Fishbein 1980; Ajzen 1988: Figure 5.2), the individual researcher will still be left with a number of decisions about how best to construct and analyse measures for any particular study.

Data are typically reported in terms of correlations between model components and multiple regressions of intentions (or expectations) on attitudes, subjective norm, perceived control and any other additional predictor variables that have been included in the study design. Sometimes attitudes and subjective norm are included at a first step, with perceived behavioural control added at a second step and other variables at subsequent steps.

6.6 Particular problems with applications of the model to food-related behaviour

While some of the general 'problems' with the TPB are addressed in the subsequent section, here we deal with a subset of those that are especially pertinent to food-related behaviours.

Perceived control and actual control?

One interesting issue that has not been fully addressed in the literature is control problems of which the person is not aware. While such problems are not designed to be included within the notion of perceived behavioural control, people's behaviour will no doubt be influenced by control problems whether or not they envisage/recognize them or not. For example, imagine we want to assess people's attitudes towards eating a low-fat diet (and we can specify what we mean by this in terms of actual fat intake); their perceptions of control may not be a good predictor of their actual behaviour if they are unaware of the control problems that they are likely to encounter. So, the addition of the perceived behavioural control construct is only likely to be of great value where people are aware of the control problems that they are likely to experience if they attempt to eat a low-fat diet. This is not really a problem for the theory but it is a potential problem for those concerned with health promotion who would wish to deal with the actual barriers and impediments to dietary change rather than merely to the perceived barriers. For example, if it were shown to be the case that food advertising had a detrimental nutritional effect on children's dietary patterns,[4] then health promoters might consider it worthwhile to refocus more of their efforts in this direction.

A second, related, issue concerns those instances where people may all report the same level of *PBC* (whether high or low). It is entirely feasible to imagine the case where there is little variability in *PBC* ratings because perceived control is uniformly low, and where *PBC* contributes no independent predictive effect on intention or behaviour measures.

Ambivalence

People may be ambivalent towards dietary change or towards particular foods. People may be attracted to certain foods because they taste nice, yet at the same time, and in some sense, would prefer to avoid those foods because of their perceived detrimental impact on health (or the waistline?). They may want to diet on the one hand because they wish to be slim, while on the other hand they may not want to diet because they do not wish to be fashion victims (White and Wetherell 1988). The issue of attitudinal ambivalence has appeared sporadically in the literature (e.g. Kaplan 1972; Katz and Hass 1988; Eagly and Chaiken 1993); however, it has not been systematically applied to dietary change issues (but see Sparks *et al.* 1992), despite the fact that food is often used in anecdotal examples of people's internal conflicts of interest (Ainslie 1986), their conflicting wants (Elster 1989), changing preferences (March 1978), impulsiveness (Herrnstein 1990) or weakness of will (Austin 1961, cited in Davidson 1970). This issue has significant implications for the TPB since that model would suggest that people arrive at their attitudes through a compensatory trade-off between expected good and bad outcomes: there is not really space within the model for people to remain 'essentially ambivalent' (see March 1978).

Affect

There is an irony in the widespread concern that affective factors have been neglected in attitude research, given that attitudes are usually conceptualized in affective terms. On the one hand there is the suggestion that the elicitation procedures for sampling 'behavioural beliefs' about specific behaviours sample an excessively cognitive subset of the influences that actually play on people's attitudes (Wilson *et al.* 1989). On the other hand it has been proposed that the way in which attitude is measured will tend to neglect affective factors. Ajzen and Timko (1986), for example, indicate that the healthy behaviours that they studied were better predicted 'from an affective than from an evaluative measure of attitude' (p. 273). Chan and Fishbein (1993) call for more attention to be paid to 'emotional reactions', which are conceived of as less 'cognitively based' than the way in which the attitude construct is usually measured within the TRA.

However, the extent to which it is the attitude concept that lacks an affective component rather than measures designed to reflect attitudes is an issue that requires a clear conceptual statement. We have already noted the work of Richard and colleagues (Richard 1993), who have drawn attention to a distinction between affect that is associated with the experience of performing a behaviour and affect that arises (or is anticipated to arise) following the completion (or non-completion) of the behaviour. Research in relation to healthy eating has produced similar effects: in one study, the inclusion of a measure of regret about eating certain foods also made a significant independent contribution to the prediction of intentions to reduce consumption of cheese, chocolate, biscuits and meat (Sparks and Shepherd, in preparation). Food consumption is a theme that is heavily affectively laden, such that developments in the assessment of affect within the TPB structure are likely to be highly pertinent.

7 Future directions

Hand in hand with the numerous 'successful' applications of the model, there are a number of criticisms of the model that warrant attention. We shall not go into these in any great detail but would direct the reader to the discussion provided by Eagly and Chaiken (1993) and to earlier criticisms of the TRA provided, for example, by Sarver (1983) and Liska (1984). In this section, we discuss just some of the issues that are likely to be of relevance for those seeking to use the TPB in applied settings. In so doing, we make a rather crude distinction between what the model does not include (sins of omission?) and what the model gets wrong (sins of commission?)!

7.1 Extending the model

While support for the model is usually adduced from significant correlations and significant beta weights in multiple regressions, serious attention needs to be paid to how much variance in intention and/or behaviour scores is being accounted for by the predictor variables. Questions then need to be asked along the lines of 'Why does the model not account for more of the variance?' 'What can be done to increase the amount of variance explained?' 'Are there better methods of data collection and analysis that might be employed?'

7.2 Compatibility

Furthermore, although we may expect some predictive power if we adhere to the demands of 'compatibility', we should consider the suggestion made by Ajzen (1988) that individuals' actions on specific occasions are not essentially what psychologists are interested in; rather, what are of interest are 'regularities in behaviour, consistent patterns of action, response tendencies' (p. 46). We have discussed the 'aggregation' of behaviour earlier. In a related way, it is not altogether clear that we would want to dispense with attitudes towards the target when we consider attitudes towards particular actions. For example, attitudes towards purchasing foods produced by certain technologies may well be affected by more general attitudes towards these technologies as well as by attitudes towards specific purchase behaviours, especially if attitudes towards purchase are focused on outcomes (Frisch and Clemen 1994) of purchase (rather than, for example, on the processes by which the foods were produced).

On a related theme, there has been the suggestion by Lord et al. (1979) that attitudes towards targets will only correspond with actual behaviours if the attitude target matches the person's representation of the attitude target. So, for example, if people's representation of a low-fat diet or of a production technology do not match their actual subsequent firsthand experience with those 'targets', then we can expect poor attitude–behaviour relationships.

7.3 Attitudes towards alternative actions

The usual applications of the TRA and TPB are in the context of single attitudes and single behaviours. One might expect better predictive power if attitudes towards alternative courses of action are assessed (see Davidson and Morrison 1982). For example, if one were interested in attitudes towards eating food A, it may well be also advisable to assess attitudes that are alternatives to eating food A (Shepherd *et al.* 1993). Such an approach is also more faithful to the subjective expected utility (SEU) underpinnings of the theory, which are concerned with choices between options, rather than on locating individuals on dimensions of attitude and behaviour for single options (as is often the case with applications of TRA and TPB).

7.4 Attitude change

The rationale for using the model by health researchers is often that identification of beliefs and values (especially beliefs) that influence attitudes in the hope that these may be addressed in communication strategies designed to promote behavioural change. But research assessing this possibility is surprisingly thin on the ground (Brubaker and Fowler 1990; van den Putte 1993). In the face of rather widespread criticism of the effect of communication strategies in promoting attitude change (Brown 1965; Jaspars 1978; Fishbein and Ajzen 1981; Billig 1987), there has been much recent interest in developments such as the elaboration likelihood model (ELM; Petty and Cacioppo 1986) and the heuristic-systematic model (HSM; Chaiken *et al.* 1989). However, an assessment of the TPB in conjunction with these types of models is to date lacking (Eagly 1992).

Moreover, Ajzen and Fishbein (1980) suggest that if one is interested in attitude change one might 'try to influence some of the beliefs that are salient in a subject population or try to introduce novel, previously nonsalient, beliefs' (p. 224). There also seems to have been little research addressing this latter issue directly, although implications for this possibility are to be found in the recent literature (e.g. Edward 1990; Millar and Millar 1990; Millar 1992).

7.5 Construct measurement

We have discussed above the issue of the measurement of the *PBC* construct and have alluded to potential problems with the standard ways in which attitude is measured. Clearly, measures need to address the concepts under consideration. This is also true of, for example, the subjective norm construct, which has long been believed to be measured in an inadequate way (Ajzen and Fishbein 1980: 246).

Of course, inter-item reliability is also likely to be poor if items do not clearly address the core of the construct. Because the notion of perceived behavioural control is a broad one, measures used to assess it have been quite diverse. Consider, for example, the measures used by Chan and

Fishbein (1993): 'My telling my partner to use a condom every time I have sexual intercourse is . . .' ('easy–difficult', 'up to me–not up to me', 'under my control–dependent upon other people or events'). The authors found an inter-item reliability of coefficient (alpha) of 0.40, removed the second item and ended up with a measure of *PBC* constructed from the two remaining items, which had a correlation of 0.30: the measure did not figure significantly in predictions of intentions!

We have discussed the issue of control and difficulty above: it is of interest to note here the suggestion by Ajzen and Timko (1986), who, while suggesting that 'easy–difficult' scales correlate well with other *PBC* items, note that 'Our measure of "perceived behavioral control" might perhaps better be labelled perceived difficulty of performing a given behavior' (p. 274). On the one hand, we believe that this is a promising direction since it narrows and clarifies the issue at stake; on the other hand, a measure based on this conceptualization may miss some important 'control' issues. For example, if we wish to assess attitudes towards consumption of chocolate, most people would report that eating chocolate was 'easy': a *PBC* measure based on an easy–difficult scale would not distinguish between those for whom *not* eating chocolate was difficult and those for whom *not* eating chocolate presented no such problem. Part of the answer may be to construct entirely new kinds of measure to capture the nature of the problem here; perhaps more systematic would be to assess attitudes towards eating chocolate in conjunction with attitudes towards avoiding eating chocolate (but this latter issue may be considered not to be a behaviour, thus raising difficulties all of its own). The consideration of overlaps with self-efficacy concepts (see Schwarzer and Fuchs, Chapter 6 in this volume) may be fruitful.

7.6 Descriptive accuracy

It seems to be fairly widely accepted that subjective expected utility is not an accurate descriptive account of how people make choices (e.g. Edwards 1992). Likewise, there has long been some concern that the method of combining behavioural beliefs and outcome evaluations is not a felicitous description of the processes by which people will form attitudes (e.g. Fischhoff *et al.* 1982; Fishbein 1993). In a similar way, it is highly unlikely that summing the products of control beliefs and power will reflect an accurate account of how perceptions of behavioural control will become established. Future research could examine whether equations which more accurately reflect the way individuals combine such information increase the predictive power of these models.

7.7 Conclusion

We have taken a rather critical stance towards the TPB since we believe that this is the best foundation on which to make progress. The TPB offers an account of how perceptions of control may influence people's intentions and behaviour. Its contribution may be seen as both significant and limited for health: significant because at one level of analysis it offers an improvement to our understanding of many health-related behaviours; limited because it deals with perceptions of control and not with actual control issues themselves. In the broad social environment there will be a number of influences on people's health and on their behaviour: any of these that do not impinge on people's perceptions of control will not be accessible to analysis via the TPB. Consumption behaviours and patterns need to be understood not only in terms of people's beliefs, values, perceived social pressure and perceived control but also in terms of the history of food consumption patterns and the broader social pressures (e.g. food advertising) that may be operating. While the TPB is concerned with proximal psychological influences on behaviour, we have to recognize the broader social structure within which these influences develop.

As far as the TPB is concerned, further developments as we see them will need to focus on the measurement issues arising out of a more careful consideration of the *PBC* construct. The nature of the control problems that people experience (or envisage) in particular contexts also needs to be identified. Some of these problems may be addressable in the same way that behavioural beliefs are thought to be amenable to persuasive communications; however, some of the perceptions of control may reflect actual control problems which are beyond the influence of the person concerned. While more detailed analysis of the control issues that are actually amenable to personal influence would be a laudable goal, health researchers should not lose sight of, or omit to address, the broader social and structural factors that give rise to perceived and actual control problems. It is here perhaps that the integration with other social science perspectives needs to be developed. As we indicate above (see Figure 5.1), demographic variables may correlate with people's beliefs and values but there may be more subtle social forces that influence beliefs, values and control problems in a (more) dynamic way.

Notes

1 Originally called the principle of correspondence (Fishbein and Ajzen 1975; Ajzen and Fishbein 1977), Ajzen (1988) suggested renaming it the principle of compatibility to distinguish it from ideas of attitude–behaviour links.
2 It has been estimated that meat (and meat products) contribute 24 per cent to average dietary fat intake in the UK; the corresponding figures for biscuits (buns, cakes and pastries) and cheese are 10 per cent and 6 per cent respectively (Gregory *et al.* 1990).
3 Of course, people have motives other than those of personal health for supporting or opposing particular technologies.
4 Although this is a contentious issue, it is worth noting that Logue (1986: 99) has suggested that children in the United States 'view an average of some 22,000 commercials per year, and more than 50 per cent of these advertise foods that are low in nutrition.'

References

Abraham, C. and Sheeran, P. (1994) Modelling and modifying young heterosexuals' HIV-preventive behaviour; a review of theories, findings and educational implications, *Patient Education and Counseling*, 23, 173–86.

Ainslie, G. (1986) Beyond microeconomics. Conflict among interests in a multiple self as a determinant of value. In J. Elster (ed.) *The Multiple Self*. Cambridge: Cambridge University Press, 133–75.

Ajzen, I. (1985) From intentions to action: a theory of planned behavior. In J. Kuhl and J. Beckman (eds) *Action Control: from Cognitions to Behaviors*. New York: Springer, 11–39.

Ajzen, I. (1988) *Attitudes, Personality and Behavior*. Milton Keynes: Open University Press.

Ajzen, I. (1991) The theory of planned behavior, *Organizational Behavior and Human Decision Processes*, 50, 179–211.

Ajzen, I. and Driver, B.L. (1991) Prediction of leisure participation from behavioral, normative, and control beliefs: an application of the theory of planned behavior, *Leisure Sciences*, 13, 185–204.

Ajzen, I. and Driver, B.L. (1992) Application of the theory of planned behavior to leisure choice, *Journal of Leisure Research*, 24, 207–24.

Ajzen, A. and Fishbein, M. (1977) Attitude–behavior relations: a theoretical analysis and review of empirical research, *Psychological Bulletin*, 84, 888–918.

Ajzen, I. and Fishbein, M. (1980) *Understanding Attitudes and Predicting Social Behavior*. Englewood Cliffs, NJ: Prentice-Hall.

Ajzen, I. and Madden, T.J. (1986) Prediction of goal directed behavior: attitudes, intentions and perceived behavioral control, *Journal of Experimental Social Psychology*, 22, 453–74.

Ajzen, A. and Timko, C. (1986) Correspondence between health attitudes and behavior, *Journal of Basic and Applied Social Psychology*, 7, 259–76.

Babrow, A.S., Black, D.R. and Tiffany, S.T. (1990) Beliefs, attitudes, intentions, and a smoking-cessation program: a planned behavior analysis of communication campaign development, *Health Communication*, 2, 145–63.

Bagozzi, R.P. (1981) Attitudes, intentions, and behavior: a test of some key hypotheses, *Journal of Personality and Social Psychology*, 41, 607–27.

Bagozzi, R.P. (1989) An investigation of the role of affective and moral evaluations in the purposeful behaviour model of attitude, *British Journal of Social Psychology*, 28, 97–113.

Bamberg, S. and Schmidt, P. (1993) Choosing between means of transportation – an application of the theory of planned behavior, *Zeitschrift für Sozialpsychologie*, 24, 25–37.

Bandura, A. (1982) Self-efficacy mechanism in human agency, *American Psychologist*, 37, 122–47.

Beale, D.A. and Manstead, A.S.R. (1991) Predicting mothers' intentions to limit frequency of infants' sugar intake: testing the theory of planned behavior, *Journal of Applied Social Psychology*, 21, 409–31.

Beck, L. and Ajzen, I. (1991) Predicting dishonest actions using the Theory of Planned Behavior, *Journal of Research in Personality*, 25, 285–301.

Bentler, P. and Speckhart, G. (1979) Models of attitude–behavior relations, *Psychological Review*, 86, 452–64.

Bentler, P. and Speckhart, G. (1981) Attitudes 'cause' behaviors: a structural equation analysis, *Journal of Personality and Social Psychology*, 40, 226–38.

Billig, M. (1987) *Arguing and Thinking: a Rhetorical Approach to Social Psychology*. Cambridge: Cambridge University Press.

Boldero, J., Moore, S. and Rosenthal, D. (1992) Intention, context, and safe sex: Australian adolescents' responses to AIDS, *Journal of Applied Social Psychology*, **22**, 1374–96.

Borgida, E., Conner, C. and Manteufel, L. (1992) Understanding living kidney donation: a behavioral decision perspective. In S. Spacapan and S. Oskamp (eds) *Helping and Being Helped: Naturalistic Studies*. Newbury Park, CA: Sage, 183–212.

Brinberg, D. and Durand, J. (1983) Eating at fast-food restaurants: an analysis using two behavioral intention models, *Journal of Applied Social Psychology*, **13**, 459–72.

Brown, R. (1965) *Social Psychology*. New York: Raven Press.

Brubaker, R.G. and Fowler, C. (1990) Encouraging college males to perform testicular self-examination: evaluation of a persuasive message based on the revised theory of reasoned action, *Journal of Applied Social Psychology*, **17**, 1411–22.

Brubaker, R.G. and Wickersham, D. (1990) Encouraging the practice of testicular self-examination: a field application of the theory of reasoned action, *Health Psychology*, **9**, 154–63.

Budd, R.J. (1986) Predicting cigarette use: the need to incorporate measures of salience in the theory of reasoned action, *Journal of Applied Social Psychology*, **16**, 663–85.

Budd, R.J. (1987) Response bias and the theory of reasoned action, *Social Cognition*, **5**, 95–107.

Budd, R.J. and Spencer, C.P. (1984) Predicting undergraduates' intentions to drink *Journal of Studies on Alcohol*, **45**, 179–83.

Cannon, G. (1992) *Food and Health: the Experts Agree*. London: The Consumers' Association.

Chaiken, S., Liberman, A. and Eagly, A.H. (1989) Heuristic and systematic information processing within and beyond the persuasion context. In J.S. Uleman and J.A. Bargh (eds) *Unintended Thought*. New York: Guilford Press, 212–52.

Chan, D.K. and Fishbein, M. (1993) Determinants of college women's intentions to tell their partners to use condoms, *Journal of Applied Social Psychology*, **23**, 1455–70.

Chassin, L., Corty, E., Presson, C.C., Olhavsky, R.W., Bensenberg, M. and Sherman, S.J. (1981) Predicting adolescents' intentions to smoke cigarettes, *Journal of Health and Social Behavior*, **22**, 445–55.

Cialdini, R.B., Kallgren, C.A. and Reno, R.R. (1991) A focus theory of normative conduct: a theoretical refinement and re-evaluation of the role of norms in human behaviour. In M.P. Zanna (ed.) *Advances in Experimental Social Psychology*, Vol. 23. San Diego: Academic Press, 201–34.

Conner, M., Povey, R., Bell, R. and Norman, P. (1994). GP intervention to produce dietary change, paper presented at the BPS Special Group in Health Psychology Annual Conference, Sheffield, 7–9 September.

Conner, M.T. and Graham, S. (1994) Situational and attitudinal influences upon students' intentions to use condoms. In H. Schroder, K. Reschke, M. Johnston and S. Maes (eds) *Health Psychology: Potential in Diversity*. Regensberg: Verlag, 91–100.

Conner, M.T. and Sherlock, K. (1993) Attitudes and ecstasy use. In *Social Psychology in Europe*. Lisbon: EAESP, 26.

Courneya, K.S. (1994) Predicting repeated behavior from intention: the issue of scale correspondence, *Journal of Applied Social Psychology*, **24**, 580–94.

Crawley, F.E. (1990) Intentions of science teachers to use investigative teaching methods: a test of the theory of planned behavior, *Journal of Research in Science Teaching*, **27**, 685–97.

Crawley, F.E. and Black, C.B. (1992) Causal modeling of secondary science students' intentions to enrol in physics, *Journal of Research in Science Teaching*, **29**, 585–99.

Crawley, F.E. and Koballa, T.R. (1992) Hispanic-American students' attitudes toward enrolling in high school chemistry – a study of planned behavior and belief-based change, *Hispanic Journal of Behavioral Sciences*, **14**, 469–86.

Davidson, A.R. and Jaccard, J.J. (1979) Variables that moderate the attitude-behavior relation: results of a longitudinal survey, *Journal of Personality and Social Psychology*, **37**, 1364–76.

Davidson, A.R. and Morrison, D.M. (1982) Predicting contraceptive behaviour from attitudes: a comparison of within- versus across-subjects procedures, *Journal of Personality and Social Psychology*, **45**, 997–1009.

Davidson, D. (1970) How is weakness of the will possible? Reprinted in D. Davidson (1980). *Essays on Actions and Events*. Oxford: Clarendon Press, 21–42.

DeVellis, B.M., Blalock, S.J. and Sandler, R.S. (1990) Predicting participation in cancer screening: the role of perceived behavioral control, *Journal of Applied Social Psychology*, **20**, 639–60.

De Vries, H. and Kok, G.J. (1986) From determinants of smoking behavior to the implications for a prevention programme, *Health Education Research*, **1**, 85–94.

Doll, J. and Ajzen, I. (1992) Accessibility and stability of predictors in the theory of planned behaviour, *Journal of Personality and Social Psychology*, **63**, 754–65.

Doll, J., Mentz, M. and Orth, B. (1991) The prediction of goal-directed behavior: attitude, subjective estimations of competence, and emotions, *Zeitschrift für Experimentelle und Angewandte Psychologie*, **38**, 539–59.

Doll, J. and Orth, B. (1993) The Fishbein and Ajzen theory of reasoned action applied to contraceptive behavior: model variants and meaningfulness, *Journal of Applied Social Psychology*, **23**, 395–415.

Dzewaltowski, D.A. Noble, J.M. and Shaw, J.M. (1990) Physical activity participation – social cognitive theory versus the theories of reasoned action and planned behavior, *Journal of Sport and Exercise Psychology*, **12**, 388–405.

Eagly, A.H. (1992) Uneven progress: social psychology and the study of attitudes, *Journal of Personality and Social Psychology*, **63**, 693–710.

Eagly, A.H. and Chaiken, S. (1993) *The Psychology of Attitudes*. Fort Worth, TX: Harcourt Brace Jovanovich.

East, R. (1993) Investment decisions and the theory of planned behavior, *Journal of Economic Psychology*, **14**, 337–75.

Edwards, K. (1990) The interplay of affect and cognition in attitude formation and change, *Journal of Personality and Social Psychology*, **59**, 202–16.

Edwards, W. (1992) *Utility Theories: Measurements and Applications*. Boston: Kluwer.

Elster, J. (1989) *Nuts and Bolts for the Social Sciences*. Cambridge: Cambridge University Press.

Evans, M.G. (1991) The problem of analyzing multiplicative composites: interactions revisited, *American Psychologist*, **46**, 6–15.

Fazio, R.H. (1986) How do attitudes guide behavior? In R.M. Sorrentino and E.T. Higgins (eds) *Handbook of Motivation and Cognition: Foundations of Social Behavior*. New York: Guilford Press, 204–43.

Fischhoff, B., Goitein, B. and Shapira, Z. (1982) The experienced utility of expected utility approaches. In N.T. Feather (ed.) *Expectations and Actions: Expectancy-value Models in Psychology.* Hillsdale, NJ: Erlbaum, 287–343.

Fishbein, M. (1967a) Attitude and the prediction of behavior. In M. Fishbein (ed.) *Readings in Attitude Theory and Measurement.* New York: Wiley, 477–92.

Fishbein, M. (1967b) A behavior theory approach to the relations between beliefs about an object and the attitude toward the object. In M. Fishbein (ed.) *Readings in Attitude Theory and Measurement.* New York: Wiley, 389–400.

Fishbein, M. (1982). Social psychological analysis of smoking behavior. In J.R. Eiser (Ed.) *Social Psychology and Behavioral Medicine.* New York: Wiley, 179–97.

Fishbein, M. (1993) Introduction. In D.J. Terry, C. Gallois and M. McCamish (eds) *The Theory of Reasoned Action: Its Application to AIDS-preventive Behaviour.* Oxford: Pergamon, xv–xxv.

Fishbein, M. and Ajzen, I. (1975) *Belief, Attitude, Intention, and Behavior.* New York: Wiley.

Fishbein, M. and Ajzen, I. (1981) Acceptance, yielding and impact: cognitive processes in persuasion. In R.E. Petty, T.M. Ostrom and T.C. Brock (eds) *Cognitive Responses in Persuasion.* Hillsdale, NJ: Lawrence Erlbaum, 339–59.

Fishbein, M., Ajzen, I. and McArdle, J. (1980) Changing the behavior of alcoholics: effects of persuasive communication. In I. Ajzen and M. Fishbein (eds) *Understanding Attitudes and Predicting Social Behavior.* Englewood Cliffs, NJ: Prentice-Hall, 217–42.

Fishbein, M., Chan, D.K.-S., O'Reilly, K., Schnell, D., Wood, R., Beeker, C. and Cohn, D. (1992) Attitudinal and normative factors as determinants of gay men's intentions to perform AIDS-related sexual behavior: a multisite analysis, *Journal of Applied Social Psychology,* **22**, 999–1011.

Fishbein, M., Middlestadt, S.E. and Chung, J. (1986) Predicting participation and choice among first time voters in US partisan elections. In S. Kraus and R. Perloff (eds) *Mass Media and Political Thoughts: an Information Processing Approach.* Beverly Hills, CA: Sage, 65–82.

Fishbein, M. and Stasson, M. (1990) The role of desires, self-predictions, and perceived control in the prediction of training session attendance, *Journal of Applied Social Psychology,* **20**, 173–98.

Frisch, D. and Clemen, R.T. (1994) Beyond expected utility: rethinking behavioral decision research, *Psychological Bulletin,* **116**, 46–54.

Godin, G. and Shepherd, R.J. (1987) Psychosocial factors influencing intentions to exercise in a group of individuals ranging from 45 to 74 years of age. In M.E. Berridge and G.R. Ward (eds) *International Perspectives on Adapted Physical Activity.* Champaign, IL: Human Kinetics Publishers, 243–9.

Godin, G., Valois, P. and Lepage, L. (1993) The pattern of influence of perceived behavioral control upon exercising behavior – an application of Ajzen theory of planned behaviour, *Journal of Behavioral Medicine,* **16**, 81–102.

Godin, G., Valois, P., Lepage, L. and Desharnais, R. (1992) Predictors of smoking behaviour – an application of Ajzen's theory of planned behaviour, *British Journal of Addiction,* **87**, 1335–43.

Godin, G., Vezina, L. and Leclerc, O. (1989) Factors influencing intentions of pregnant women to exercise after giving birth, *Public Health Reports,* **104**, 188–95.

Goodman, D. and Redclift, M. (1991) *Refashioning Nature: Food, Ecology and Culture.* London: Routledge.

Gregory, J., Foster, K., Tyler, H. and Wiseman, M. (1990) *The Dietary and Nutritional Survey of British Adults*. London: HMSO.

Grube, J.W., Morgan, M. and McGree, S.T. (1986) Attitudes and normative beliefs as predictors of smoking intentions and behaviours: a test of three models, *British Journal of Social Psychology*, **25**, 81–93.

Herrnstein, R.J. (1990) Rational choice theory: necessary but not sufficient, *American Psychologist*, **45**, 356–67.

Holbrook, M.B. and Hulbert, J.M. (1975) Multi-attribute attitude models: a comparative analysis. In M.J. Schlinger (ed.) *Advances in Consumer Research, Volume 2*. Ann Arbor, MI: Association for Consumer Research, 375–88.

Hounsa, A.M., Godin, G., Alihonou, E. and Valois, P. (1993) An application of Ajzen's theory of planned behaviour to predict mothers' intention to use oral rehydration therapy in a rural area of Benin, *Social Science and Medicine*, **37**, 253–61.

Jaccard, J.J., Brinberg, D. and Ackerman, L.J. (1986) Assessing attribute importance: a comparison of six methods. *Journal of Consumer Research*, **12**, 463–8.

Jaspars, J.M.F. (1978) Determinants of attitudes and attitude change. In H. Tajfel and C. Fraser (eds) *Introducing Social Psychology*. Harmondsworth: Penguin, 277–301.

Kaplan, K.J. (1972) On the ambivalence-indifference problem in attitude theory and measurement: a suggested modification of the semantic differential technique, *Psychological Bulletin*, **77**, 361–72.

Katz, I. and Hass, R.G. (1988) Racial ambivalence and American value conflict: correlational and priming studies of dual cognitive structures, *Journal of Personality and Social Psychology*, **55**, 893–905.

Kimiecik, J. (1992) Predicting vigorous physical activity of corporate employees: comparing the theories of reasoned action and planned behavior, *Journal of Sport and Exercise Psychology*, **14**, 192–206.

Kinket, B., Paans, L. and Verplanken, B. (1992) Patient education by general practitioners: application of the theory of planned behavior, *Gedrag – Gezondheid Tijdschrift voor Psychologie – Gezondheid*, **20**, 187–95.

Krosnick, J.A., Boninger, D.S., Chuang, Y.C., Berent, M.K. and Carnot, C.G. (1994) Attitude strength: one construct or many related constructs?, *Journal of Personality and Social Psychology*, **65**, 1132–51.

Lauver, D. and Chang, A. (1991) Testing theoretical explanations of intention to seek care for a breast cancer symptom, *Journal of Applied Social Psychology*, **21**, 1440–58.

Lay, C.H. and Burns, P. (1991) Intentions and behavior in studying for an examination: the role of trait procrastination and its interaction with optimism, *Journal of Social Behavior and Personality*, **6**, 605–17.

Lewis, C.J., Sims, L.S. and Shannon, B. (1989) Examination of specific nutrition/ health behaviors using a social cognitive model, *Journal of the American Dietetic Association*, **81**, 194–202.

Liska, A.E. (1984) A critical examination of the causal structure of the Fishbein/ Ajzen attitude–behavior model, *Social Psychology Quarterly*, **47**, 61–74.

Lloyd, H.M., Paisley, C.M. and Mela, D.J. (1993) Changing to a low fat diet: attitudes and beliefs of UK consumers, *European Journal of Clinical Nutrition*, **47**, 361–73.

Logue, A.W. (1986) *The Psychology of Eating and Drinking*. New York: Freeman.

London, F.B. (1982) Attitudinal and social normative factors as predictors of intended alcohol abuse among fifth- and seventh-grade students, *Journal of School Health*, **52**, 244–9.

Lord, C.G., Ross, L. and Lepper, M. (1979) Biased assimilation and attitude polarization: The effects of prior theories on subsequently considered evidence, *Journal of Personality and Social Psychology*, **37**, 2098–109.

McCarty, D. (1981) Changing contraceptive usage intentions: a test of the Fishbein model of intention, *Journal of Applied Social Psychology*, **11**, 192–211.

McCaul, K.D., Sandgren, A.K., O'Neill, H.K. and Hinsz, V.B. (1993) The value of the theory of planned behavior, perceived control, and self-efficacy expectations for predicting health-protective behaviors, *Basic and Applied Social Psychology*, **14**, 231–52.

Madden, T.J., Ellen, P.S. and Ajzen, I. (1992) A comparison of the theory of planned behavior and the theory of reasoned action, *Personality and Social Psychology Bulletin*, **18**, 3–9.

Manstead, A.S.R., Plevin, C.E. and Smart, J.L. (1983) Predicting and understanding mothers' infant-feeding intentions and behavior, *Journal of Personality and Social Psychology*, **44**, 657–71.

Manstead, A.S.R., Plevin, C.E. and Smart, J.L. (1984) Predicting mothers' choice of infant feeding method, *British Journal of Social Psychology*, **23**, 223–31.

March, J.G. (1978) Bounded rationality, ambiguity, and the engineering of choice, *Bell Journal of Economics*, **9**, 587–608.

Marin, B., Marin, G., Perez-Stable, E.J., Otero-Sabogal, R. and Sabogal, F. (1990) Cultural differences in attitudes towards smoking: developing messages using the theory of reasoned action, *Journal of Applied Social Psychology*, **20**, 478–93.

Millar, M.G. (1992) Effects of experience on matched and mismatched arguments and attitudes, *Social Behavior and Personality,* **20**, 47–56.

Millar, M.G. and Millar, K.U. (1990) Attitude change as a function of attitude type and argument type, *Journal of Personality and Social Psychology*, **59**, 217–28.

Miniard, P.W. and Cohen, J.B. (1981) An examination of the Fishbein-Ajzen behavioural-intentions model's concepts and measures, *Journal of Experimental Social Psychology*, **17**, 309–39.

Nash, R., Edwards, H. and Nebauer, M. (1993) Effects of attitudes, subjective norms and perceived control on nurses' intention to assess patients' pain, *Journal of Advanced Nursing*, **18**, 941–7.

Netemeyer, R.G. and Burton, S. (1990) Examining the relationship between voting behavior, intention, perceived behavioral control and expectation, *Journal of Applied Social Psychology*, **20**, 661–80.

Netemeyer, R.G., Burton, S. and Johnston, M. (1991) A comparison of two models for the prediction of volitional and goal-directed behaviors: a confirmatory analysis approach, *Social Psychology Quarterly*, **54**, 87–100.

Norman, P. and Conner, M.T. (1993) The role of social cognition models in predicting attendance at health checks, *Psychology and Health*, **8**, 447–62.

Norman, P. and Smith, L. (1995). The theory of planned behaviour and exercise: an investigation into the role of prior behaviour, behavioural intentions and attitude variability, *European Journal of Social Psychology*, **25**, 403–15.

Nucifora, J., Gallois, C. and Kashima, Y. (1993) Influences on condom use among undergraduates: testing the theories of reasoned action and planned behaviour. In D.J. Terry, C. Gallois and M. McCamish (eds) *The Theory of Reasoned Action: Its Application to AIDS-Preventive Behaviour*. Oxford: Pergamon, 47–64.

O'Keefe, D. (1990) *Persuasion*. London: Sage.

Olson, J.M. and Zanna, M.P. (1993) Attitudes and attitude change, *Annual Review of Psychology*, **44**, 117–54.

Osgood, C.E., Suci, G.J. and Tannenbaum, P.H. (1957) *The Measurement of Meaning*. Urbana: University of Illinois Press.

Pagel, M.D. and Davidson, A.R. (1984) A comparison of three social-psychological models of attitude and behavioral plan: prediction of contraceptive behavior, *Journal of Personality and Social Psychology*, **47**, 517–33.

Paisley, C.M. (1994). Barriers to the adoption and maintenance of reduced-fat diets, unpublished doctoral dissertation, University of Reading.

Parker, D., Manstead, A.S.R., Stradling, S.G., Reason, J.T. and Baxter, J.S. (1992a) Intention to commit driving violations – an application of the theory of planned behavior, *Journal of Applied Psychology*, **77**, 94–101.

Parker, D., Manstead, A.S., Stradling, S.G. and Reason, J.T. (1992b) Determinants of intention to commit driving violations, *Accident Analysis and Prevention*, **24**, 117–31.

Parker, D., Manstead, A.S. and Stradling, S.G. (1995). Extending the theory of planned behaviour: the role of personal norm, *British Journal of Social Psychology*, **34**, 127–37.

Peak, H. (1955) Attitude and motivation. In M.R. Jones (ed.) *Nebraska Symposium on Motivation, Volume 3*. Lincoln: University of Nebraska Press, 149–88.

Petty, R.E. and Cacioppo, J.T. (1986) *Communication and Persuasion: Central and Peripheral Routes of Attitude Change*. New York: Springer Verlag.

Prislin, R. (1993) Effect of direct experience on the relative importance of attitudes, subjective norms and perceived behavioral control for the prediction of intentions and behavior, *Psychology*, **30**, 51–8.

Prislin, R. and Kovrlija, N. (1992) Predicting behavior of high and low self-monitors – an application of the theory of planned behavior, *Psychological Reports*, **70**, 1131–8.

Raats, M.M., Shepherd, R. and Sparks, P. (1995) Including moral dimensions of choice within the structure of the theory of planned behavior. *Journal of Applied Social Psychology*, **25**, 484–94.

Randall, D.M. and Gibson, A.M. (1991) Ethical decision making in the medical profession – an application of the theory of planned behaviour, *Journal of Business Ethics*, **10**, 111–22.

Randall, D.M. and Wolff, J.A. (1994) The time interval in the intention-behaviour relationship: meta-analysis, *British Journal of Social Psychology*, **33**, 405–18.

Richard, R. (1993) Reğret is what you get, unpublished doctoral dissertation, University of Amsterdam.

Richard, R., van der Pligt, J. and de Vries, N. (1995) Anticipated affective reactions and prevention of AIDS, *British Journal of Social Psychology*, **34**, 9–21.

Rutter, D.R. and Bunce, D.J. (1989) The theory of reasoned action of Fishbein and Ajzen: a test of Towriss's amended procedure for measuring beliefs, *British Journal of Social Psychology*, **28**, 39–46.

Sarver, V.T. Jr (1983) Ajzen & Fishbein's 'theory of reasoned action': a critical assessment, *Journal for the Theory of Social Behaviour*, **13**, 155–63.

Schifter, D.B. and Ajzen, I. (1985) Intention, perceived control, and weight loss: an application of the theory of planned behavior, *Journal of Personality and Social Psychology*, **49**, 843–51.

Schlegel, R.P., Crawford, C.A. and Sanborn, M.D. (1977) Correspondence and mediational properties of the Fishbein model: an application to adolescent alcohol use, *Journal of Experimental Social Psychology*, **13**, 421–30.

Schlegel, R.P., D'Avernas, J.R., Zanna, M.P. and DeCourville, N.H. (1992) Problem drinking: a problem for the theory of reasoned action?, *Journal of Applied Social Psychology*, **22**, 358–85.

Schwarz, N. and Sudman, S. (1992) *Context Effects in Social and Psychological Research*. New York: Springer.

Schwarzer, R. (1992), Self-efficacy in the adoption and maintenance of health behaviors: theoretical approaches and a new model. In R. Schwarzer (ed.) *Self-efficacy: Thought Control of Action*. London: Hemisphere, 217–43.

Secretary of State for Health (1992) *The Health of the Nation*. London: HMSO.

Sejwacz, D., Ajzen, I. and Fishbein, M. (1980) Predicting and understanding weight loss. In I. Ajzen and M. Fishbein (eds) *Understanding Attitudes and Predicting Social Behavior*. Englewood Cliffs, NJ: Prentice-Hall, 101–12.

Sheeran, P. and Orbell, S. (1995) How confidently can we infer health beliefs from questionnaire responses?, *Psychology and Health*.

Shepherd, R., Sparks, P., Bellier, S. and Raats, M.M. (1993) The effects of information on sensory ratings and preferences: the importance of attitudes, *Food Quality and Preference*, **3**, 147–55.

Sheppard, B.H., Hartwick, J. and Warshaw, P.R. (1988) The theory of reasoned action: a meta-analysis of past research with recommendations for modifications and future research, *Journal of Consumer Research*, **15**, 325–39.

Sherman, S.J., Presson, C.C., Chassin, L., Bensenberg, M., Corty, E. and Olshavsky, R.W. (1982) Smoking intention in adolescents: direct experience and predictability, *Personality and Social Psychology Bulletin*, **8**, 376–83.

Sparks, P. (1994) Attitudes towards food: applying, assessing and extending the 'theory of planned behaviour'. In D.R. Rutter and L. Quine (eds) *Social Psychology and Health: European Perspectives*. Aldershot: Avebury Press, 25–46.

Sparks, P., Hedderley, P. and Shepherd, R. (1992) An investigation into the relationship between perceived control, attitude variability and the consumption of two common foods, *European Journal of Social Psychology*, **22**, 55–71.

Sparks, P. and Shepherd, R. (1992) Self-identity and the theory of planned behavior – assessing the role of identification with green consumerism, *Social Psychology Quarterly*, **55**, 388–99.

Sparks, P. and Shepherd, R. (in preparation). Attitudes towards dietary change: an assessment of the theory of planned behaviour and the proximal antecedents of perceived behavioural control.

Sparks, P., Shepherd, R., Wieringa, N. and Zimmermanns, N. (1995) Perceived behavioural control, unrealistic optimism and dietary change: an exploratory study. *Appetite*, **24**, 243–55.

Stephen, A.M. and Wald, N.J. (1990) Trends in individual consumption of dietary fat in the United States, 1920–1984, *American Journal of Clinical Nutrition*, **52**, 457–69.

Sutton, S. (1989) Smoking attitudes and behaviour: an application of Fishbein and Ajzen's theory of reasoned action to predicting and understanding smoking decisions. In T. Ney and A. Gale (eds) *Smoking and Human Behaviour*. Chichester: Wiley, 289–312.

Terry, D.A., Galligan, R.F. and Conway, V.J. (1993a) The prediction of safe sex behaviour: the role of intentions, attitudes, norms and control beliefs, *Psychology and Health*, **8**, 355–68.

Terry, D.J., Gallois, C. and McCamish, M. (1993b) *The Theory of Reasoned Action: Its Application to AIDS-preventive Behaviour*. Oxford: Pergamon.

Terry, D.J., Gallois, C. and McCamish, M. (1993c) The theory of reasoned action and health care behaviour. In D.J. Terry, C. Gallois and M. McCamish (eds) *The Theory of Reasoned Action: Its Application to AIDS-preventive Behaviour*. Oxford: Pergamon, 1–27.

Tesser, A. and Shaffer, D.R. (1990) Attitudes and attitude change, *Annual Review of Psychology*, **41**, 479–523.

Theodorakis, Y. (1992) Prediction of athletic participation – a test of planned behavior theory, *Perceptual and Motor Skills*, **74**, 371–9.

Theodorakis, Y. (1994) Planned behaviour, attitude strength, role identity, and the prediction of exercise behaviour, *The Sport Psychologist*, **8**, 149–65.

Theodorakis, Y., Doganis, G., Bagiatis, K. and Gouthas, M. (1991) Preliminary study of the ability of the reasoned action model in predicting exercise behaviour of young children, *Perceptual and Motor Skills*, **72**, 51–8.

Towler, G. and Shepherd, R. (1992) Modification of Fishbein and Ajzen's theory of reasoned action to predict chip consumption. *Food Quality and Preference*, **3**, 37–45.

Traen, B. and Nordlund, S. (1993) Visiting public drinking places in Oslo: an application of the theory of planned behaviour, *Addition*, **88**, 1215–24.

Valois, P., Desharnais, R., Godin, G., Perron, J. and Lecomte, C. (1993) Psychometric properties of a perceived behavioral control multiplicative scale developed according to Ajzen theory of planned behavior, *Psychological Reports*, **72**, 1079–83.

Van den Putte, H. (1993) On the theory of reasoned action, unpublished doctoral dissertation, University of Amsterdam.

Van-Ryn, M. and Vinokur, A.D. (1992) How did it work? An examination of the mechanisms through which an intervention for the unemployed promoted job-search behavior, *American Journal of Community Psychology*, **20**, 577–97.

Werner, P.D. and Middlestadt, S.E. (1979) Factors in the use of oral contraceptives by young women, *Journal of Applied Social Psychology*, **9**, 537–47.

White, S. and Wetherell, M. (1988) Fear of fat: a study of discourses concerning eating patterns and body shape, paper presented to BPS Social Psychology Section Annual Conference.

Wilson, D., Zenda, A., McMaster, J. and Lavelle, S. (1992) Factors predicting Zimbabwean students' intentions to use condoms, *Psychology and Health*, **7**, 99–114.

Wilson, T.D., Dunn, D.S., Kraft, D. and Lisle, D.J. (1989) Introspection, attitude change, and attitude–behaviour consistency: the disruptive effects of explaining why we feel the way we do. In L. Berkowitz (ed.) *Advances in Experimental Social Psychology*, Vol. 22. New York: Academic Press, 287–343.

Yordy, G.A. and Lent, R.W. (1993) Predicting aerobic exercise participation – social cognitive, reasoned action, and planned behavior models, *Journal of Sport and Exercise Psychology*, **15**, 363–74.

Young, H.M., Lierman, L., Powell-Cope, G. and Kasprzyk, D. (1991) Operationalizing the theory of planned behaviour, *Research in Nursing and Health*, **14**, 137–44.

| 6 | RALF SCHWARZER AND REINHARD FUCHS |

SELF-EFFICACY AND HEALTH BEHAVIOURS

1 General background

Self-referent thought has become an issue that pervades psychological research in many domains. In 1977, the famous psychologist Albert Bandura at Stanford University introduced the concept of perceived self-efficacy in the context of cognitive behaviour modification. It has been found that a strong sense of personal efficacy is related to better health, higher achievement and more social integration. This concept has been applied to such diverse areas as school achievement, emotional disorders, mental and physical health, career choice and sociopolitical change. It has become a key variable in clinical, educational, social, developmental, health and personality psychology. The present chapter refers to its influence on the adoption, initiation and maintenance of health behaviours. It represents the key construct in social cognitive theory (Bandura 1977, 1986, 1991, 1992).

Behavioural change is facilitated by a personal sense of control. If people believe that they can take action to solve a problem instrumentally, they become more inclined to do so and feel more committed to this decision. While outcome expectancies refer to the perception of the possible consequences of one's action, perceived self-efficacy pertains to personal action control or agency (Maddux 1991, 1993; Bandura 1992; Wallston 1994). A person who believes in being able to cause an event can conduct a more active and self-determined life course. This 'can do' cognition mirrors a sense of control over one's environment. It reflects the belief in being able to master challenging demands by means of adaptive action. It can also be regarded as an optimistic view of one's capacity to deal with stress.

Self-efficacy makes a difference in how people feel, think and act. In terms of feeling, a low sense of self-efficacy is associated with depression, anxiety and helplessness. Such individuals also have low self-esteem and harbour pessimistic thoughts about their accomplishments and personal development. In terms of thinking, a strong sense of competence facilitates cognitive processes and academic performance. Self-efficacy levels can enhance or impede the motivation to act. Individuals with high self-efficacy choose to perform more challenging tasks. They set themselves higher goals and stick to them (Locke and Latham 1990). Actions are pre-shaped in thought, and people anticipate either optimistic or pessimistic scenarios in line with their level of self-efficacy. Once an action has been taken, high self-efficacious persons invest more effort and persist longer than those with low self-efficacy. When setbacks occur, the former recover more quickly and maintain the commitment to their goals. Self-efficacy also allows people to select challenging settings, explore their environments or create new situations. A sense of competence can be acquired by mastery experience, vicarious experience, verbal persuasion or physiological feedback (Bandura 1977). Self-efficacy, however, is not the same as positive illusions or unrealistic optimism, since it is based on experience and does not lead to unreasonable risk taking. Instead, it leads to venturesome behaviour that is within reach of one's capabilities.

2 Description of the model

According to social cognitive theory, human motivation and action are extensively regulated by forethought. This anticipatory control mechanism involves three types of expectancies: (a) situation-outcome expectancies, in which consequences are cued by environmental events without personal action; (b) action-outcome expectancies, in which outcomes flow from personal action; and (c) perceived self-efficacy, which is concerned with people's beliefs in their capabilities to perform a specific action required to attain a desired outcome.

Situation-outcome expectancies represent the belief that the world changes without one's own personal engagement. Risks are perceived, and persons may feel more or less vulnerable towards critical events that they anticipate. Individuals may sit and wait for things to happen, but illusions about the future may help one cope with threat. When, for example, people anticipate a disease, they may distort its likelihood of occurrence. This can be seen as a defensive optimism. Defences can be made in terms of social comparison bias, e.g. 'I am less vulnerable than others to illness.' On the other hand, action-outcome expectancies and self-efficacy expectancies include the option to change the world and to cope instrumentally with health threats by taking preventive action. These action beliefs and personal resource beliefs reflect a functional optimism. Empirically, the distinction of the latter two is hard to confirm because the second does not operate without the first. In making judgements about health-related goals, people usually unite personal agency with means. Perceived self-efficacy implicitly includes some degree of outcome expectancies because individuals believe they can produce the responses necessary for desired outcomes.

Adopting health-promoting behaviours and refraining from health-impairing behaviours is difficult. Most people have a hard time making the decision to change and, later on, maintaining the adopted changes when they face temptations. The likelihood that people will adopt a valued health behaviour (such as physical exercise) or change a detrimental habit (such as quitting smoking) may therefore depend on three sets of cognitions: (a) the expectancy that one is at risk ('My risk of getting cancer from smoking is above average'); (b) the expectancy that behavioural change would reduce the threat ('If I quit smoking, I will reduce my risk'); and (c) the expectancy that one is sufficiently capable of adopting a positive behaviour or refraining from a risky habit ('I am capable of quitting smoking permanently'). In order to initiate and maintain health behaviours, it is not sufficient to perceive an action-outcome contingency. One must also believe that one has the capability to perform the required behaviour. A large body of research has examined the role of optimistic self-beliefs as a predictor of behaviour change in the health domain (for an overview see Bandura 1992; O'Leary 1992; Schwarzer 1992; Maddux 1993). Behavioural change goals exert their effect through optimistic self-beliefs. These beliefs slightly overestimate perceived coping capabilities rather than simply reflect the existing ones.

Both outcome expectancies and efficacy beliefs play influential roles in adopting health behaviours, eliminating detrimental habits and maintaining change. In adopting a desired behaviour, individuals first form an intention and then attempt to execute the action. Outcome expectancies are important determinants in the formation of intentions, but are less so in action control. Self-efficacy, on the other hand, seems to be crucial in both stages of the self-regulation of health behaviour. Positive outcome expectancies encourage the decision to change one's behaviour. Thereafter, outcome expectancies may be dispensable because a new problem arises, namely the actual performance of the behaviour and its maintenance. At this stage, perceived self-efficacy continues to operate as a controlling influence.

Perceived self-efficacy represents the belief that one can change risky health behaviours by personal action, e.g. by employing one's skills to resist temptation. Behaviour change is seen as dependent on one's perceived capability to cope with stress and boredom and to mobilize one's resources and take the courses of action required to meet the situational demands. Efficacy beliefs affect the intention to change risk behaviour, the amount of effort expended to attain this goal and the persistence to continue striving despite barriers and setbacks that may undermine motivation. Perceived self-efficacy has become a widely applied theoretical construct in models of addiction and relapse (e.g. Marlatt and Gordon 1985; Donovan and Marlatt 1988; Marlatt *et al.* 1994). This view suggests that success in coping with high-risk situations depends partly on people's beliefs that they operate as active agents of their own actions and that they possess the necessary skills to reinstate control should a slip occur. The common denominator of relapse prevention theory and the model to be described later refers to the assumption of distinct stages and the claim that specific self-efficacy operates at these stages.

3 Summary of research

In this section, the relationship between self-efficacy and specific health behaviours is reviewed. A number of studies on adoption of health practices have measured self-efficacy to assess its potential influences in initiating behaviour change. As people proceed from considering precautions in a general way towards shaping a behavioural intention, contemplating detailed action plans and actually performing a health behaviour on a regular basis, they begin to crystallize beliefs in their capabilities to initiate change. In an early study, Beck and Lund (1981) exposed dental patients to a persuasive communication designed to alter their beliefs about periodontal disease. Neither perceived disease severity nor outcome expectancy were predictive of adoptive behaviour when perceived self-efficacy was controlled. Perceived self-efficacy emerged as the best predictor of the intention to floss ($r = 0.69$) and of the actual behaviour, frequency of flossing ($r = 0.44$). Seydel *et al.* (1990) report that outcome expectancies as well as perceived self-efficacy are good predictors of intention to engage in behaviours to detect breast cancer (such as breast self-examination) (see also Meyerowitz and Chaiken 1987; Rippetoe and Rogers 1987). Perceived self-efficacy was found to predict outcomes of a controlled drinking programme (Sitharthan and Kavanagh 1990). Perceived self-efficacy has also proven to be a powerful personal resource in coping with stress (Lazarus and Folkman 1987). There is evidence that perceived self-efficacy in coping with stressors affects immune function (Wiedenfeld *et al.* 1990). Subjects with high efficacy beliefs are better able to control pain than those with low self-efficacy (Manning and Wright 1983; Litt 1988; Altmaier *et al.* 1993). Self-efficacy has been shown to affect blood pressure, heart rate and serum catecholamine levels in coping with challenging or threatening situations (Bandura *et al.* 1982, 1985, 1988). Recovery of cardiovascular function in post-coronary patients is similarly enhanced by beliefs in one's physical and cardiac efficacy (Taylor *et al.* 1985). Cognitive-behavioural treatment of patients with rheumatoid arthritis enhanced their efficacy beliefs, reduced pain and joint inflammation and improved psychosocial functioning (O'Leary *et al.* 1988). Obviously, perceived self-efficacy predicts degree of therapeutic change in a variety of settings (Bandura 1992).

3.1 Sexual risk behaviour

Perceived self-efficacy has been studied with respect to prevention of unprotected sexual behaviour, e.g. the resistance of sexual coercion and the use of contraceptives to avoid unwanted pregnancies. For example, teenage women with a high rate of unprotected intercourse have been found to use contraceptives more effectively if they believe they can exercise control over their sexual activities (Levinson 1982). Gilchrist and Schinke (1983) taught teenagers through modelling and role-playing how to deal with pressures and ensure the use of contraceptives. This mode of treatment significantly raised their sense of perceived efficacy and protective skills. Sexual risk-taking behaviour, such as not using condoms to protect against sexually transmitted disease, has also been studied among homosexual men with multiple partners and intravenous drug users. Beliefs in one's capability to negotiate safer sex practices emerged as the most important predictor of such behaviours (McKusick *et al.* 1990; Basen-Engquist 1992; Basen-Engquist and Parcel 1992; Kasen *et al.* 1992; O'Leary *et al.* 1992).

Influencing health behaviours that contribute to the prevention of AIDS has become an urgent issue. Perceived self-efficacy has been shown to play a role in such behaviours. Kok *et al.* (1991) reported a study from their Dutch laboratory that analysed the use of condoms and clean needles by drug addicts. Intentions and behaviours were predicted by attitudes, social norms and especially by efficacy beliefs. Perceived self-efficacy correlated with the intention to use clean needles (0.35), reported clean needle use (0.46), the intention to use condoms (0.74) and reported condom use (0.67) (Paulussen *et al.* 1989). Bandura (1994) has summarized a large body of research relating perceived self-efficacy to the exercise of control over HIV infection.

Condom use requires not only some technical skills, but interpersonal negotiation as well (Coates 1990; Brafford and Beck 1991; Bandura 1994). Convincing a resistant partner to comply with safer sex practices can call for a high sense of efficacy to exercise control over sexual activities. Programmes were launched to enhance self-efficacy and to build self-protective skills in various segments of the population to prevent the spread of the HIV virus. In particular, studies with homosexual men have focused on their perceived efficacy to adopt safer sex (Ekstrand and Coates 1990; McKusick *et al.* 1990). Jemmott and his associates have conducted a number of interesting intervention studies designed to raise self-regulatory efficacy (Jemmott *et al.* 1992a, b).

3.2 Physical exercise

Motivating people to do regular physical exercise depends on several factors, among them optimistic self-beliefs of being able to perform appropriately. Perceived self-efficacy has been found to be a major instigating force in forming intentions to exercise and in maintaining the practice for an extended time (Weiss *et al.* 1989; Dzewaltowski *et al.* 1990; Feltz and Riessinger 1990; McAuley 1992, 1993; Shaw *et al.* 1992; Weinberg *et al.* 1992). Dzewaltowski (1989) has compared the predictiveness of the theory of reasoned action (Fishbein and Ajzen 1975) and social cognitive theory in the field of exercise motivation. The exercise behaviour of 328 students was recorded for seven weeks and then related to prior measures of different cognitive factors. Behavioural intention was measured by asking the individuals the likelihood that they would perform exercise behaviour. Attitude towards physical exercise, perceived behavioural control and beliefs about the subjective norm concerning exercise were assessed. The theory of reasoned action fit the data, as indicated by a path analysis. Exercise behaviour correlated with intention (0.22), attitude (0.18) and behavioural control beliefs (0.13). In addition, three social cognitive variables were assessed: (a) strength of self-efficacy to participate in an exercise programme when faced with impediments; (b) 13 expected outcomes multiplied by the evaluation of those outcomes; and (c) self-satisfaction or dissatisfaction with their level of activities and with the multiple outcomes of exercise. Exercise behaviour was correlated with perceived self-efficacy (0.34), outcome expectancies (0.15) and dissatisfaction (0.23), as well as with the interactions of these factors. The higher the three social cognitive constructs were at the onset of the programme, the more days the students exercised per week. Persons who were confident that they could adhere to the strenuous exercise programme were dissatisfied with their present level of physical activity and expected positive outcomes, and they exercised more. The variables in the theory of reasoned action did not account for any unique variance in exercise behaviour after the influence of the social cognitive factor was controlled for. These findings indicate that social cognitive theory provides powerful explanatory constructs.

The role of efficacy beliefs in initiating and maintaining a regular programme of physical exercise has also been studied by Desharnais *et al.* (1986), Sallis *et al.* (1986, 1992), Wurtele and Maddux (1987), Long and Haney (1988) and Fuchs (1995). Endurance in physical performance was found to be dependent on experimentally created efficacy beliefs in a series of experiments on competitive efficacy by Weinberg *et al.* (1979, 1980, 1981). In terms of competitive performance, tests of the role of efficacy beliefs in tennis performance revealed that perceived efficacy was related to 12 rated performance criteria (Barling and Abel 1983).

Patients with rheumatoid arthritis were motivated to engage in regular physical exercise by enhancing their perceived efficacy in a self-management programme (Holman and Lorig 1992). In applying self-efficacy theory to recovery from heart disease, patients who had suffered a myocardial infarction were prescribed a moderate exercise regimen (Ewart 1992). Ewart found that efficacy beliefs predicted both under-exercise and over-exertion during programmed exercise. Patients with chronic obstructive pulmonary diseases tend to avoid physical exertion owing to experienced discomfort, but rehabilitation programmes insist on compliance with an exercise regimen (Toshima *et al.* 1992). Compliance with medical regimens improved after patients suffering from chronic obstructive pulmonary disease received a cognitive-behavioural treatment designed to raise confidence in their capabilities. Efficacy beliefs predicted moderate exercise (r = whereas perceived control did not (Kaplan *et al.* 1984).

3.3 Nutrition and weight control

Dieting and weight control are health-related behaviours that can also be governed by self-efficacy beliefs (Chambliss and Murray 1979; Weinberg *et al.* 1984; Bernier and Avard 1986; Glynn and Ruderman 1986; Slater 1989; Hofstetter *et al.* 1990; Shannon *et al.* 1990). Chambliss and Murray (1979) found that overweight individuals were most responsive to behavioural treatment where they had a high sense of efficacy and an internal locus of control. Other studies on weight control have been published by Sallis *et al.* (1988) and Bagozzi and Warshaw (1990). It has been found that self-efficacy operates best in concert with general lifestyle changes, including physical exercise and provision of social support. Self-confident clients of intervention programmes were less likely to relapse to their previous unhealthy diet.

In sum, perceived self-efficacy has been found to predict intentions and actions in different domains of health functioning. The intention to engage in a certain health behaviour and the actual behaviour itself are positively associated with beliefs in one's personal efficacy. Efficacy beliefs determine appraisal of one's personal resources in stressful encounters and contribute to the forming of behavioural intentions. The stronger people's efficacy beliefs, the higher are the goals they set for themselves, and the firmer their commitment to engage in the intended behaviour, even in the face of failures (Locke and Latham 1990).

3.4 Self-efficacy approaches to addictive behaviours _

Another area in the health field where perceived self-efficacy has been studied extensively is smoking. Quitting the habit requires optimistic self-beliefs which can be instilled in smoking cessation programmes (Baer and Lichtenstein 1988; Devins and Edwards 1988; Carmody 1992; Haaga and Stewart 1992; Ho 1992; Karanci 1992; Kok *et al.* 1992). Efficacy beliefs to resist temptation to smoke predict reduction in the number of cigarettes smoked ($r = -0.62$), the amount of tobacco per smoke ($r = -0.43$) and the nicotine content ($r = -0.30$) (Godding and Glasgow 1985). Pre-treatment self-efficacy does not predict relapse, but post-treatment self-efficacy does (Kavanagh *et al.* 1993). Mudde *et al.* (1989) found that efficacy beliefs increased after treatment, and those who had acquired the highest levels of self-efficacy remained successful quitters as assessed in a one-year period (see also Kok *et al.* 1991). Various researchers have verified relationships between perceived self-regulatory efficacy and relapse occurrence or time of relapse, with correlations ranging from -0.34 to -0.69 (Condiotte and Lichtenstein 1981; Colletti *et al.* 1985; DiClemente *et al.* 1985; Garcia *et al.* 1990; Wilson *et al.* 1990). Hierarchies of tempting situations correspond to hierarchies of self-efficacy: the more a critical situation induces craving, the greater the perceived efficacy needed to prevent relapse (Velicer *et al.* 1990). In a programme of research on smoking prevention with Dutch adolescents, Kok *et al.* (1992) conducted several studies on the influence of perceived self-efficacy on non-smoking intentions and behaviours. Cross-sectionally, they could explain 64 per cent of the variance of intentions as well as of behaviour, which was owing to the overwhelming predictive power of perceived self-efficacy ($r = 0.66$ for intention, $r = 0.71$ for reported behaviour) (DeVries *et al.* 1988). These relationships were replicated longitudinally, although with somewhat less impressive coefficients (DeVries *et al.* 1989). Moreover, studies of the onset of smoking in teenagers have shown that perceived self-efficacy mediates peer social influence on smoking (Stacy *et al.* 1992).

Overcoming addictive behaviours such as substance use, alcohol consumption and smoking poses a major challenge for those who are dependent on these substances as well as for professional helpers. Smoking, for example, remains the number one public health problem in spite of declining prevalence rates (Shiffman 1993). Almost one hundred scientific publications per year deal with the issue of smoking cessation. Clinical approaches include multisession, multicomponent counselling or therapy programmes where individuals or small groups receive abstinence and relapse prevention training, often combined with medical treatment. The most promising pharmaceutical aid is the use of a nicotine patch that achieves a transdermal nicotine substitute to help counteract withdrawal symptoms.

On the other end of the treatment continuum lie community interventions, including worksite cessation programmes. This acknowledges the fact that only one-tenth of smokers make use of formal clinical programmes. In contrast, most are self-quitters who need only minimal assistance (Cohen *et al.* 1989; Curry 1993; Orleans *et al.* 1993). While relapse rates after professional treatment lie typically between 70 and 90 per cent, those of self-quitters are even higher. Nevertheless, investments in the public health approach are more cost-effective because it reaches a much larger target population and, thus, results in higher overall numbers of persons quitting (Lichtenstein and Glasgow 1992).

The community-wide minimal treatment programmes benefit from what was learned in clinical settings, although it is not yet clear what the most effective ingredients really are. It seems as if more is better, i.e. treatment packages that consist of many heterogeneous components are superior to theory-based single strategy approaches.

It has also been found that readiness to quit makes a difference. In clinical settings, most clients are self-referred and therefore highly motivated for behavioural change. Public health messages, in contrast, have to be addressed to smokers who are at different stages of motivation (DiClemente *et al.* 1991). Pre-contemplators who do not consider quitting at all need a different message from contemplators who struggle with the pros and cons of quitting. Furthermore, those who are ready for action need different kinds of assistance from those who just have quit and face a relapse crisis.

From a social-cognitive viewpoint, the key ingredients of any psychological treatment should be: (a) the identification of high-risk situations that stimulate smoking; (b) the development and cultivation of perceived self-efficacy; and (c) the application of adequate coping strategies. This can be described as a competent self-regulation process where individuals monitor their responses to taxing situations, observe similar others facing similar demands, appraise their coping resources, create optimistic self-beliefs, plan a course of action, perform the critical action and evaluate its outcomes.

Marlatt *et al.* (1994) propose five categories of self-efficacy that are related to stages of motivation and prevention pertaining to addictive behaviours.

Primary and secondary prevention:
(a) resistance self-efficacy;
(b) harm-reduction self-efficacy.
Self-change, treatment, and relapse prevention:
(c) action self-efficacy;
(d) coping self-efficacy;
(e) recovery self-efficacy.

Resistance self-efficacy pertains to the confidence in one's ability to avoid substance use prior to its first use. This implies resistance against peer pressure to smoke, drink or take drugs. It has been repeatedly found that the combination of peer pressure and low self-efficacy predicts the onset of smoking and substance use in adolescents (Conrad *et al.* 1992). Ellickson and Hays (1991) studied the determinants of future substance use in 1138 eighth and ninth graders in ten junior high schools. As potential predictors of onset, they analysed pro-drug social influence, resistance self-efficacy and perception of drug-use prevalence. Social influence or exposure to drug users combined with low self-efficacy for drug resistance turned out to predict experimentation with drugs nine months later. Interestingly, resistance self-efficacy was no longer predictive in the subsample of students who were already involved with drugs.

In a study on smoking onset, Stacy *et al.* (1992) examined pro-smoking social influence and resistance self-efficacy in a sample of 1245 Californian high school students. Perceived self-efficacy moderated the effect of peer pressure. As expected, many adolescents succumbed to pro-smoking influence, but those high in resistance self-efficacy were less vulnerable to interpersonal power.

With these findings in mind, one would expect that the training of resistance skills would raise resistance self-efficacy, which in turn would reduce future drug use. However, intervention studies that have included such a training have not yet been very promising (Hansen *et al.* 1991; Ellickson *et al.* 1993).

Harm-reduction self-efficacy pertains to one's confidence in being able to reduce the risk after having become involved with tobacco or drugs. Once a risk behaviour has commenced, the notion of resistance loses its significance. It is then of greater importance to control further damage and to strengthen the belief that one is capable of minimizing the risk. This is particularly useful since most adolescents at least experiment with cigarettes and alcohol, which can be regarded as a normal stage in puberty when youngsters face developmental tasks including self-regulation in tempting situations. Substance use can be seen as being normative rather than deviant and might reflect a healthy exploratory behaviour and a constructive learning process (Newcomb and Bentler 1988; Shedler and Block 1990). The conflict here is between solving normative developmental tasks on the one hand, and, on the other, initiating a risk behaviour that might accumulate and habitualize to a detrimental lifestyle pattern. Thus, the question is, how can a drug be curiously explored without becoming the gateway drug? The answer lies in the notion of harm-reduction self-efficacy. The individual must acquire not only the competence and skills, but also the optimistic belief in control of the impending risk. The aim of secondary prevention is to let adolelscents experiment while at the same time empowering them to minimize and eliminate substance use later on.

An intervention study to accomplish this goal has been conducted at the Addictive Behaviors Research Center at the University of Washington (Baer *et al.* 1992; Baer 1993). College students received one of three treatments: (a) an alcohol information class dealing with negative consequences of alcohol; (b) a moderation-oriented cognitive-behavioural skills training class; and (c) an assessment-only control group. The second treatment group was trained to enhance their harm-reduction self-efficacy, which indeed resulted in the greatest decrease in alcohol consumption.

The above two types of self-efficacy are related to prevention. When, however, it comes to behaviour change for those who are already addicted, the focus turns to action, coping and recovery. *Action self-efficacy* concerns confidence in attaining one's desired abstinence goal (or controlled use). If, for example, someone sets a date for quitting, then a commitment is made, moving the person beyond the mere contemplation stage. When intentions to quit are translated into preparatory acts, the individual needs optimistic self-beliefs to make detailed plans of how to refrain from the substance, imagine success scenarios and take instrumental actions. This applies to unaided cessation as well as to formal treatment settings. Action self-efficacy has been found to predict attempts to quit smoking (Marlatt *et al.* 1988; Sussman *et al.* 1989). From as early as 1981, many smoking cessation studies have included self-efficacy to predict abstinence (Condiotte and Lichtenstein 1981; Colletti *et al.* 1985; DiClemente *et al.* 1985; Godding and Glasgow 1985; Baer *et al.* 1986; Garcia *et al.* 1990; Wilson *et al.* 1990; Ho 1992; Karanci 1992; Kok *et al.* 1992). These findings corroborate consistently the beneficial influence of optimistic self-beliefs, but this effect is restricted to post-treatment self-efficacy. Typically, pre-treatment self-efficacy does not predict relapse, but post-treatment self-efficacy does. This generalizes, by the way, to a broad range of domains of human functioning (Kok *et al.* 1992; Kavanagh *et al.* 1993; Marlatt *et al.* 1994). Pre-treatment self-efficacy is not based on personal experience with quitting and is, therefore, inappropriate for the prediction of treatment outcomes. During the cessation training, self-efficacy is being developed with a realistic sense of one's capabilities, resulting in more accurate self-knowledge that allows one to foresee one's most likely reactions in tempting situations.

Coping self-efficacy relates to anticipatory coping with relapse crises. After one has made a successful attempt to quit, long-term maintenance is at stake. At this stage, quitters are confronted with high-risk situations, such as experiencing negative affect or temptations in positive social situations. Lapses are likely to occur unless the quitter can mobilize alternative coping strategies. Believing in one's coping reservoir assists in making sound judgements and in initiating adaptive coping responses. Relapse prevention training aims at making use of a variety of situation-tailored coping strategies, which in turn enhance coping self-efficacy (Marlatt and Gordon 1985; Curry 1993; Gruder *et al.* 1993). This includes behavioural as well as cognitive coping modes.

Recovery self-efficacy is closely related to coping self-efficacy, but the two tap different aspects within the maintenance stage (similar to the distinction between resistance and harm-reduction self-efficacy in the prevention stage). If a lapse occurs, individuals can fall prey to the 'abstinence violation effect', i.e. they attribute their lapse to internal, stable and global causes, dramatize the event and interpret it as a full-blown relapse (Marlatt and Gordon 1985). High self-efficacious individuals, however, avoid this effect by making a high-risk situation responsible and by finding ways to control the damage and to restore hope. Self-efficacy for recovery of abstinence after an initial lapse has been found to promote long-term maintenance. Clinical interventions focus on specific recovery strategies after setbacks, such as reviewing and reattributing the situation, balancing alternative ways of coping and making an immediate plan for recovery (e.g. renew initial commitment to quit, mobilize social support, reframe the lapse as a normal event within a productive learning process) (Curry and Marlatt 1987). This restores self-efficacy and helps a quick return to the path of maintenance. However, Haaga and Stewart (1992) found that not high but moderate self-efficacy for recovery leads to the best survival rates (continuation of abstinence). If this finding can be replicated in further research, it would reflect an 'overconfidence effect', since too high a self-efficacy would embolden trials of risk behaviours.

As these examples from research on addictive behaviours demonstrate, it is essential to identify several stages at which self-efficacy operates in different manners. Specific kinds of self-efficacy are protective as the individual moves through the process of peer influence, substance experimentation, cessation and abstinence maintenance. Psychological interventions have to be stage-tailored.

4 Developments

Over the years, the notion of self-efficacy has become so appealing to health psychologists that it has been adopted as part of most health behaviour theories. Becker and Rosenstock (1987) have incorporated it into their health belief model, mainly by reinterpreting what used to be 'barriers' to action. Ajzen (1988, 1991) has extended the theory of reasoned action to the theory of planned behaviour by adding a predictor labelled 'perceived behavioural control', which is about the same as self-efficacy (see Conner and Sparks, Chapter 5 in this volume). Maddux and Rogers (1983) have incorporated self-efficacy as one major determinant of intentions in their protection motivation theory (see also Maddux 1993; Boer and Seydel, Chapter 4 in this volume). These theories are described in more detail in other chapters of this book (see also Schwarzer 1992; Weinstein 1993; Wallston 1994). Thus, 'self-efficacy models' are no longer really distinct from other approaches since the key construct that was originally developed within Bandura's social cognitive theory has meanwhile proven to be an essential component in all major models.

In this section, we describe our own extensions of previous models, the health action process approach (HAPA), which is in particular influenced by social cognitive theory. Its basic notion is that the adoption, initiation and maintenance of health behaviours must be explicitly conceived as a process that consists of at least two stages, a motivation phase and a volition phase. The latter might be further subdivided into a planning phase, action phase and maintenance phase. It is claimed that self-efficacy plays a crucial role at all stages, while in contrast other cognitions are of limited scope. For example, risk perceptions serve predominantly to set the stage for a contemplation process early in the motivation phase but do not extend beyond. Similarly, outcome expectancies are chiefly important in the motivation phase when individuals balance the pros and cons of certain consequences of behaviours, but they lose their predictive power after a personal decision has been made. However, if one does not believe in one's capability to perform a desired action, one will fail to adopt, initiate and maintain it.

Behavioural intentions are far from being sufficient to initiate a difficult action such as refraining from smoking or switching to a diet. There is a post-intentional and pre-actional process that can be called a 'volitional process', or simply a planning stage (Heckhausen and Gollwitzer 1987; Bagozzi 1992; Karoly 1993; Kuhl and Beckmann 1993). Several authors have suggested stage models that may account for this phenomenon. Prochaska and DiClemente (1983, 1984), for example, have put forward their transtheoretical model of change, which starts with pre-contemplation where individuals have not thought at all about the health issue. In the subsequent contemplation stage they develop a motivation to change. Afterwards, they enter a preparation stage before the actual behaviour is finally performed. This preparation stage reflects a post-intentional pre-actional state.

Similarly, Weinstein and Sandman (1992) have suggested a six-stage model. They distinguish individuals who are unaware of the issue or unengaged by it from those who are just deciding about acting. Before they finally initiate the new behaviour they have 'decided to act'. Again, this is a post-intentional pre-actional state that deserves further scientific attention.

In the health action process approach (HAPA; Schwarzer 1992; see Figure 6.1) this critical state is also explicitly considered as part of a volition process. It is labelled 'action plans' – individuals prepare for the intended behaviour by imagining scenarios of how and under which circumstances they could perform specific acts. In this stage, self-efficacy plays a crucial role because individuals rely more or less on optimistic self-beliefs when facing self-imposed challenges. Subsequent performance then represents a successful outcome of cognitive activities in the planning and preparation stage. The association between self-efficacy and performance thus reflects intermediate cognitive processes that have been left unmeasured in past research. The post-intentional pre-actional state is influenced by self-referent thought about how to prepare and initiate a novel health behaviour which, then, is reflected in individual differences in subsequent health behaviours.

4.1 The motivation phase

In the motivation phase, the individual forms an intention either to adopt a precaution measure or to change risk behaviours in favour of other behaviours. This has also been conceived as a decision-making stage by some authors (Fishbein and Ajzen 1975; Eiser and Sutton 1977; Eiser 1983). Today, it is known that self-efficacy and outcome expectancies are the major predictors of intentions. Most previous models treat these two as being unrelated predictors. However, there might be a temporal and causal order among them. Bandura (1989: 1180) has underscored that their interrelationship should also be taken into consideration:

> the effects of outcome expectancies on performance motivation are partly governed by self-beliefs of efficacy. There are many activities that, if performed well, guarantee valued outcomes, but they are not pursued if people doubt they can do what it takes to succeed . . . Self-perceived inefficacy can thus nullify the motivating potential of alluring outcome expectations . . . When variations in perceived self-efficacy are partialed out, the outcomes expected for given performances do not have much of an independent effect on behaviour.

Outcome expectancies can be seen as precursors of self-efficacy because people usually make assumptions about the possible consequences of behaviours before enquiring whether they can take the action themselves. If self-efficacy is specified as a mediator between outcome expectancies and intention, the direct influence of outcome expectancy on intention may

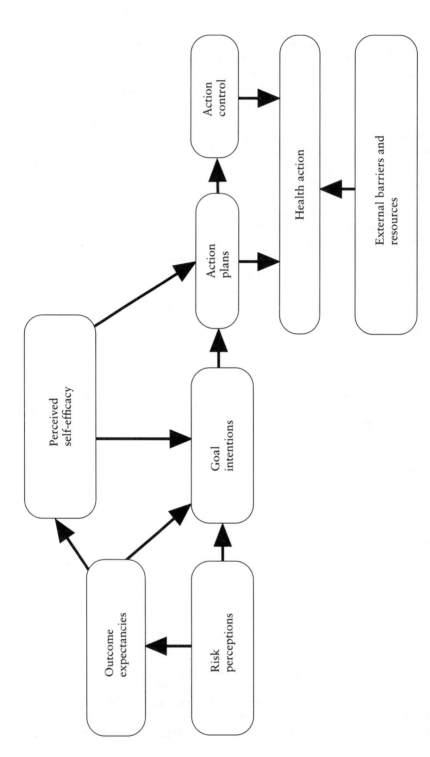

Figure 6.1 The health action process approach.

dissipate. But the research findings on this issue are very inconsistent, rendering both cognitions primary candidates for motivating change. Under conditions where individuals have no experience with the behaviour they are contemplating, we assume that outcome expectancies may have a stronger direct influence. Only after a sufficient level of experience is attained does self-efficacy receive the lion's share of the intention variance.

A specific subset of outcome expectancies, namely social outcome expectancies, should also be considered explicitly as determinants within the motivation phase, as proposed in the theory of reasoned action and the theory of planned behaviour, where this has been called subjective norm or normative beliefs. People often develop intentions because they perceive social pressures to do so. Individuals comply with the perceived expectations of significant others in order to receive gratifications or to avoid conflicts or disregard, or because of naive trust in the opinion of others. Previous findings on the predictive value of the subjective norm (or normative beliefs) have not been overwhelming, which is possibly because of limited measurement and theoretical elaboration. The perceived social expectation factor should be viewed from two additional vantage points: (a) from a social comparison perspective which suggests that our intentions and actions are governed by our desire to maintain or enhance self-esteem or self-consistency within normative reference groups (see Wood 1989; Wills 1990); and (b) from a social support perspective which suggests that people draw on their social networks and resources when making decisions, e.g. the intention to quit smoking being facilitated by a network of non-smokers (Cohen *et al.* 1988). The link between social outcome expectancies and intentions has to be reconsidered with these research perspectives in mind.

The interplay between perceived severity of an illness, perceived vulnerability and the resulting threat, as hypothesized in the health belief model, is still undetermined. The influential role of threat or risk perception in the motivation and volition process has been overestimated in past research and interventions. Fear appeals are of limited value; the message has to be framed in a way that allows individuals to draw on their coping resources and to exercise skills in order to control health threats. In persuasive communications, a focus should be made on self-percepts of personal coping capabilities to manage effective precaution strategies (Bandura 1991). This suggests a causal order where threat is specified as a distal antecedent that helps to stimulate outcome expectancies which further stimulate self-efficacy. A minimum level of threat or concern must exist before people start contemplating the benefits of possible actions and ruminate on their competence actually to perform them. The direct path from threat to intention may become negligible if expectancies are already well established.

In establishing a rank order among the three direct paths that lead to intention, it is assumed that self-efficacy dominates, followed by outcome expectancies, whereas threat (or risk perceptions) may fail to contribute any additional direct influence. As an indirect factor, however, threat may be of considerable significance within the motivation phase. As mentioned above, the context and one's personal experience play a role and may change the pattern of weights.

4.2 The action phase

It is common knowledge that good intentions do not necessarily guarantee corresponding actions. Correlations between intentions and behaviours vary tremendously. The previously mentioned theories refer more generally to barriers or costs as the reasons for this gap, and they list a number of impediments, such as situational constraints or lack of willpower. The theory of planned behaviour, which was designed for the case of incomplete control over behaviour, makes an attempt to quantify this problem by specifying a direct link between perceived behavioural control and behaviour, thus circumventing the intention. More theoretical elaborations are required, however, to understand better the processes involved. Relapse prevention theory (Marlatt and Gordon 1985), volition theory (Kuhl 1983; Heckhausen 1991), and self-efficacy theory (Bandura 1977, 1986) have sparked the following ideas.

In the motivation phase what people choose to do is described, and in the subsequent action or volition phase how hard they try and how long they persist are described. The right-hand part of Figure 6.1 consists of three levels: cognitive, behavioural and situational. The focus is on cognitions that instigate and control the action, i.e. a volitional or self-regulative process which is subdivided into action plans and action control.

When a preference for a particular health behaviour has been shaped, the intention has to be transformed into detailed instructions on how to perform the desired action. If, for example, someone intends to lose weight, he or she has to plan how to do it, i.e. what foods to buy, when and how often to eat which amounts, when and where to exercise, and perhaps even whether to give up smoking as well. Thus, a global intention can be specified by a set of subordinate intentions and action plans that contain proximal goals and algorithms of action sequences. The volition process is barely influenced by outcome expectancies, but more strongly by self-efficacy, since the number and quality of action plans are dependent on one's perceived competence and experience. Self-efficacy beliefs influence the cognitive construction of specific action plans, for example by visualizing scenarios that may guide goal attainment. These post-decisional pre-actional cognitions are necessary because otherwise the person would act impulsively in a trial-and-error fashion and would not know where to allocate the available resources.

Once an action has been initiated, it has to be controlled by cognitions in order to be maintained. The action has to be protected from being interrupted and abandoned prematurely owing to incompatible competing intentions which may become dominant while a behaviour is being performed. Meta-cognitive activity is needed to complete the primary action and to suppress distracting secondary action tendencies. Daily physical exercise, for example, requires self-regulatory processes in order to secure effort and persistence and to keep other motivational tendencies at a distance (such as the desire to eat, socialize or sleep) until these tendencies can prevail for a limited time period.

When an action is being performed, self-efficacy determines the amount of effort invested and the perseverance. People with self-doubts are more inclined to anticipate failure scenarios, worry about possible performance deficiencies and abort their attempts prematurely. People with an optimistic sense of self-efficacy, however, visualize success scenarios that guide the action and let them persevere in face of obstacles. When running into unforeseen difficulties they quickly recover.

Performing an intended health behaviour is an action, just as is refraining from a risk behaviour. The suppression of health-detrimental actions requires effort and persistence as well, and therefore is also guided by a volitional process that includes action plans and action control. If one intends to quit smoking or drinking, one has to plan how to do it. For example, it is important to avoid high-risk situations where the pressures to relapse are overwhelming. Attaining proximal subgoals helps to increase the difficulty level of situations until one can resist under all possible circumstances. If someone is craving a cigarette or a drink, action control helps him or her to survive the critical situation. For example, individuals can make favourable social comparisons, refer to their self-concept or simply pull themselves together. The more these meta-cognitive skills and internal coping dialogues are developed and the better they are matched to specific risk situations, the more easily the urges can be controlled. Self-efficacy helps to re-establish the perseverance efforts needed for the accomplishment of self-imposed goals.

One of the major action control paradigms is the delay of gratification pattern. Children already possess the meta-cognitive skills to suppress the craving for a small piece of candy if they are promised a bigger piece at a later time; they apply cognitive distraction and other techniques for this purpose (Mischel 1973; Mischel and Moore 1980). A similar paradigm can be found in disease prevention. If children comply with brushing and flossing their teeth regularly, they are promised that they will not suffer from tooth decay or periodontal disease several decades later. Evidently, it requires an immense volitional strength (after the necessary intention is given) to obtain this kind of gratification, which can hardly be expected from the majority of human beings. After a circumscribed action has been completed, the individual evaluates it as successful or failing and attributes the perceived outcome to possible causes. Dependent on this cognitive event, emotions and expectancies are varied, and the volitional strength may be increased or decreased for subsequent similar actions. Self-reinforcement is seen as a favourable meta-cognitive strategy.

Finally, situational barriers as well as opportunities have to be considered.

If situational cues are overwhelming, meta-cognitive skills fail to protect the individual and the temptation cannot be resisted. Actions are not only a function of intentions and cognitive control, but also influenced by the perceived and the actual environment. For example, a social network that ignores the coping process of a quitter, by smoking in his presence, creates a difficult stress situation which taxes the quitter's volitional strength. If, on the other hand, a spouse decides to quit too, then a social support situation is created that enables the quitter to remain abstinent in spite of lower levels of volitional strength.

In sum, the action phase can be described along three levels: cognitive, behavioural and situational. The cognitive level refers to self-regulatory processes that mediate between the intentions and the actions. This volitional process contains action plans and action control and is strongly influenced by self-efficacy expectancies, but also by perceived situational barriers and support.

5 Operationalization of the model

The three major cognitions that operate during the motivation phase can be assessed by single items such as the following:

Risk perception

My risk of getting lung cancer is

very low   *low*   *high*   *very high*

compared to the average person of my age and sex.

Outcome expectancy

If I stopped smoking, then it would reduce my risk of lung cancer.

not at all true   *barely true*   *somewhat true*   *very true*

Perceived self-efficacy

I am certain that I can resist smoking even when I drink alcohol with my friends.

not at all true   *barely true*   *somewhat true*   *very true*

It is of note that the first kind of cognition, risk perception, need not be the same as threat experience, and the relationship between the two still awaits theoretical and empirical elaboration. To make test construction simple, one can keep in mind that outcome expectancies are best worded as '*if–then*' statements, and self-efficacy items as *confidence*-statements. The semantic structure of outcome expectancies is:

If (*behaviour*), then (*consequences*).

For self-efficacy the corresponding wording could be:

I am confident that I can (*perform something*), even if (*barrier*).

This rule need not be applied rigidly, but should serve as a heuristic. It is suggested that a variety of outcome expectancies are assessed, including positive and negative ones. People have many reasons why they should quit smoking or why they find it better to continue. The test items should cover the scope of pros and cons that an individual balances. It is also suggested that the different constructs not be neatly separated in the questionnaire, but rather scrambled so that the respondents do not realize at first glance what this is all about.

However, there is no way to determine the reliability of single items, and therefore one might want to consider using psychometric scales that consist of a number of items. These scales are, of course, less economical, but they often help to assure that the theoretical constructs are tapped by the sum score and are measured more reliably. Self-efficacy scales that are more or less adequate have been published for all kinds of health behaviours.

Various psychometric instruments have been developed to assess self-efficacy for physical activities, such as the diving efficacy scale of Feltz *et al.* (1979), the physical self-efficacy scale of Ryckman *et al.* (1982), the exercise self-efficacy scale of Garcia and King (1991) and others (Barling and Abel 1983; Woolfolk *et al.* 1985; Fruin *et al.* 1991; Marcus and Owen 1992; Godin *et al.* 1993; Fuchs and Schwarzer 1994). Physical exercise self-efficacy scales for patients coping with chronic disease were designed by Holman and Lorig (1992) and Toshima *et al.* (1992).

In the field of nutrition and weight control, Stotland *et al.* (1991) came up with a situation-based dieting self-efficacy scale that presents 25 risk situations and measures adherence to a diet in these situations. Clark *et al.* (1991) devised a 20-item weight efficacy lifestyle questionnaire with five situational factors, namely negative emotions, availability of foods, social pressure, physical discomfort and positive activities.

There are two basic methods for designing a risk-behaviour self-efficacy scale. One is to confront the individual with a list or hierarchy of tempting situations and to assess situation-specific self-efficacy in line with these demands. The second approach aims at the restricted use of substances, asking subjects whether in general they feel competent to control the behaviour in question (irrespective of specific risk situations). In the domain of *smoking*, for example, the first method has been chosen by Colletti *et al.* (1985) and Velicer *et al.* (1990). In research on drinking, it has been preferred by Annis (1982), DiClemente *et al.* (1985), Annis and Davis (1988) and Miller *et al.* (1989). The second approach was chosen by Godding and Glasgow (1985), for example, to assess smoking self-efficacy. For alcohol consumption, instruments were presented by Sitharthan and Kavanagh (1990), Young *et al.* (1991) and Rychtarik *et al.* (1992). A third attempt to assess self-efficacy has been published by Haaga and Stewart (1992), who developed an 'articulated thoughts technique' to measure recovery self-efficacy after a setback from smoking abstinence.

Scales for self-efficacy for smoking, dieting, physical exercise, condom use, cancer screening and social support provision can be found in Schwarzer

---

Each rung on this ladder represents where various smokers are in their thinking about quitting. Circle the number that indicates where you are now.

10 → Taking action to quit (e.g. cutting down, enrolling in a programme).

9

8 → Starting to think about how to change my smoking patterns.

7

6

5 → Think I should quit but not quite ready.

4

3

2 → Think I need to consider quitting someday.

1

0 → No thought about quitting.

Figure 6.2   The contemplation ladder.

(1993). These scales are available in English, Spanish and German. A generalized self-efficacy scale is available in more languages.

In addition to the assessment of risk perception, outcome expectancies and self-efficacy, it is essential to identify the individual's motivation stage. A unique way to arrive at some idea about one's stage is given by a single-item self-report measure, the 'contemplation ladder' (Biener and Abrams 1991): see Figure 6.2.

Inconsistency in research findings is partly owing to heterogeneous designs of the assessment methods. The present recommendations might help to standardize the construction rationales, but not the inventories themselves.

6 Application of the model

To explore the interplay between self-efficacy, outcome expectancies and risk perceptions, a longitudinal data set of about 800 citizens of Berlin, Germany, was analysed. In the summer of 1992, participants (18–70 years of age) were asked to fill out a self-administered questionnaire on health cognitions and behaviours. A second wave of measurement took place six months later. Multiple regression analyses presented here are based on the following measures. Self-efficacy towards healthy eating behaviour was assessed by a scale consisting of six items (internal consistency: alpha = 0.76). A typical item was: 'If I commit myself to eating healthy foods, then I can persist with it' (1–4). Positive outcome expectancies regarding a healthy eating behaviour were measured by seven items, such as 'If I stick to a low-fat diet, my risk of a myocardial infarction will be reduced' (1–5). Negative outcome expectancies (five items) had the same format, but referred to undesired consequences of a healthy eating behaviour, such as 'If I stick

Table 6.1 Prediction of the intention to eat healthy foods

Predictor	Men (n = 534) Beta	Women (n = 664) Beta
Prior eating behaviour	0.16**	0.16**
Risk perception	−0.02	−0.03
Self-efficacy	0.16**	0.13**
Positive outcome expectancy	0.40**	0.37**
Negative outcome expectancy	−0.04	−0.10*
Risk perception × self-efficacy	−0.07	0.03
Pos. outc. exp. × self-efficacy	0.00	−0.03
Neg. outc. exp. × self-efficacy	0.07	0.03
Pos. outc. exp. × risk percept.	−0.06	−0.04
Neg. outc. exp. × risk percept.	−0.05	0.07
	$R = 0.55$	$R = 0.54$
	(adj. $R^2 = 0.29$)	(adj. $R^2 = 0.28$)

to a low-fat diet then I need to spend more time preparing the meals'. Risk perception (perceived vulnerability) was assessed by two items: (a) 'Compared to other persons of my age and sex, my risk of suffering a heart attack or stroke is' (much smaller . . . the same as that of the others . . . much higher; 1–7), and (b) 'How likely do you think it is that you will get a heart attack or stroke in the future?' (very unlikely . . . very likely; 1–7). The healthy eating behaviour index was based on frequency responses to 13 items with the format: 'How often do you usually eat salad or raw vegetables (red meat; cake or cookies; nuts or chips; fresh fruit; sausage (salami, ham, etc.); whole milk . . .)?' Items were classified into three groups of products (foods high in fat/cholesterol, high in sugar and high in fibre) and were summed up within each group separately. Finally, these group scores were used to calculate the 'healthy eating behaviour' index (the higher the value, the more health-conscious the eating behaviour). The intention to eat healthy foods was measured by two items of the type 'I intend to eat as healthfully as possible during the next few months' (1–7).

Hierarchical regression analyses were computed where interaction terms were entered at the second step after all main effects had been considered. The first analysis aimed at the prediction of the intention. Table 6.1 shows the results separately for men and women.

Results are similar for both sexes. Health-related cognitions and prior behaviour jointly account for about 28–29 per cent of the intention variance, with positive outcome expectancies being most influential. Risk perceptions and all interactions did not contribute to the prediction. The same kind of analysis has been replicated, with intentions being measured half a year later, but no substantial differences from the above results emerged. Thus, an interaction model of intention prediction was not supported by the present data.

Next, the same three social-cognitive predictors were used to determine

Table 6.2 Prediction of healthy eating behaviour half a year later (wave 2)

Predictor	Men (n = 353) Beta	Women (n = 462) Beta
Intention to eat healthy foods	0.24**	0.12*
Risk perception	0.07	−0.01
Self-efficacy	0.23**	0.28**
Positive outcome expectancy	0.19**	0.19**
Negative outcome expectancy	0.01	−0.10*
Risk perception × self-efficacy	−0.07	−0.05
Pos. outc. exp. × self-efficacy	−0.03	0.02
Neg. outc. exp. × self-efficacy	0.00	−0.01
Pos. outc. exp. × risk percept.	0.03	0.02
Neg. outc. exp. × risk percept.	−0.08	−0.02
	$R = 0.48$	$R = 0.47$
	(adj. $R^2 = 0.21$)	(adj. $R^2 = 0.20$)

their possible influence at the volition stage of health behaviour. The intention was added as a predictor of healthy eating behaviour half a year later. Table 6.2 shows the results of the regression analysis.

Sex differences emerged here. For men, intention was a markedly better predictor of future eating behaviour than for women. Most interestingly, self-efficacy was the best predictor in the data set of the women. Women who believed they could persist in eating healthy foods consumed less fat and cholesterol and ate more fruit and vegetables than those who did not share this belief.

In the theory of planned behaviour (Ajzen 1988), perceived behavioural control (that is, about the same as perceived self-efficacy) is expected to influence behaviour through intentions, but it can also influence behaviour directly. The explanation for the latter case is that behaviour may not be under volitional control. If an action cannot be performed owing to a lack of resources or opportunities then the best intentions are worthless. If, for example, people intend to eat healthfully, but perceive realistically that no health foods are available in a certain situation, perceived behavioural control would be a good direct predictor of the behaviour.

To clarify further the role of self-efficacy, outcome expectancies and risk perception in predicting intention and behaviour, a more complex analysis was computed. Since no interactions had turned out to be of importance, a structural equation model was specified that was limited to main effects, which can be subdivided into direct and indirect effects. This kind of path analysis is appropriate in particular for testing mediator hypotheses. Each latent variable was associated with two observed variables. The model was tested using the LISREL 8 program (Jöreskog and Sörbom 1993).

The path model in Figure 6.3 refers to the subsample of 353 men and obtains a rather good data fit ($\chi^2 = 47.9$, d.f. = 41, $p = 0.21$, RMR = 0.049, GFI = 0.98). Intention was predicted by positive outcome expectancies

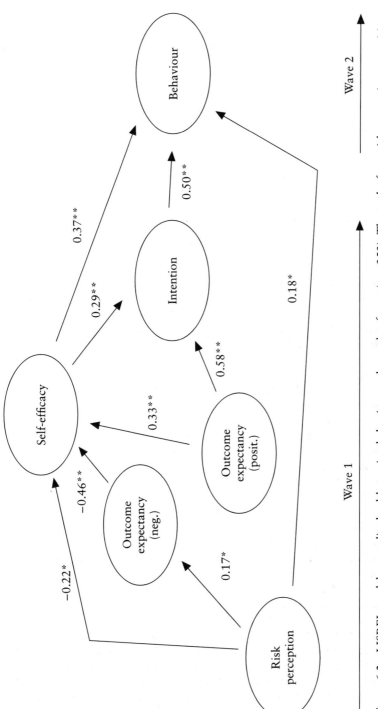

Figure 6.3 LISREL model to predict healthy eating behaviour: subsample of men (*n* = 353). The paths from risk perception to positive outcome expectancy, from risk perception to intention and from negative outcome expectancy to intention were also specified, but turned out to be not significant. Positive and negative outcome expectancies were correlated at 0.15. *Path coefficient significant at *p* < 0.05, **p* < 0.01.

(0.58) and self-efficacy (0.29), whereas behaviour was mainly predicted by intention (0.50) and self-efficacy (0.37). For women, the same structural model also obtained a reasonable data fit; however, the key difference was found in a significant path (−0.34) from negative outcome expectancy to intention. In sum, these results not only suggest that self-efficacy cognitions are important in establishing a strong readiness to eat healthy foods, but also support the notion that self-efficacy beliefs are crucial for those volitional processes that transform dietary intentions into corresponding actions.

7 Future directions

Theoretical process approaches to the adoption and maintenance of health behaviours should include distinct stages of motivation and volition as well as the construct of self-efficacy, which has turned out to be the most powerful single resource factor. However, self-efficacy is not the 'magic bullet' to solve all problems that can arise in the prediction and treatment of behavioural change. Peer pressure usually appears to have higher predictive value, and its counterpart, social support, also has a high potential as a resource factor (Schwarzer and Leppin 1991). On the other hand, social influence is not unconfounded by self-efficacy. The degree to which peer pressure makes a difference also depends on the individual's resistance self-efficacy; the degree to which social support operates also rests on one's self-efficacy to build, maintain and mobilize social networks.

An open question refers to the optimal degree of specificity or generality of the self-efficacy construct. According to Bandura, perceived self-efficacy should always be as situation-specific as possible. This specificity issue can even be further subdivided into a formal and a substantial facet. In a formal sense, Marlatt *et al.* (1994) have conceptualized five kinds of self-efficacy that reflect different stages. In a substantial sense, one has to tailor the questions to the situation, such as smoking cessation or condom use. Although there is nothing wrong with more and more specificity, there still exist generalized measures that have considerable predictive value (Snyder *et al.* 1991; Wallston 1992; Mittag and Schwarzer 1993). Self-efficacy can be a generalized trait reflecting a personal resource factor to cope with stress in various life domains. In this sense, it mirrors optimistic self-beliefs that relate to confidence in one's overall coping resources. There are a few theoretical differences between dispositional optimism (as understood by Scheier and Carver 1992) and generalized self-efficacy, but the empirical association is above 0.60 (Schwarzer 1994). Optimism is a broader construct that can be further subdivided into defensive and functional optimism (Taylor 1989). Most people are unrealistically optimistic when they assess situation-outcome relationships. They feel less vulnerable towards health threats than they should, and they believe that their reference group is at greater risk for diseases than themselves (Weinstein 1982). Moreover, most people believe that their actions will produce positive outcomes and that they are personally capable of coping with their life demands. The former has been called defensive optimism, the latter functional optimism. Functional optimism relies not only on positive outcome expectancies, but more so on personal coping resources, including self-efficacy. If perceptions are distorted, then it is likely that some people overestimate their capabilities. Evidence has only been found by Haaga and Stewart (1992), whose high-efficacy subjects did not recover as well from lapses as their moderate-efficacy subjects. Perceived self-efficacy has to be optimistic to generate motivational power and should be somewhat overly optimistic, not exceeding a certain limit where unrealistic optimism leads to disappointment or harm. Previous interventions have focused on risk communication to lower defensive optimism. The idea was to let people understand how much they really are at risk. This intervention strategy was obviously not very successful. Social cognitive theory would emphasize the opposite strategy by making people understand what they are able to change. Resource communication might be met with more acceptance. Individuals should not only be threatened by what they may lose, they should also be challenged by what they could gain.

References

Ajzen, I. (1988) *Attitudes, Personality and Behavior*. Milton Keynes: Open University Press.

Ajzen, I. (1991) The theory of planned behavior, *Organizational Behavior and Human Decision Processes*, 50, 179–211.

Altmaier, E.M., Russell, D.W., Kao, C.F., Lehmann, T.R. and Weinstein, J.N. (1993) Role of self-efficacy in rehabilitation outcome among chronic low back pain patients, *Journal of Counseling Psychology*, 40, 335–9.

Annis, H.M. (1982) *Inventory of Drinking Situations*. Ontario: Addiction Research Foundation.

Annis, H.M. and Davis, C.S. (1988) Assessment of expectancies. In D.M. Donovan and G.A. Marlatt (eds) *Assessment of Addictive Behaviors*. New York: Guilford, 84–111.

Baer, J.S. (1993) Etiology and secondary prevention of alcohol problems with young adults. In J.S. Baer, G.A. Marlatt and R.J. McMahon (eds) *Addictive Behaviors Across the Lifespan: Prevention, Treatment, and Policy Issues*. Newbury Park, CA: Sage, 111–37.

Baer, J.S., Holt, C.S. and Lichtenstein, E. (1986) Self-efficacy and smoking reexamined: construct validity and clinical utility, *Journal of Consulting and Clinical Psychology*, 54, 846–52.

Baer, J.S. and Lichtenstein, E. (1988) Classification and prediction of smoking relapse episodes: an exploration of individual differences, *Journal of Consulting and Clinical Psychology*, 56, 104–10.

Baer, J.S., Marlatt, G.A., Kivlahan, D.R., Fromme, K., Larimer, M.E. and Williams, E. (1992) An experimental test of three methods of alcohol risk reduction with young adults, *Journal of Consulting and Clinical Psychology*, 60, 974–9.

Bagozzi, R.P. (1992) The self-regulation of attitudes, intentions, and behavior, *Social Psychology Quarterly*, 55, 178–204.

Bagozzi, R.P. and Warshaw, P.R. (1990) Trying to consume, *Journal of Consumer Research*, **17**, 127–40.

Bandura, A. (1977) Self-efficacy: toward a unifying theory of behavioral change, *Psychological Review*, **84**, 191–215.

Bandura, A. (1986) *Social Foundations of Thought and Action*. Englewood Cliffs, NJ: Prentice Hall.

Bandura, A. (1989) Self-efficacy mechanism in physiological activation and health-promoting behavior. In J. Madden, S. Matthysse and J. Barchas (eds) *Adaptation, Learning and Affect*. New York: Raven, 1169–88.

Bandura, A. (1991) Self-efficacy conception of anxiety. In R. Schwarzer and R.A. Wicklund (eds) *Anxiety and Self-focused Attention*. New York: Harwood, 89–110.

Bandura, A. (1992) Self-efficacy mechanism in psychobiologic functioning. In R. Schwarzer (ed.), *Self-efficacy: Thought Control of Action*. Washington, DC: Hemisphere, 355–94.

Bandura, A. (1994) *Self-efficacy. The Exercise of Control*. New York: Freeman.

Bandura, A., Cioffi, D., Taylor, C.B. and Brouillard, M.E. (1988) Perceived self-efficacy in coping with cognitive stressors and opioid activation, *Journal of Personality and Social Psychology*, **55**, 479–88.

Bandura, A., Reese, L. and Adams, N.E. (1982) Micro-analysis of action and fear arousal as a function of differential levels of perceived self-efficacy, *Journal of Personality and Social Psychology*, **43**, 5–21.

Bandura, A., Taylor, C.B., Williams, S.L., Mefford, I.N. and Barchas, J.D. (1985) Catecholamine secretion as a function of perceived coping self-efficacy, *Journal of Consulting and Clinical Psychology*, **53**, 406–14.

Barling, J. and Abel, M. (1983) Self-efficacy and tennis performance, *Cognitive Therapy and Research*, **7**, 265–72.

Basen-Engquist, K. (1992) Psychosocial predictors of 'safer-sex' behaviors in young adults, *Aids Education and Prevention*, **4**, 120–34.

Basen-Engquist, K. and Parcel, G.S. (1992) Attitudes, norms, and self-efficacy: a model of adolescents' HIV-related sexual risk behavior, *Health Education Quarterly*, **19**, 263–77.

Beck, K.H. and Lund, A.K. (1981) The effects of health threat seriousness and personal efficacy upon intentions and behavior, *Journal of Applied Social Psychology*, **11**, 401–15.

Becker, M.H. and Rosenstock, I.M. (1987) Comparing social learning theory and the health belief model. In W.B. Ward (ed.) *Advances in Health Education and Promotion*, Vol. 2. Greenwich, CT: JAI, 245–9.

Bernier, M. and Avard, J. (1986) Self-efficacy, outcome and attrition in a weight reduction program, *Cognitive Therapy and Research*, **10**, 319–38.

Biener, L. and Abrams, D.B. (1991) The contemplation ladder: validation of a measure of readiness to consider smoking cessation, *Health Psychology*, **10**, 360–5.

Brafford, L.J. and Beck, K.H. (1991) Development and validation of a condom self-efficacy scale for college students, *Journal of American College Health*, **39**, 219–25.

Carmody, T.P. (1992) Preventing relapse in the treatment of nicotine addiction: current issues and future directions, *Journal of Psychoactive Drugs*, **24**, 131–58.

Chambliss, C.A. and Murray, E.J. (1979) Efficacy attribution, locus of control, and weight loss, *Cognitive Therapy and Research*, **3**, 349–53.

Clark, M.M., Abrams, D.B., Niaura, R.S., Eaton, C.A. and Rossi, J.S. (1991) Self-efficacy in weight management, *Journal of Consulting and Clinical Psychology*, **59**, 739–44.

Coates, T.J. (1990) Strategies for modifying sexual behavior for primary and secondary prevention of HIV disease, *Journal of Consulting and Clinical Psychology*, **58**, 57–69.

Cohen, S., Lichtenstein, E., Mermelstein, R., Kingsolver, K., Baer, J.S. and Kamarck, T.W. (1988) Social support interventions for smoking cessation. In B.H. Gottlieb (ed.) *Marshaling Social Support. Formats, Processes, and Effects*. Beverly Hills, CA: Sage, 211–40.

Cohen, S., Lichtenstein, E., Prochaska, J.O., Rossi, J.S., Gritz, E.R., Carr, C.R., Orleans, C.T., Schoenbach, V.J., Biener, L., Abrams, D., DiClemente, C., Curry, S., Marlatt, G.A., Cunnings, K.M., Emont, S.L., Giovino, G. and Ossip-Klein, D. (1989) Debunking myths about self-quitting: evidence from 10 prospective studies of persons who attempt to quit smoking by themselves, *American Psychologist*, **44**, 1355–65.

Colletti, G., Supnick, J.A. and Payne, T.J. (1985) The smoking self-efficacy questionnaire (SSEQ): preliminary scale development and validation, *Behavioral Assessment*, **7**, 249–60.

Condiotte, M.M. and Lichtenstein, E. (1981) Self-efficacy and relapse in smoking cessation programs, *Journal of Consulting and Clinical Psychology*, **49**, 648–58.

Conrad, K.M., Flay, B.R. and Hill, D. (1992) Why children start smoking cigarettes: predictors of onset, *British Journal of Addiction*, **87**, 1711–24.

Curry, S.J. (1993) Self-help interventions for smoking cessation, *Journal of Consulting and Clinical Psychology*, **61**, 790–803.

Curry, S. and Marlatt, G.A. (1987) Building self-confidence, self-efficacy, and self-control. In W.M. Cox (ed.) *Treatment and Prevention of Alcohol Problems*. New York: Academic Press, 117–38.

Desharnais, R., Bouillon, J. and Godin, G. (1986) Self-efficacy and outcome expectations as determinants of exercise adherence, *Psychological Reports*, **59**, 1155–9.

Devins, G.M. and Edwards, P.J. (1988) Self-efficacy and smoking reduction in chronic obstructive pulmonary disease, *Behaviour Research and Therapy*, **26**, 127–35.

De Vries, H., Dijkstra, M. and Kok, G.J. (1989) Self-efficacy as a determinant of the onset of smoking and interventions to prevent smoking in adolescents, paper presented at the First European Congress of Psychology, Amsterdam.

De Vries, H., Dijkstra, M. and Kuhlman, P. (1988) Self-efficacy: the third factor besides attitude and subjective norm as a predictor of behavioural intentions, *Health Education Research*, **3**, 273–82.

DiClemente, C.C., Prochaska, J.O., Fairhurst, S.K., Velicer, W.F., Velasquez, M.M. and Rossi, J.S. (1991) The process of smoking cessation: an analysis of precontemplation, contemplation, and preparation stages of change, *Journal of Consulting and Clinical Psychology*, **59**, 295–304.

DiClemente, C.C., Prochaska, J.O. and Gibertini, M. (1985) Self-efficacy and the stages of self-change of smoking, *Cognitive Therapy and Research*, **9**, 181–200.

Donovan, D.M. and Marlatt, G.A. (eds) (1988) *Assessment of Addictive Behaviors*. New York: Guilford Press.

Dzewaltowski, D.A. (1989) Toward a model of exercise motivation, *Journal of Sport and Exercise Psychology*, **11**, 251–69.

Dzewaltowski, D.A., Noble, J.M. and Shaw, J.M. (1990) Physical activity participation: social cognitive theory versus the theories of reasoned action and planned behavior, *Journal of Sport and Exercise Psychology*, 12, 388–405.

Eiser, J.R. (1983) Smoking, addiction and decision-making, *International Review of Applied Psychology*, 32, 11–28.

Eiser, J.R. and Sutton, S.R. (1977) Smoking as a subjectively rational choice, *Addictive Behaviors*, 2, 129–34.

Ekstrand, M. and Coates, T.J. (1990) Maintenance of safer sexual behaviors and predictors of risky sex: the San Francisco Men's Health Study, *American Journal of Public Health*, 80, 973–7.

Ellickson, P.L., Bell, R.M. and McGuigan, K. (1993) Preventing adolescent drug use: long-term results of a junior high program, *American Journal of Public Health*, 83, 856–61.

Ellickson, P.L. and Hays, R.D. (1991) Beliefs about resistance self-efficacy and drug prevalence: do they really affect drug use?, *International Journal of the Addictions*, 25, 1353–78.

Ewart, C.K. (1992) The role of physical self-efficacy in recovery from heart attack. In R. Schwarzer (ed.) *Self-efficacy: Thought Control of Action*. Washington, DC: Hemisphere, 287–304.

Feltz, D.L., Landers, D.M. and Raeder, V. (1979) Enhancing self-efficacy in high-avoidance tasks: a comparison of modeling techniques, *Journal of Sport Psychology*, 1, 112–22.

Feltz, D.L. and Riessinger, C.A. (1990) Effects of in vivo emotive imagery and performance feedback on self-efficacy and muscular endurance, *Journal of Sport and Exercise Psychology*, 12, 132–43.

Fishbein, M. and Ajzen, I. (1975) *Belief, Attitude, Intention, and Behavior: an Introduction to Theory and Research*. Reading, MA: Addison-Wesley.

Fruin, D.J., Pratt, C. and Owen, N. (1991) Protection Motivation Theory and adolescents' perceptions of exercise, *Journal of Applied Psychology*, 22, 55–69.

Fuchs, R. (1995). Causal models of physical exercise participation: testing the predictive power of the construct 'pressure to change', *Journal of Applied Social Psychology*.

Fuchs, R. and Schwarzer, R. (1994) Selbstwirksamkeit zur sportlichen Aktivität: Reliabilität und Validität eines neuen Meßinstruments (Self-efficacy toward physical exercise: Reliability and validity of a new instrument), *Zeitschrift für Differentielle und Diagnostische Psychologie*, 15.

Garcia, A.W. and King, A.C. (1991) Predicting long-term adherence to aerobic exercise: a comparison of two models, *Journal of Sport and Exercise Psychology*, 13, 394–410.

Garcia, M.E., Schmitz, J.M. and Doerfler, L.A. (1990) A fine-grained analysis of the role of self-efficacy in self-initiated attempts to quit smoking, *Journal of Consulting and Clinical Psychology*, 58, 317–22.

Gilchrist, L.D. and Schinke, S.P. (1983) Coping with contraception: cognitive and behavioral methods with adolescents, *Cognitive Therapy and Research*, 7, 379–88.

Glynn, S.M. and Ruderman, A.J. (1986) The development and validation of an eating self-efficacy scale, *Cognitive Therapy and Research*, 10, 403–20.

Godding, P.R. and Glasgow, R.E. (1985) Self-efficacy and outcome expectations as predictors of controlled smoking status, *Cognitive Therapy and Research*, 9, 583–90.

Godin, G., Valois, P. and Lepage, L. (1993) The pattern of influence of perceived behavioral control upon exercising behavior: an application of Ajzen's Theory of Planned Behavior, *Journal of Behavioral Medicine*, 16, 81–102.

Gruder, C.L., Mermelstein, R.J., Kirkendol, S., Hedeker, D., Wong, S.C., Schreckengost, J., Warnecke, R.B., Burzette, R. and Miller, T.Q. (1993) Effects of social support and relapse prevention training as adjuncts to a televised smoking-cessation intervention, *Journal of Consulting and Clinical Psychology*, 61, 113–20.

Haaga, D.A.F. and Stewart, B.L. (1992) Self-efficacy for recovery from a lapse after smoking cessation, *Journal of Consulting and Clinical Psychology*, 60, 24–8.

Hansen, W.B., Graham, J.W., Wolkenstein, B.H. and Rohrbach, L.A. (1991) Program integrity as a moderator of prevention program effectiveness: results for fifth-grade students in the adolescent alcohol prevention trial, *Journal of Studies on Alcohol*, 52, 568–79.

Heckhausen, H. (1991) *Motivation and Action*. Berlin: Springer.

Heckhausen, H. and Gollwitzer, P.M. (1987) Thought contents and cognitive functioning in motivational vs. volitional states of mind, *Motivation and Emotion*, 11, 101–20.

Ho, R. (1992) Cigarette health warnings: the effects of perceived severity, expectancy of occurrence, and self-efficacy on intentions to give up smoking, *Australian Psychologist*, 27, 109–13.

Hofstetter, C.R., Sallis, J.F. and Hovell, M.F. (1990) Some health dimensions of self-efficacy: Analysis of theoretical specificity, *Social Science and Medicine*, 31, 1051–6.

Holman, H.R. and Lorig, K. (1992) Perceived self-efficacy in self-management of chronic disease. In R. Schwarzer (ed.) *Self-efficacy: Thought Control of Action*. Washington, DC: Hemisphere, 305–23.

Jemmott, J.B., Jemmott, L.S. and Fong, G.T. (1992a) Reducing the risk of sexually transmitted HIV infection: attitudes, knowledge, intentions, and behavior, *American Journal of Public Health*, 82, 371–8.

Jemmott, J.B., Jemmott, L.S., Spears, H., Hewitt, N. *et al.* (1992b) Self-efficacy, hedonistic expectancies, and condom use intentions among inner-city Black adolescent women: a social cognitive approach to AIDS risk behavior, *Journal of Adolescent Health*, 13, 512–19.

Jöreskog, K.G. and Sörbom, D. (1993) *New features in LISREL 8*. Chicago: Scientific Software.

Kaplan, R.M., Atkins, C.J. and Reinsch, S. (1984) Specific efficacy expectations mediate exercise compliance in patients with COPD, *Health Psychology*, 3, 223–42.

Karanci, N.A. (1992) Self efficacy-based smoking situation factors: the effects of contemplating quitting vs. relapsing in a Turkish sample, *International Journal of Addictions*, 27, 879–86.

Karoly, P. (1993) Mechanisms of self-regulation: a system view, *Annual Review of Psychology*, 44, 23–52.

Kasen, S., Vaughn, R.D. and Walter, H.J. (1992) Self-efficacy for AIDS preventive behaviors among tenth grade students, *Health Education Quarterly*, 19, 187–202.

Kavanagh, D.J., Pierce, J., Lo, S.K. and Shelley, J. (1993) Self-efficacy and social support as predictors of smoking after a quit attempt, *Psychology and Health*, 8, 231–42.

Kok, G., de Vries, H., Mudde, A.N. and Strecher, V.J. (1991) Planned health education and the role of self-efficacy: Dutch research, *Health Education Research*, **6**, 231–8.

Kok, G., Den Boer, D., DeVries, H., Gerards, F., Hospers, H.J. and Mudde, A.N. (1992) Self-efficacy and attribution theory in health education. In R. Schwarzer (ed.) *Self-efficacy: Thought Control of Action*. Washington, DC: Hemisphere, 245–62.

Kuhl, J. (1983) *Motivation, Konflikt und Handlungskontrolle* (*Motivation, Conflict and Action Control*). Berlin: Springer.

Kuhl, J. and Beckmann, J. (eds) (1993) *Volition and Personality: Action versus State Orientation*. Göttingen/Toronto: Hogrefe.

Lazarus, R.S. and Folkman, S. (1987) Transactional theory and research on emotions and coping, *European Journal of Personality*, **1**, 141–70.

Levinson, R.A. (1982) Teenage women and contraceptive behavior: focus on self-efficacy in sexual and contraceptive situations, unpublished doctoral dissertation, Stanford University.

Lichtenstein, E. and Glasgow, R.E. (1992) Smoking cessation: what have we learned over the past decade?, *Journal of Consulting and Clinical Psychology*, **60**, 518–27.

Litt, M.D. (1988) Self-efficacy and perceived control: cognitive mediators of pain tolerance, *Journal of Personality and Social Psychology*, **54**, 149–60.

Locke, E.A. and Latham, G.P. (1990) *A Theory of Goal Setting and Task Performance*. Englewood Cliffs, NJ: Prentice Hall.

Long, B.C. and Haney, C.J. (1988) Coping strategies for working women: aerobic exercise and relaxation interventions, *Behavior Therapy*, **19**, 75–83.

McAuley, E. (1992) The role of efficacy cognitions in the prediction of exercise behavior in middle-aged adults, *Journal of Behavioral Medicine*, **15**, 65–88.

McAuley, E. (1993) Self-efficacy and the maintenance of exercise participation in older adults, *Journal of Behavioral Medicine*, **16**, 103–13.

McKusick, L., Coates, T.J., Morin, S.F., Pollack, L. and Hoff, N. (1990) Longitudinal predictors of reductions in unprotected anal intercourse among gay men in San Francisco – the AIDS Behavioral Research Project, *American Journal of Public Health*, **80**, 978–83.

Maddux, J.E. (1991) Self-efficacy. In C.R. Snyder and D.R. Forsyth (eds) *Handbook of Social and Clinical Psychology: the Health Perspective*. New York: Pergamon Press, 57–78.

Maddux, J.E. (ed.) (1993) *Self-efficacy, Adaptation, and Adjustment: Theory, Research, and Application*. New York: Plenum.

Maddux, J.E. and Rogers, R.W. (1983) Protection motivation and self-efficacy: a revised theory of fear appeals and attitude change, *Journal of Experimental Social Psychology*, **19**, 469–79.

Manning, M.M. and Wright, T.L. (1983) Self-efficacy expectancies, outcome expectancies, and the persistence of pain control in childbirth, *Journal of Personality and Social Psychology*, **45**, 421–31.

Marcus, B.H. and Owen, N. (1992) Motivational readiness, self-efficacy and decision-making for exercise, *Journal of Applied Social Psychology*, **22**, 3–16.

Marlatt, G.A., Baer, J.S. and Quigley, L.A. (1994) Self-efficacy and addictive behavior. In A. Bandura (ed.) *Self-efficacy in Changing Societies*. Marbach: Johann Jacobs Foundation.

Marlatt, G.A., Curry, S. and Gordon, J.R. (1988) A longitudinal analysis of unaided smoking cessation, *Journal of Consulting and Clinical Psychology*, **56**, 715–20.

Marlatt, G.A. and Gordon, J.R. (eds) (1985) *Relapse Prevention*. New York: Guilford.

Meyerowitz, B.E. and Chaiken, S. (1987) The effect of message framing on breast self-examination attitudes, intentions, and behavior, *Journal of Personality and Social Psychology*, 52, 500–10.

Miller, P.J., Ross, S.M., Emmerson, R.Y. and Todt, E.H. (1989) Self-efficacy in alcoholics: clinical validation of the Situational Confidence Questionnaire, *Addictive Behaviors*, 14, 217–24.

Mischel, W. (1973) Toward a cognitive social learning reconceptualization of personality, *Psychological Review*, 80, 252–83.

Mischel, W. and Moore, B. (1980) The role of ideation in voluntary delay for symbolically presented rewards, *Cognitive Therapy and Research*, 4, 211–21.

Mittag, W. and Schwarzer, R. (1993) Interaction of employment status and self-efficacy on alcohol consumption: a two-wave study on stressful life transitions, *Psychology and Health*, 8, 77–87.

Mudde, A., Kok, G. and Strecher, V. (1989) Self-efficacy and success expectancy as predictors of the cessation of smoking, paper presented at the First European Congress of Psychology, Amsterdam.

Newcomb, M.D. and Bentler, P.M. (1988) *Consequence of Adolescent Drug Use: Impact on the Lives of Young Adults*. Beverly Hills, CA: Sage.

O'Leary, A. (1992) Self-efficacy and health: behavioral and stress-physiological mediation, *Cognitive Therapy and Research*, 16, 229–45.

O'Leary, A., Goodhart, F., Jemmott, L.S. and Boccher-Lattimore, D. (1992) Predictors of safer sex on the college campus: a social cognitive theory analysis, *Journal of American College Health*, 40, 254–63.

O'Leary, A., Shoor, S., Lorig, K. and Holman, H.R. (1988) A cognitive-behavioral treatment for rheumatoid arthritis, *Health Psychology*, 7, 527–42.

Orleans, C.T., Kristeller, J.L. and Gritz, E.R. (1993) Helping hospitalized smokers quit: new directions for treatment and research, *Journal of Consulting and Clinical Psychology*, 61, 778–89.

Paulussen, T., Kok, G.J., Knibbe, R. and Kramer, T. (1989) AIDS en intraveneus druggebruik (AIDS and IV-drug use), *Tijdschrift voor Sociale Gezondheitszorg (Dutch Journal of Social Health Care)*, 68, 129–36.

Prochaska, J.O. and DiClemente, C.C. (1983) Stages and processes of self-change of smoking: toward an integrative model of change, *Journal of Consulting and Clinical Psychology*, 51, 390–5.

Prochaska, J.O. and DiClemente, C.C. (1984) *The Transtheoretical Approach: Crossing Traditional Boundaries of Change*. Homewood, IL: Irwin.

Rippetoe, P.A. and Rogers, R.W. (1987) Effects on components of protection motivation theory on adaptive and maladaptive coping with a health threat, *Journal of Personality and Social Psychology*, 52, 596–604.

Rychtarik, R.G., Prue, D.M., Rapp, S.R. and King, A.C. (1992) Self-efficacy, aftercare and relapse in a treatment program for alcoholics, *Journal of Studies on Alcohol*, 53, 435–40.

Ryckman, R.M., Robbins, M.A., Thornton, B. and Cantrell, P. (1982) Development and validation of a physical self-efficacy scale, *Journal of Personality and Social Psychology*, 42, 891–900.

Sallis, J.F., Haskell, W.L., Fortmann, S.P., Vranizan, K.M. *et al.* (1986) Predictors of adoption and maintenance of physical activity in a community sample, *Preventive Medicine*, 15, 331–41.

Sallis, J.F., Hovell, M.F., Hofstetter, C.R. and Barrington, E. (1992) Explanation of vigorous physical activity during two years using social learning variables, *Social Science and Medicine*, 34, 25–32.

Sallis, J.F., Pinski, R.B., Grossman, R.M., Patterson, T.L. and Nader, P.R. (1988) The development of self-efficacy scales for health-related diet and exercise behaviors, *Health Education Research*, 3, 283–92.

Scheier, M.F. and Carver, C.S. (1992) Effects of optimism on psychological and physical well-being: theoretical overview and empirical update, *Cognitive Therapy and Research*, 16, 201–28.

Schwarzer, R. (1992) Self-efficacy in the adoption and maintenance of health behaviors: Theoretical approaches and a new model. In R. Schwarzer (ed.) *Self-efficacy: Thought Control of Action*. Washington, DC: Hemisphere, 217–42.

Schwarzer, R. (1993) *Measurement of Perceived Self-efficacy: Psychometric Scales for Cross-cultural Research*. Berlin: Freie Universität Berlin, Institut für Psychologie.

Schwarzer, R. (1994) Optimism, vulnerability, and self-beliefs as health-related cognitions: a systematic overview, *Psychology and Health*, 9, 161–80.

Schwarzer, R. and Leppin, A. (1991) Social support and health: a theoretical and empirical overview, *Journal of Social and Personal Relationships*, 8, 99–127.

Seydel, E., Taal, E. and Wiegman, O. (1990) Risk-appraisal, outcome and self-efficacy expectancies: cognitive factors in preventive behavior related to cancer, *Psychology and Health*, 4, 99–109.

Shannon, B., Bagby, R., Wang, M.Q. and Trenkner, L. (1990) Self-efficacy: a contributor to the explanation of eating behavior, *Health Education Research*, 5, 395–407.

Shaw, J.M., Dzewaltowski, D.A. and McElroy, M. (1992) Self-efficacy and causal attributions as mediators of perceptions of psychological momentum, *Journal of Sport and Exercise Psychology*, 14, 134–47.

Shedler, J. and Block, J. (1990) Adolescent drug use and psychological health: a longitudinal inquiry, *American Psychologist*, 45, 612–30.

Shiffman, S. (1993) Assessing smoking patterns and motives, *Journal of Consulting and Clinical Psychology*, 61, 732–42.

Sitharthan, T. and Kavanagh, D.J. (1990) Role of self-efficacy in predicting outcomes from a programme for controlled drinking, *Drug and Alcohol Dependence*, 27, 87–94.

Slater, M.D. (1989) Social influences and cognitive control as predictors of self-efficacy and eating behavior, *Cognitive Therapy and Research*, 13, 231–45.

Snyder, C.R., Harris, C., Anderson, J.R., Holleran, S.A., Irving, L.M., Sigmon, S.T., Yoshinobu, L., Gibb, J., Langelle, C. and Harney, P. (1991) The will and the ways: development and validation of an individual-differences measure of hope, *Journal of Personality and Social Psychology*, 60, 570–85.

Stacy, A.W., Sussman, S., Dent, C.W., Burton, D. and Flay, B.R. (1992) Moderators of peer social influence in adolescent smoking, *Personality and Social Psychology Bulletin*, 18, 163–72.

Stotland, S., Zuroff, D.C. and Roy, M. (1991) Situational dieting self-efficacy and short-term regulation of eating, *Appetite*, 17, 81–90.

Sussman, S., Whitney Saltiel, D.A., Budd, R.J., Spiegel, D. *et al.* (1989) Joiners and non-joiners in worksite smoking treatment: pretreatment smoking, smoking by significant others, and expectation to quit as predictors, *Addictive Behaviors*, 14, 113–19.

Taylor, C.B., Bandura, A., Ewart, C.K., Miller, N.H. and DeBusk, R.F. (1985) Exercise testing to enhance wives' confidence in their husbands' cardiac capability soon after clinically uncomplicated acute myocardial infarction, *American Journal of Cardiology*, 55, 635–8.

Taylor, S.E. (1989) *Positive Illusions: Creative Self-deception and the Healthy Mind.* New York: Basic Books.

Toshima, M.T., Kaplan, R.M. and Ries, A.L. (1992) Self-efficacy expectancies in chronic obstructive pulmonary disease rehabilitation. In R. Schwarzer (ed.) *Self-efficacy: Thought Control of Action.* Washington, DC: Hemisphere, 325–54.

Velicer, W.F., DiClemente, C.C., Rossi, J.S. and Prochaska, J.O. (1990) Relapse situations and self-efficacy: an integrative model, *Addictive Behaviors*, 15, 271–83.

Wallston, K.A. (1992) Hocus-pocus, the focus isn't strictly on locus: Rotter's social learning theory modified for health, *Cognitive Therapy and Research*, 16, 183–99.

Wallston, K.A. (1994) Theoretically based strategies for health behavior change. In M.P. O'Donnell and J.S. Harris (eds) *Health Promotion in the Workplace*, 2nd edn. Albany, NY: Delmar Publishers, 185–203.

Weinberg, R.S., Gould, D. and Jackson, A. (1979) Expectations and performance: an empirical test of Bandura's self-efficacy theory, *Journal of Sport Psychology*, 1, 320–31.

Weinberg, R.S., Gould, D., Yukelson, D. and Jackson, A. (1981) The effect of preexisting and manipulated self-efficacy on competitive muscular endurance task, *Journal of Sport Psychology*, 4, 345–54.

Weinberg, R., Grove, R. and Jackson, A. (1992) Strategies for building self-efficacy in tennis players: a comparative analysis of Australian and American coaches, *Sport Psychologist*, 6, 3–13.

Weinberg, R.S., Hughes, H.H., Critelli, J.W., England, R. and Jackson, A. (1984) Effects of preexisting and manipulated self-efficacy on weight loss in a self-control program, *Journal of Research in Personality*, 18, 352–8.

Weinberg, R.S., Yukelson, D. and Jackson, A. (1980) Effects of public and private efficacy expectations on competitive performance, *Journal of Sport Psychology*, 2, 340–9.

Weinstein, N.D. (1982) Unrealistic optimism about susceptibility to health problems, *Journal of Behavioral Medicine*, 5, 441–60.

Weinstein, N.D. (1993) Testing four competing theories of health-protective behavior, *Health Psychology*, 12, 324–33.

Weinstein, N.D. and Sandman, P.M. (1992) A model of the precaution adoption process: evidence from home radon testing, *Health Psychology*, 11, 170–80.

Weiss, M.R., Wiese, D.M. and Klint, K.A. (1989) Head over heels with success: the relationship between self-efficacy and performance in competitive youth gymnastics, *Journal of Sport and Exercise Psychology*, 11, 444–51.

Wiedenfeld, S.A., O'Leary, A., Bandura, A., Brown, S., Levine, S. and Raska, K. (1990) Impact of perceived self-efficacy in coping with stressors on components of the immune system, *Journal of Personality and Social Psychology*, 59, 1082–94.

Wills, T.A. (1990) Multiple networks and substance use. Special issue: social support in social and clinical psychology, *Journal of Social and Clinical Psychology*, 9, 78–90.

Wilson, D.K., Wallston, K.A. and King, J.E. (1990) Effects of contract framing, motivation to quit, and self-efficacy on smoking reduction, *Journal of Applied Social Psychology*, **20**, 531–47.

Wood, J. (1989) Theory and research concerning social comparisons of personal attributes, *Psychological Bulletin*, **106**, 231–48.

Woolfolk, R.L., Murphy, S.M., Gottesfeld, D. and Aitken, D. (1985) Effects of mental rehearsal of task motor activity and mental depiction of task outcome on motor skill performance, *Journal of Sport Psychology*, **7**, 191–7.

Wurtele, S.K. and Maddux, J.E. (1987) Relative contributions of protection motivation theory components in predicting exercise intentions and behavior, *Health Psychology*, **6**, 453–66.

Young, R.M., Oei, T.P.S. and Crook, G.M. (1991) Development of a drinking self-efficacy questionnaire, *Journal of Psychopathology and Behavioral Assessment*, **13**, 1–15.

| 7 | PAUL NORMAN AND MARK CONNER |

THE ROLE OF SOCIAL COGNITION MODELS IN PREDICTING HEALTH BEHAVIOURS: FUTURE DIRECTIONS

1 Introduction

Psychologists have long been interested in the factors that underlie the performance of health behaviour. As the research reviewed in this book testifies, social cognition models provide one important framework for increasing our understanding of the determinants of a wide range of health behaviours. In the preceding chapters five of the most influential social cognition models in this area were presented and evaluated: the health belief model (HBM), health locus of control (HLC), protection motivation theory (PMT), the theory of reasoned action/theory of planned behaviour (TRA/TPB) and social cognitive theory/self-efficacy (SCT/SET). While these models represent five fairly distinct approaches to the study of health behaviour, it is also clear that considerable overlap exists between their constructs and that they share similar shortcomings (see Conner and Norman, Chapter 1 in this volume). In this final chapter we first consider work that has attempted to compare the models, on an empirical and a conceptual level. Second, we present a number of new directions for research with social cognition models which are currently engaging researchers in this area. Finally, we outline some of the basic requirements for an integrative social cognition model of health behaviour.

2 Comparisons

2.1 Empirical comparisons

Despite a substantial volume of empirical work using the main social cognition models to predict a range of health behaviours, there has been little empirical work comparing the predictive power of the different models

(Stroebe and Stroebe 1995). As Weinstein (1993) notes, the lack of comparison studies means that there is little consensus on whether some variables are more influential than others and whether some models of health behaviour are more predictive than others. However, while this criticism of research with social cognition models is clearly valid, it is also evident that those studies which have attempted to compare different models have been important in helping to identify the key predictors of health behaviour. A number of these studies are reviewed below.

Hill *et al.* (1985) compared the HBM (i.e. susceptibility, severity, benefits, barriers, health motivation) with the TRA (i.e. attitude, subjective norm) in their study on the determinants of womens' intentions to perform breast self-examination and to have a Pap test. Both models were found to predict intentions, explaining between 17 and 20 per cent of the variance in breast self-examination intentions and 26 and 32 per cent of the variance in Pap test intentions. The HBM was found to predict slightly more of the variance in each case but, as Hill *et al.* (1985) point out, this may be because of the greater number of constructs measured in the HBM.

Similar results have been reported by Mullen *et al.* (1987). They examined the ability of the TRA and the HBM to predict changes in a range of health behaviours over an eight-month period. Again, both models were found to produce significant predictions of changes in the health behaviours, with the HBM explaining slightly more of the variance. Mullen *et al.* (1987) also reported that the HBM was more economical in predicting behaviour change in that it only required an average of 23 items to measure its constructs, compared with the 32 needed to measure the constructs of the TRA. However, it should be noted that Mullen *et al.* (1987) used both direct and indirect measures of the attitude and subjective norm components of the TRA. While the above studies show the HBM to be a slightly superior model when compared with the TRA, a couple of further studies have suggested the opposite conclusion. For example, Oliver and Berger (1979) found the TRA to be a superior predictor of inoculation behaviour, and Rutter (1989) found it superior in relation to AIDS-preventive behaviour. More recently, a couple of studies have attempted to compare the TPB and the HBM. Conner and Norman (1994) examined the determinants of attendance at a health check and found the models to predict intentions and behaviour to a similar level, while Bakker *et al.* (1994) found the TPB to be more predictive of condom use among heterosexuals.

A number of studies have examined the role of self-efficacy in relation to the main social cognition models and have identified it as a key social cognitive variable. For example, Seydel *et al.* (1990) compared a restricted HBM (susceptibility, severity, outcome expectancies) with the PMT (susceptibility, severity, outcome expectancies, self-efficacy) and found outcome expectancies and self-efficacy to be the most important predictors of cancer-related preventive intentions and behaviour. Dzewaltowski (1989) has also highlighted the importance of self-efficacy in a study comparing the TRA and SCT. The study examined the predictors of exercise behaviour measured seven weeks later, and found SCT to provide a better prediction of exercise behaviour than the TRA ($R^2 = 0.14$ versus 0.06), with self-efficacy emerging as the most important single predictor. Ajzen (1988) has recently added the concept of perceived behavioural control to the TRA with good effect (see Conner and Sparks, Chapter 5 in this volume). However, given the close similarity between perceived behavioural control and self-efficacy, Schwarzer (1992) has suggested that perceived behavioural control be replaced with the self-efficacy construct. A number of researchers have followed this suggestion, producing encouraging results (DeVries and Kok 1986; DeVries *et al.* 1988; Kok *et al.* 1991). However, it is still not entirely clear to what extent concepts of 'difficulty', which characterize some perceived behavioural control measures, are equivalent to measures of self-efficacy, which focus on one's confidence to perform the behaviour (see Conner and Sparks, Chapter 5 in this volume).

On the basis of the above review of work which has sought to compare the predictive power of the social cognition models, it is possible to draw two main conclusions. First, many of the comparisons have shown the models to perform to a similar level, suggesting that there may be little to choose between them. Second, the self-efficacy construct appears to be a key predictor of health behaviour, providing a strong case for its inclusion in social cognition models of health behaviour.

2.2 Theoretical comparisons

A number of authors have commented on the similarities between the various social cognition models at a conceptual level. As Cummings *et al.* (1980) have noted, there is considerable overlap between the various constructs contained within the models; where differences do appear, they may represent differences in labelling rather than differences in the underlying constructs. In this section we consider some of the main constructs outlined in social cognition models of health behaviour and the extent to which they may overlap.

First, with the exception of HLC, models that have been developed specifically to predict health behaviour (i.e. HBM, PMT) focus on the notion of threat as measured by perceived susceptibility and perceived severity. In addition, SCT focuses on expectancies about environmental cues (i.e. risk perception) (Rosenstock *et al.* 1988). In contrast, the TPB does not explicitly cater for emotional or arousal variables, leading some authors to suggest that the TPB may be limited to the rational part of a health decision (Oliver and Berger 1979). Weinstein (1993) argues against this viewpoint, pointing out that perceptions of severity may be tapped indirectly by the evaluation component of behavioural beliefs, while perceptions of severity may be tapped by belief strength. For example, a behavioural belief may focus on the perceived likelihood that continued smoking may lead to lung cancer (i.e. perceived susceptibility) and an evaluation of this consequence (i.e. perceived severity). However, while perceptions of susceptibility and severity may be tapped by a consideration of behavioural beliefs, it may be advantageous to maintain the distinction between threat perception and behavioural beliefs.

Second, most social cognition models of health behaviour focus on the perceived consequences of performing a health behaviour (Rosenstock *et al.* 1988; Weinstein 1993; Conner and Norman 1994; van der Pligt 1994). For example, in the TPB the focus is on behavioural beliefs, in the HBM it is on the benefits and costs of performing a health behaviour, while in SCT it is on outcome expectancies and in PMT it is on response efficacy. Of the models covered in this book, only HLC fails to consider the perceived consequences of performing a health behaviour, as it is a generalized expectancy of the relationship between one's actions and health outcomes.

Third, considerable attention has focused on the importance of perceptions of control following Ajzen's (1988) introduction of the construct of perceived behavioural control into the TPB. According to Ajzen (1988) perceived behavioural control refers to the individual's perception of the ease or difficulty of performing a behaviour. This concept can be contrasted with Rotter's (1966) earlier concept of locus of control, inasmuch as locus of control is a generalized expectancy that is seen to be relatively stable across different situations, whereas perceived behavioural control is behaviour-specific and therefore can be seen to vary considerably. Thus, it is possible to make the distinction between one's general control beliefs and one's control beliefs in a specific situation. A similar distinction can be made in relation to health locus of control beliefs that, while specific to health, are seen to cut across different situations (e.g. exercise, smoking, dietary choice). However, where behaviour-specific health locus of control scales have been developed, the distinction between health locus of control and perceived behavioural control becomes less clear-cut (see Norman and Bennett, Chapter 3 in this volume). The most common comparison, though, is made between perceived behavioural control and self-efficacy (Ajzen 1991). In fact, Schwarzer (1992) has argued that perceived behavioural control should simply be relabelled as self-efficacy and considered as such. Self-efficacy is a well-established and well-researched construct that is firmly embedded within SCT (Schwarzer and Fuchs, Chapter 6 in this volume) and can be contrasted with the still exploratory nature of the perceived behavioural control construct. However, as noted above, there may be some advantage in distinguishing between perceptions of the ease or difficulty of performing a behaviour (i.e. perceived behavioural control) and one's confidence in performing the behaviour (i.e. self-efficacy).

A number of the models focus on specific control issues or barriers to the performance of health behaviour. Thus, a similarity can be noted between control beliefs in the TPB and the perceived barriers dimension of the HBM (Conner and Norman 1994; van der Pligt 1994). Rosenstock *et al.* (1988) have further considered the overlap between the perceived barriers dimension of the HBM and self-efficacy. They consider the perceived barriers dimension to be a 'catch-all' term for all the potential barriers to action, both internal and external. As a result, they argue for the inclusion of self-efficacy as a separate construct within the HBM, highlighting two important consequences: first, it would help to delimit the scope of the barriers dimension; second, it would add to the predictive power of the HBM. Hochbaum (1983) has similarly argued for the inclusion of self-efficacy in the HBM.

Fourth, normative influences on behaviour are not explicitly covered by social cognition models of health behaviour (Conner and Norman 1994), with the exception of the TPB, which includes the subjective norm construct and underlying normative beliefs. In the HBM, normative influences are simply listed as one of many potential cues to action. In SCT, normative influences may be covered by outcome expectancies that focus on the perceived social consequences of behaviour. However, Schwarzer (1992) has questioned the extent to which it is necessary to differentiate between social outcome expectancies and other expectancies in SCT, and Weinstein (1993) has put forward a similar argument in relation to normative beliefs and behavioural beliefs in the TPB. Nevertheless, there may be some merit in limiting the scope of outcome expectancies or behavioural beliefs so that the independent influence of normative influences can be considered in more detail.

Fifth, both the TPB and PMT include an intervening variable which is seen to mediate the relationship between other social cognitive variables and behaviour (Weinstein 1993). In the TPB this variable is behavioural intention, while in PMT it is labelled protection motivation, although Prentice-Dunn and Rogers (1986) state that protection motivation is most appropriately assessed by behavioural intention measures. The other social cognition models considered here do not include a measure of behavioural intention, although a number of researchers have called for the addition of behavioural intention to the HBM to act as a mediating variable between the HBM variables and behaviour (Becker *et al.* 1977; King 1982; Calnan 1984; Norman and Fitter 1989). Finally, both the TPB and PMT also postulate a direct relationship between self-efficacy (or perceived behavioural control) and behaviour in addition to the one between intention and behaviour.

Four main conclusions can be drawn from the above comparisons. First, there is considerable overlap between the constructs included in the models. For example, most focus on outcome expectancies or the consequences of performing a behaviour. Second, some of the models may usefully be expanded to consider normative influences and perceived threat. Third, there is a strong case for including self-efficacy in all models of health behaviour. Fourth, behavioural intention may act as a mediating variable between other social cognitive variables and behaviour.

3 Future directions

While the social cognition models outlined in this book have provided an important framework for considering the social psychological determinants of health behaviour, it is clear that in some instances they only account for a small amount of the variance in health behaviour. For example, Sheppard *et al.* (1988) noted that about 10 per cent of studies using the TRA reported correlations between behavioural intentions and behaviour below 0.2. There are a number of plausible reasons for this poor predictive performance (Marteau 1989; Conner 1993; Conner and Norman 1994), which are considered below together with suggestions for new directions for research with social cognition models in health psychology. First, we outline various measurement issues surrounding the use of social cognition models to predict health behaviour. Second, the addition of new variables to the models is considered. Third, the role of past behaviour as a predictor of behaviour and its potential role as a moderator of attitude–behaviour relations is discussed. Fourth, spontaneous processing models of the relationship between social cognitive variables and behaviour are introduced. Fifth, the need to develop stage models of health behaviour is highlighted. Finally, some of the social cognitive variables that may help to translate intentions into actions are considered.

3.1 Measurement issues

Ajzen and Fishbein (1974) have highlighted the importance of measuring attitudes and behaviour at the same level of specificity in order to obtain strong correlations. In short, there is a need to match measures of attitudes and behaviour with respect to the target, the action, the time frame and the context (Ajzen and Fishbein 1977). Such considerations are likely to apply to the use of many social cognitive variables as predictors of health behaviour. The main implication of this position is that general measures of social cognitive variables are unlikely to be strong predictors of specific behaviours, but when there is a close match between social cognitive measures and the corresponding behaviour, stronger correlations are to be expected. For example, Davidson and Jaccard (1979) reported that a general measure of attitudes towards birth control was unrelated ($r = 0.08$) to women's use of birth control pills over a two year period. However, a more specific attitude measure towards birth control pills was found to correlate highly ($r = 0.57$) with the subsequent use of birth control pills. Hence, specificity may be an important issue in many studies of health behaviour and may help to account for a number of weak relationships between social cognitive variables and behaviour reported in the literature. This may be particularly relevant to studies which employ the HLC construct (Wallston *et al.* 1978). Being a generalized measure of control expectancies, it is perhaps not surprising that it has been found to be a poor predictor of specific health behaviours. In contrast, Ajzen's (1988) TPB and Bandura's (1986) SCT place a greater emphasis on the need to measure cognitions that are specific to the behaviour in question and, as a result, have generally been found to produce good predictions of specific health behaviours.

A number of researchers have focused in more detail on when and how behaviour is measured. This has important implications for the strength of the relationship between social cognitive variables and behaviour. First, there is often a large time gap between the completion of questionnaires assessing social cognitive variables and the assessment of the target behaviour (Norman 1993). This large time gap may weaken the predictive power of the social cognitive variables given that change in these variables may occur in the intervening period (Ajzen 1985), although Randall and Wolff (1994) found little evidence for a weakening of the intention–behaviour relationship over time. Second, Conner and Norman (1994) have argued that more attention should be paid to the measurement of health behaviour. Frequently behaviour is measured on a single occasion in a single context (e.g. attendance or non-attendance at a health check, use or non-use of a condom with a new sexual partner). The problems of using single-item scales to measure social psychological constructs is well known and has led to the informed use of multi-item scales. However, this psychometric principle has not been applied in general to the measurement of behaviour (Epstein 1979). Performance of a behaviour on a specific occasion may be open to a whole range of idiosyncratic influences, which may mean that the observed behaviour is atypical. This will therefore tend to underestimate the strength of the relationship between social cognitive variables and behaviour. One solution to this problem is to assess the target behaviour over several occasions or situations (Fishbein and Ajzen 1974), which coincides with Ajzen's (1988) argument that psychologists should study behavioural tendencies rather than single instances of behaviour.

A number of researchers have expressed concern with the way in which certain constructs are measured or operationalized. This concern is particularly relevant to the HBM, where a multitude of operational definitions have been used across studies, with little attention given to the reliability and validity of the measures (Champion 1984; Sheeran and Abraham, Chapter 2 in this volume). For example, Harrison *et al.* (1992) found only 16 studies out of a sample of 234 which had measured the four main dimensions of the HBM satisfactorily. The use of unreliable scales will serve to weaken correlations between social cognitive variables and behaviour.

Further interest has focused on the measurement of beliefs within the TPB, although the implications of this work are also relevant to other models. Towriss (1984) noted that respondents are normally presented with modal salient beliefs based on pilot work, following the procedures outlined by Ajzen and Fishbein (1980). However, this procedure has two main disadvantages. First, the TPB is primarily concerned with individuals' beliefs and how they relate to behaviour. The supplying of beliefs by researchers may not adequately capture the beliefs salient to the individual. For example, the researcher may present beliefs that are not salient to all individuals, or not include beliefs that are. In response to this possibility, a couple of studies have attempted to allow respondents to generate their own beliefs (Rutter and Bunce 1989; Rosin *et al.* 1992). For example, in a study on milk consumption, Rutter and Bunce (1989) found that allowing respondents to generate their own beliefs led to a better prediction of intention and current behaviour than the usual procedure of supplying modal salient beliefs, although the opposite pattern of results was found with follow-up behaviour measured eight weeks later. Some of the problems surrounding the use of modal salient beliefs has also been investigated by van der Pligt and Eiser (1984). They noted that in some studies respondents have been presented with in excess of 20 belief statements to rate. This is despite evidence from cognitive psychology which suggests that individuals have quite poor information processing capabilities and are therefore very unlikely to consider all the presented beliefs when making their decisions. Van der Pligt and Eiser (1984) argued that researchers should investigate the beliefs that are most salient to specific individuals or groups and put forward a variant of the usual procedure for assessing beliefs. They suggested that when respondents are presented with a common set of beliefs to rate, they should also be asked to indicate the personally most salient beliefs. Budd (1986) followed this approach when looking at students' attitudes towards cigarette smoking. In this study respondents were presented with 18 belief items to rate and were then asked to choose the five most salient beliefs to them. It was found that belief–attitude correlations with the five most salient beliefs were stronger ($r = 0.62$) than correlations with the 13 least salient beliefs ($r = 0.07$).

A second problem with the use of modal salient beliefs concerns the actual elicitation procedure. Sparks (1994) argues that asking a pilot sample of respondents to generate the possible consequences, or advantages and disadvantages, of performing a behaviour may lead to a biased set of belief items. In particular, it is argued that this procedure may lead to the elicitation of predominantly cognitive influences on behaviour as these are more easily articulated. As a result, other influences (e.g. affective, moral) on behaviour may not be assessed even though they may be important determinants of behaviour.

Another point worth noting is that tests of the models outlined in this book are typically based on 'between-subjects' comparisons; that is, individuals who have a positive attitude towards performing a behaviour are seen to be more likely than other individuals, who have a less positive attitude, to perform the behaviour in question. However, while this type of analysis may be useful in distinguishing between individuals who do or do not perform a behaviour, it tells us very little about how *individuals* come to their decisions. Instead, a number of authors have argued that a more appropriate type of analysis is to consider individuals' attitudes towards other competing actions (e.g. Schuman 1972; Davidson and Morrison 1983; Fishbein *et al.* 1986; Sheppard *et al.* 1988; van den Putte 1993). Thus, it is not the strength of one's attitude towards performing a behaviour that is important, but its relative strength in relation to attitudes towards other competing actions. For example, Michelle may have a positive attitude towards going to the gym on a Monday evening (which is more positive than other respondents' attitudes), but she may have an even more positive attitude towards watching football on television with friends in a bar. Not only is a 'within-subjects' analysis likely to lead to a better prediction of behaviour, it is also more in line with the (often implicit) assumption that individuals are faced with behavioural alternatives when considering whether or not to perform a behaviour and it is the choice between these alternatives which determines behaviour. For example, Ajzen and Fishbein (1980) argue that when a behaviour represents a choice between two or more alternatives, the components of the TRA and the TPB should be assessed in relation to each alternative.

There are few studies that have attempted to compare between- and within-subjects approaches to the analysis of attitude data. Davidson and Morrison (1983), for example, compared these approaches when considering the determinants of contraceptive behaviour. The attitudes of 349 married couples towards four contraceptive methods (oral, IUD, diaphragm, condoms) were assessed and related to contraceptive behaviour over a one-year period. The within-subjects analysis was found to produce significantly stronger predictions of contraceptive behaviour than the between-subjects analysis. Similar results have been reported by Ajzen and Driver (1992) in relation to leisure time exercise behaviour.

Assessing individuals' beliefs and attitudes towards the full range of behavioural alternatives in each context may result in an unacceptably long questionnaire or interview schedule. Another possible approach taken by some researchers has been to assess respondents' attitudes towards a restricted number of behavioural alternatives. This may simply involve assessing respondents' attitudes towards performing or not performing the behaviour or towards two clear alternatives (Fishbein *et al.* 1986; Raats 1992; Shepherd *et al.* 1993; van den Putte 1993). For example, Shepherd *et al.* (1993) examined people's attitudes towards two flavoured milks and found the attitude–intention correlation to be higher ($r = 0.73$) when differential scores were used (e.g. the difference between the attitudes towards the two milks) than when separate attitude–intentions correlations were considered for each milk separately ($rs = 0.53, 0.58$). Raats (1992) has reported similar results when considering attitudes towards milk of different fat contents.

3.2 New variables

A range of additional social cognitive variables have been suggested as potential predictors of health behaviour, including self-predictions, moral norms, anticipated regret and self-identity. The case for each of these variables is considered in turn.

First, Sheppard *et al.* (1988) have argued for the need to consider both behavioural intentions and self-predictions when predicting behaviour. This argument stems from the work of Warshaw and Davis (1985), which focused on the measurement of behavioural intentions. They noted a number of different ways in which this construct had been measured, and distinguished measures of behavioural intentions (e.g. 'I intend to perform behaviour x') from measures of self-predictions (e.g. 'How likely is it that you will perform behaviour x?'). This distinction is important when considering the prediction of health behaviour, because while, for example, David might intend to take up regular exercise, he might also think that it is unlikely that he will do so. Sheppard *et al.* (1988) went on to argue that self-predictions should provide better predictions of behaviour as they are likely to include a consideration of those factors which may facilitate or inhibit performance of a behaviour as well as a consideration of the likely choice of other competing behaviours. The results of Sheppard *et al.*'s (1988) meta-analysis of the TRA support this view; measures of self-predictions were found to have stronger relationships with behaviour than behavioural intention measures. However, Norman and Smith (1995) found no difference in the extent to which the two measures correlated with exercise behaviour. Furthermore, they noted that the measures of behavioural intentions and self-predictions were moderately correlated, suggesting that while it may be possible to make the conceptual distinction between behavioural intentions and self-predictions, the discriminant validity for the concepts may be weak. Clearly, more work is needed to disentangle further these and other related constructs, such as planning and commitment (Bagozzi 1992, 1993).

Second, a number of researchers have argued that in addition to assessing the perceived social pressures to perform a behaviour, as in the TRA, attention should also be paid to the influence of personal, or moral, norms (that is, the individual's perception of the moral correctness or incorrectness of performing a behaviour) (Ajzen 1991; Sparks 1994). Moral norms should have an important influence on the performance of those behaviours which can be seen to have a moral or ethical dimension (Gorsuch and Ortberg 1983; Beck and Ajzen 1991). A number of studies have found measures of moral norms to be predictive of blood donating behaviour (Pomazal and Jaccard 1976; Zuckerman and Reiss 1978) as well as intentions to donate organs (Schwartz and Tessler 1972), eat genetically produced food (Sparks *et al.* 1995a), buy milk (Raats 1992), and commit driving violations (Parker *et al.* 1995). The above research suggests that studies focusing on the prediction of health behaviours that may have important moral or ethical considerations may be enhanced by the inclusion of variables tapping moral norms.

Third, anticipated feelings associated with the performance or nonperformance of a behaviour may also be an important determinant of behaviour (Triandis 1977), especially in situations where the consequences of performing or not performing the behaviour are unpleasant or negatively affectively laden. Recent research has focused on the influence of anticipated regret (Richard and van der Pligt 1991; Richard *et al.* 1993; Parker *et al.* 1995). It is argued that if an individual anticipates feeling regret after performing a behaviour then he/she will be unlikely to perform the behaviour. Richard and van der Pligt (1991) investigated the role of anticipated regret in relation to condom use among adolescents and found such feelings to be an important predictor of previous behaviour. In a more recent study, Richard *et al.* (1993) examined the influence of anticipated regret on subsequent behaviour. Participants in their experiment were asked to either focus on their anticipated feelings following safe and unsafe sexual behaviour or on their present feelings about these behaviours. At follow-up, participants in the anticipated feelings condition were more likely to have used condoms in casual sexual encounters in the intervening five months. This study suggests that anticipated feelings may have an important influence on behaviour. However, in terms of developing social cognition models of health behaviour it is possible to argue that such anticipated affective reactions may be incorporated into constructs that focus on the consequences of behaviour (e.g. behavioural beliefs in the TPB).

Fourth, the concept of self-identity has been put forward as a potential predictor of behaviour (Biddle *et al.* 1987; Charng *et al.* 1988; Eagly and Chaiken 1993). For example, it can be argued that the extent to which an individual thinks of him or herself as a 'healthy eater' should predict his or her dietary intentions and behaviour. In support of this argument, Sparks and Shepherd (1992) found that respondents who thought of themselves as 'green consumers' had stronger intentions to consume organic vegetables. Sparks (1994) noted that self-identity may simply be a proxy for past behaviour, although Sparks and Shepherd (1992) found that the relationship between self-identity and future intentions remained when past consumption of organic vegetables was controlled for. Self-identity as someone who is concerned about the health consequences of one's diet has also been related to intentions to reduce fat consumption (Sparks *et al.* 1995b), although in an earlier study Sparks *et al.* (1992) failed to find an independent effect for self-identity. Future work needs to assess the influence of self-identity across a range of behaviours. As with the consideration of moral norms, it may be the case that self-identity is only important in a restricted range of situations.

3.3 The role of past behaviour

The role of past behaviour with regard to current behaviour in social cognition models is an issue that has attracted a great deal of attention in the literature. In short, it is argued that many health behaviours are determined not by social cognitive variables, as outlined in this book, but rather by one's previous behaviour. This argument is based on the results of a number of studies showing past behaviour to be the best predictor of future behaviour. For example, Mullen *et al.* (1987) used the TRA and the HBM to examine changes in the consumption of sweet and fried foods, smoking behaviour and exercise behaviour over an eight-month period. In each case, initial behaviour was found to be the strongest predictor of later behaviour. Similar results have been reported in relation to drug use (Bentler and Speckhart 1979), exercise (Valois *et al.* 1988; Godin *et al.* 1993; Norman and Smith 1995), attendance at health checks (Norman and Conner 1994) and seat belt use (Sutton and Hallett 1989). Such results have led some researchers to call for past behaviour to be considered as an independent predictor of future behaviour (Bentler and Speckhart 1979; Fredricks and Dossett 1983).

However, there are problems with this position. Ajzen (1988) has argued that the effects of past behaviour on future behaviour should be mediated by the variables included in social cognition models; past behaviour shapes individuals' beliefs about the behaviour in question, and it is these cognitions that determine subsequent behaviour. In particular, Ajzen (1988) has suggested that the effect of past behaviour in the TPB should primarily be mediated by the perceived behavioural control construct, which is consistent with Bandura's (1986) claim that past behaviour provides an important source of information about a person's sense of control. Thus, past behaviour is only important to the extent to which it influences social cognitive variables, which in turn determine behaviour. When past behaviour is found to have a direct effect on future behaviour it is because key social cognitive variables have not been considered (Ajzen 1991).

Even when all the relevant social cognitive variables have been considered it is likely that past behaviour will still have a small, independent, effect on future behaviour. This is because measures of past and future behaviour are likely to have common method variance not shared by the social cognitive variables (Ajzen, 1991). In short, while the social cognitive variables are likely to be assessed via questionnaires, behaviour may be assessed by observation at both time points. Even when behaviour is assessed by self-report questionnaires, the response format is likely to be different from those used to measure the social cognitive variables. As a result, the strength of the relationship between measures of past and future behaviour may be inflated.

Ajzen (1987) has further argued that past behaviour cannot be considered as a causal factor in the same way as social cognitive variables as it has no independent, explanatory value. Arguing from a trait perspective, he states that when 'the "trait" used to predict a behavior is the tendency to perform that very behavior, its explanatory power is completely lost' (p. 41). For example, Robin is unlikely to go jogging tomorrow *because* he went jogging today. When past behaviour is seen to have an independent effect on future behaviour, it is usually explained by reference to habit. Repeated performance of a behaviour is believed to lead to the formation of a habit. Behaviour at follow-up is therefore seen to be habitual in nature and, as such, is not seen to require the mediation of social cognitive variables.

Despite the predictive power of past behaviour and the reference to habit, few social cognition models have attempted to incorporate habit as a predictor variable. A notable exception is the Triandis (1977) attitude–behaviour model, which states that behaviour is a function of three key variables: intention, facilitating conditions and habit. In particular, Triandis (1977) argues that it is possible to make a distinction between habitual behaviour and intentional behaviour and that, for relatively novel behaviours, behaviour will be primarily determined by intention, while for repeated behaviours, behaviour will be primarily determined by habit. A similar position has been put forward by Ronis *et al.* (1989), who made the distinction between habits and decisions, arguing that the performance of repeated behaviour is determined by habit rather than by social cognitive variables. For example, Dishman (1982) distinguished between the initiation and maintenance of behaviour in relation to clinical exercise programmes and found that only the initiation of exercise behaviour was predicted by social cognitive variables. So, given that many health behaviours are repeated over time, it is possible to argue that habit may have a major role to play in the prediction of health behaviour.

According to Ronis *et al.* (1989), habits are automatic in nature; when a behaviour is habitual, its performance does not require conscious thought. It is therefore important to disentangle the influences of habit and past behaviour. Triandis (1977) suggests that habit should be simply measured as the number of times the behaviour has been performed in the past by the individual. However, as Ajzen (1991), argues, past behaviour cannot be taken as a valid measure of habit. Past behaviour may lead to habitual responses so that behaviour is performed without conscious thought, or alternatively it may lead to reasoned responses where, for example, past behaviour can be used to provide information about the ease or difficulty of performing a behaviour. Ronis *et al.* (1989) suggest that measures of habit need to be developed that show discriminant validity with respect to frequency of past behaviour. Measures of habit need to focus on the special characteristics of habitual responses; for example, the lack of conscious thought.

Finally, Sutton (1994) has proposed that a distinction should be made between habits and routines, arguing that many health behaviours which are commonly considered to be habitual in nature may be more appropriately considered as routines. Sutton (1994) describes a routine as a sequence of behaviours which is repeated on a regular basis. However, what distinguishes them from habits is their need to be supported by self-reminders. For example, going jogging every morning may appear habitual in nature, but it is not performed without conscious thought. Instead, it requires repeated self-reminders to maintain the behaviour. Sutton's (1994) analysis suggests that many repeated health behaviours are most appropriately considered as routines which require some amount of conscious thought to maintain them.

In summary, more work is needed to outline the influences of past behaviour on current and future behaviour. It may be possible to make the distinction between occasions when the influence of past behaviour is mediated by social cognitive variables and those occasions when it is seen to have a direct influence via habitual responses. In particular, future work should develop measures of habit that are discriminable from frequency of past behaviour and outline the processes through which habit determines behaviour.

3.4 Spontaneous processing models

One important implication of Ronis et al.'s (1989) distinction between habits and decisions is the suggestion that social cognition models may only predict health behaviour under certain conditions. This issue has been studied in detail by Fazio (1990) in the development of a spontaneous processing model of the attitude–behaviour relationship. As Fazio (1990) notes, the main social cognition models all view the individual as an essentially rational decision-maker who systematically uses and deliberates upon available information to form a behavioural intention. For example, in the HBM the individual is believed to perform a cost–benefit analysis of the pros and cons of performing a behaviour. Similarly, in the TPB the individual is seen to consider the various consequences of performing a behaviour. These models can therefore be labelled as deliberative process-ing models as they assume that, to some extent, behaviour results from a process of cognitive deliberation. However, Fazio (1990) argues that individuals may only make a behavioural decision in such a manner when they have the opportunity and motivation to do so (see also Kruglanski 1989). The implication of this position is that social cognitive variables will only predict behaviour in the way outlined in the models presented in this book when these conditions are met (Sanbonmatsu and Fazio 1990); under other conditions, it is argued that behaviour may be determined by highly accessible attitudes in a spontaneous fashion (Fazio et al. 1989).

Fazio (1990) has outlined a spontaneous processing model of the atti-tude–behaviour relationship to account for the way in which attitudes may have an impact on relatively spontaneous behaviour which is not mediated by the deliberate processing of information. Fazio uses the distinction between attitudes towards objects or targets and attitudes towards beha-viours, and argues that it is the former that are important in determining behaviour via spontaneous processing. According to the spontaneous processing model, an attitude towards an object/target may be *automatically* activated from memory following the presentation of relevant cues, with the likelihood of activation determined by the accessibility of the attitude. Attitude accessibility is, in turn, a function of the strength of the relationship between the attitude object and its evaluation in memory. Once activated, the attitude shapes the perception of the attitude object in an automatic, attitude-congruent, fashion. For example, if a positive attitude is activated then this will lead the individual to attend to and notice the positive qual-ities of the attitude object. This automatic process of selective percep-tion will therefore shape the individual's definition of the event, and thus determine behaviour. For example, if the event is defined on the basis of positive perceptions of the attitude object then approach behaviours will follow. In addition, it is argued that normative guidelines (e.g. social norms or rules) may also influence the definition of the event and thus may help to determine behaviour in some situations.

One important feature of the spontaneous processing model is that it outlines one way in which social cognitive variables (i.e. highly accessible attitudes) may determine behaviour *without* systematic deliberation. To date, there has been little research on Fazio's model, although it has been successfully shown that the accessibility of relevant attitudes influences the strength of the relationship between attitudes and behaviour (Fazio and Williams 1986) and that highly accessible attitudes can lead to selective perception (Fazio and Williams 1986; Houston and Fazio 1989). Both these findings are consistent with the spontaneous processing model.

The distinction made by Fazio (1990) between deliberative and spontaneous models of behaviour has clear overlaps with recent work on attitude change and the processing of persuasive communications. For example, Petty and Cacioppo (1986), in their elaboration likelihood model, argue that there is a central route and a peripheral route to persuasion which can be distinguished by the amount of issue-relevant thinking that occurs in response to a persuasive communication. Chaiken *et al.* (1989) have made a similar distinction between systematic and heuristic processing of information. It has been argued that the depth of processing is determined by the individual's motivation and ability to process persuasive communications systematically (Petty and Cacioppo 1986). Similarly, Ronis *et al.* (1989) suggest that conscious decision-making (i.e. deliberate, central or systematic processing of information) is more likely to occur in novel situations or in familiar situations when new problems arise.

The above work has important implications for the use of social cognition models to predict health behaviour. The social cognition models outlined in this book can be viewed as deliberative processing models inasmuch as they focus on the conscious processing of information and fail to consider more spontaneous or automatic influences on behaviour. For this reason, current social cognition models may provide only a partial account of the social cognitive determinants of behaviour. In short, they may only be applicable in situations where the individual has the ability and motivation to engage in such deliberative processing of information (Conner 1993). For many behavioural decisions, simplified or spontaneous decision-making rules may be employed instead (Norman and Conner 1993). Fazio's (1990) spontaneous model has considerable potential in helping to provide a full account of the cognitive influences on behaviour. However, it is clear that most of the empirical work to date has focused on issues surrounding the activation of attitudes and their influence on perception; later components of the model have received less attention (Stroebe and Stroebe 1995).

3.5 Stage models of health behaviour

As argued in the previous section, the main social cognition models can be characterized as deliberative models of health behaviour and, as such, are primarily concerned with the influences on people's decisions to perform health behaviours. However, recent work has suggested that there may be qualitatively different stages in the initiation and maintenance of health behaviour, and that to obtain a full understanding of the determinants of health behaviour it is necessary to conduct a detailed analysis of the nature of these stages. From a social cognitive perspective, an important implication of this position is that different cognitions may be important at different stages in promoting health behaviour.

One of the first stage models was put forward by Prochaska and DiClemente (1984) in their transtheoretical model of change. While initially developed in relation to addictive behaviour, their model has been widely applied to analyse the process of change in alcoholism treatment (DiClemente and Hughes 1990), smoking cessation (DiClemente *et al.* 1991), head injury rehabilitation (Lam *et al.* 1988) and psychotherapy (McConnaughly *et al.* 1989). In its most recent form DiClemente *et al.* (1991) identify five stages of change: pre-contemplation, contemplation, preparation, action and maintenance. Individuals are seen to progress through each of the stages in order to achieve successful maintenance of a new behaviour. Taking the example of smoking cessation, it is argued that in the pre-contemplation stage the smoker is unaware that his or her behaviour constitutes a problem and therefore has no intention to quit. In the contemplation stage the smoker starts to think about changing his or her behaviour, but as yet is not committed to try to quit. It is in the preparation stage that the smoker has an intention to quit and starts to make plans about how to quit. The action stage is characterized by active attempts to quit and after six months of successful abstinence the individual moves into the maintenance stage, which is characterized by attempts to prevent relapse and to consolidate the newly acquired non-smoking status.

Heckhausen (1991) has identified four phases in the initiation and maintenance of behaviour: the pre-decisional, post-decisional, actional and evaluative phases, which follow a similar progressive sequence to that outlined by Prochaska and DiClemente (1984). It is further suggested that different types of cognitions are important in each of these phases. So in the pre-decisional phase, cognitions about the desirability and feasibility of the behaviour are believed to be important determinants of a desire to perform the behaviour in question. This phase ends with the formation of an intention to change. In contrast, the decisional phase focuses on the development of plans and ends with the successful initiation of the behaviour. In the actional phase the individual focuses on effectively achieving performance of the behaviour and ends with the conclusion of the behaviour. In the final, evaluative, phase the individual compares achieved outcomes with initial goals in order to regulate and maintain behaviour. While this four-phase model of behaviour was not developed specifically for the prediction of health behaviour, the potential of its application to this area is clear.

Other stage models have recently been developed, including the health action process approach (Schwarzer 1992; Schwarzer and Fuchs, Chapter 6 in this volume), the precaution-adoption process (Weinstein 1988; Weinstein and Sandman 1992) and goal setting theory (Bagozzi 1992, 1993). There are two important themes running through each of the stage models. First, they all emphasize a temporal perspective such that there are different stages of behaviour change. While the models postulate different numbers of stages, they all follow the same basic pattern from a pre-contemplation stage through a motivation stage to the initiation and maintenance of behaviour. The important point to make is that these models are dynamic in nature; people move from one stage to another over time. Second, these stage models imply that different cognitions are important at different stages (Sandman and Weinstein 1993). For example, in the earlier stages information may be processed about the costs and benefits of performing a behaviour, while in the later stages cognitions become more focused on the development of plans of action to initiate and support the maintenance of a behaviour. Clearly, a detailed analysis of the social cognitive variables that are important in encouraging movement through the various stages is required to provide a full account of the determinants of health behaviour.

3.6 Volitional processes

The main social cognition models of health behaviour can be seen to be primarily concerned with people's motivations to perform a health behaviour and, as such, can be considered to provide strong predictions of behavioural intentions (e.g. the end of a motivation stage). Ajzen (1991), for example, reports an average multiple correlation of 0.71 between variables in the TPB and behavioural intention. However, strong intentions do not always lead to corresponding actions. Studies examining the intention–behaviour relationship have reported a wide range of correlations. In their meta-analysis of the TRA, Sheppard *et al.* (1988) reported intention–behaviour correlations ranging from 0.10 to 0.94. It is clear that many people who intend to perform a behaviour fail to do so. However, the social cognition models considered in this book generally do not directly address the issue of translating intentions into action. They can be conceptualized as relatively static models that stop at the formation of an intention; they do not go on to distinguish between intenders who become performers and those who do not. As Bagozzi (1993) argues, the variables outlined in the main social cognition models are necessary, but not sufficient, determinants of behaviour. In other words, they can provide good predictions of people's intentions (or motivation) to perform a health behaviour, but not their actual behaviour. In this section we consider the social cognitive variables that are seen to be important in translating intentions into action. This constitutes a move away from a concentration on motivational processes to a consideration of volitional processes (Kuhl and Beckman 1985).

At present, relatively little detailed attention has focused on the cognitive processes underlying the successful implementation of intentions. The main social cognition models contain few measures that account for the intention–behaviour gap (Abraham and Sheeran 1993). The TPB attempts to do this by proposing a direct link between perceived behavioural control and behaviour. Thus, people's perceptions about the amount of control they have over a behaviour influence the likely performance of behaviour independently of their intentions, although this is only seen to apply when perceived behavioural control reflects actual control. Self-efficacy is similarly able to predict behaviour independently of intention and has been related to planning, effort and persistence (Bandura 1989), all activities that are likely to increase the likelihood of successful enactment of an intention. However, it is clear that a more detailed analysis of the volitional processes underlying health behaviour is required, and a number of researchers have started to focus attention on this issue (e.g. Kuhl 1985; Weinstein 1988; Schwarzer 1992). In the rest of this section we concentrate on Gollwitzer's (1993) work on implementation intentions and Bagozzi and Warshaw's (1990) theory of trying, in order to highlight the social cognitive variables that may be important in the initiation and maintenance of behaviour.

Gollwitzer (1993) made the distinction between goal intentions and implementation intentions. While the former is concerned with intentions to perform a behaviour or achieve a goal (i.e. 'I intend to achieve x'), the latter is concerned with plans as to when, where and how the goal intention is to be translated into behaviour (i.e. 'I intend to initiate the goal-directed behaviour x when situation y is encountered'). The important point about implementation intentions is that they commit the individual to a specific course of action when certain environmental conditions are met; in so doing they help to translate goal intentions into action. Take the example of going swimming: an individual may have the intention to go swimming, but this may not be translated into behaviour if he or she does not have an implementation intention which specifies when, where and how he or she will go swimming. Gollwitzer (1993) argues that by making implementation intentions individuals pass over control to the environment. The environment therefore acts as a cue to action, such that when certain conditions are met, the performance of the intended behaviour follows. These ideas have similarities with Weinstein's (1988) 'messy desk' analogy, whereby people may have intentions to achieve a number of goals (i.e. 'projects') which get 'lost' on the 'messy desk'. Which project is actually worked upon is determined by environmental factors in a similar way, as outlined by Gollwitzer (1993).

Gollwitzer (1993) has compiled a range of experimental evidence to support the view that the making of implementation intentions can aid the performance of intended behaviour. To date, Gollwitzer's (1993) ideas have not been applied to the prediction of health behaviour, although an exception is a study by Orbell and Hodgkins (1994) on breast self-examination among female undergraduates. At the end of a question-naire about breast self-examination, half the women were asked to indicate when and where in the next month they intended to perform breast self-examination. A one-month follow-up found that 64 per cent of these women had performed breast self-examination that month compared with only 16 per cent of women who hadn't made an implementation intention, despite no difference in goal intentions. This suggests that the making of an implementation intention can significantly increase the likely performance of a behaviour. In an earlier study on exercise behaviour, Kendzierski (1990) found that respondents were more likely to implement their intentions to exercise when they had engaged in some prior planning. Further work needs to be conducted to establish the utility of implementation intentions in predicting health behaviour. However, initial findings are encouraging and suggest that those who make such plans of action are more likely to initiate and maintain behaviour.

Gollwitzer's (1993) work is important in that it identifies one way in which goal intentions may be translated into behaviour. A similar, but more comprehensive, approach has been put forward by Bagozzi and Warshaw (1990) in their theory of trying. They focus on goal-directed behaviour and argue that to initiate behaviour an individual needs first to form an 'intention to try' to achieve his or her desired goal. Once an intention to try has been formed, the individual then focuses on the means, or instru-mental acts, by which he or she will attempt to achieve the desired goal. Considering the example of condom use, a number of instrumental acts can be identified, including buying condoms, carrying them, raising con-dom use with a new sexual partner and so on. Bagozzi (1993) argues that for each of these instrumental acts, three appraisal tasks are performed. First, the individual considers the extent to which he or she is confident that he or she could perform the instrumental act (i.e. specific self-efficacies). Second, the likelihood that the instrumental act will help in achieving the desired goal is assessed (i.e. instrumental beliefs). Third, the individual considers his or her affective response towards the instrumental act (i.e. affect towards means). So, individuals are likely to engage in goal-directed behaviour if they can identify instrumental acts that they believe will lead to goal achievement, that they are confident they can perform and that they feel positive towards.

Once an individual initiates efforts to achieve a goal, there are a number of cognitive activities that can support the successful initiation and main-tenance of goal-directed behaviour. First, the individual can develop plans in order to ensure that instrumental acts are performed. This involves identifying the situation or triggering conditions under which the instru-mental act is performed (Bagozzi and Warshaw 1990). This idea that cer-tain environmental conditions may trigger behaviour has a clear overlap with Gollwitzer's (1993) work on implementation intentions and Weinstein's (1988) 'messy desk' analogy. One way in which plans are more likely to be acted upon is through the development of scripts, or cognitive rehearsal, whereby the individual imagines him or herself performing the instrumental act (Anderson 1983). Bagozzi (1993) also proposes that ongoing behaviour has to be monitored to ensure, for example, that the instrumental acts achieve their objectives. If any unforeseen impediments are encountered then these need to be taken into consideration and any future plans modified accordingly. These ideas overlap with Kuhl's (1985) theory of action control, which identifies seven aspects of the action control process. Finally, goal-directed behaviour is likely to be stronger and more persistent if the individual has a strong sense of commitment to both the decision to try to achieve the goal and the means to achieve it.

To date, Bagozzi and Warshaw's (1990) theory of trying has not been fully operationalized or tested, although Bagozzi (1993) reviews a number of studies that have produced support for different aspects of the theory. However, it is clear that the variables outlined above are likely to be important in helping individuals to translate their intentions into action. While developed in relation to consumer behaviour, the theory has important implications for the understanding of volitional processes underlying health behaviour.

The above review highlights one way in which the main social cognition models can be seen to fall short of a full account of the social cognitive determinants of health behaviour. In short, the formation of a behavioural intention may not be sufficient for the successful enactment of behaviour. In many cases, further cognitive activity is required to ensure that intentions are translated into action. This may involve the consideration of potential instrumental acts and the formation of implementation intentions. In addition, ongoing behaviour needs to be monitored and evaluated to ensure the successful behavioural enactment.

4 Future directions for social cognition models of health behaviour

The work reviewed in this chapter can be seen to have three important ramifications for the future development of social cognition models of health behaviour. First, there may be a restricted number of key predictors of health behaviour given the substantial overlap between many of the constructs contained within the main social cognition models. Second, there is a need to develop further stage models of the contemplation, initiation and maintenance of behaviour, with particular emphasis on the cognitions that aid the translation of intentions into behaviour. Third, behaviour is not always guided by cognitive variables in the way envisaged by the main social cognition models. As a result, there is a need to develop spontaneous processing models of behaviour and to identify the conditions under which behaviour is determined by spontaneous and deliberative processes. In this section we outline possible directions for the future development of an integrative social cognition model of health behaviour and in doing so outline some of the basic requirements for such a model.

It is clear that in order fully to explain health behaviour it is necessary to develop a more dynamic approach that examines different stages or phases in the contemplation, initiation and maintenance of behaviour. Though the stage models considered in this chapter have suggested differing numbers of stages, it is likely that an integrative model should address at least four or five main stages. First, there is the *pre-contemplation* stage during which the individual is not thinking about the performance of a new health behaviour. This stage may be brought to an end by various cues to action which cause the individual to start thinking about adopting a new behaviour. The second stage is a decision-making or *motivation* stage in which the individual thinks about the pros and cons of performing a new behaviour. This stage is brought to an end by the formation of an intention. In the third stage, the *planning* stage, the individual is concerned with the making of plans to initiate behaviour. This stage is brought to an end by the successful initiation of behaviour. The fourth stage is an *action* stage in which the individual is concerned with monitoring and controlling behaviour. This stage ends with the successful completion of behaviour. Finally, for ongoing behaviours there is a *maintenance* stage in which the individual is concerned with ensuring that the behaviour is successfully repeated, as in the fourth stage.

One implication of the identification of different stages is that different cognitive variables may be important in ensuring movement from one stage to the next. In the first stage the individual is not thinking about making a change to his or her behaviour. However, this stage may be brought to an end by a range of cues to action, as outlined in the HBM, which may motivate the individual to start thinking about performing a health-related behaviour. One such cue to action may be perceived threat (i.e. perceived susceptibility and perceived severity). While perceived susceptibility and perceived severity are seen to be important determinants of behaviour in the HBM, research with these dimensions has tended to show that they are relatively weak predictors of behaviour. However, as Schwarzer (1992) has argued, it may be more appropriate to consider these variables to have an indirect, or more distal, influence on behaviour. Thus they may act as a cue to action, motivating the individual to start deliberating over performing a health-related behaviour, and thus ensuring movement from the first to the second stage.

In the second stage, the individual is thinking about adopting a new behaviour, and the stage ends when the individual forms an intention to perform the behaviour. To date, most social cognition models have been primarily concerned with this stage. As highlighted earlier, these models may be tapping overlapping constructs. In short, it may be possible to distinguish between three distinct determinants of individuals' intentions to perform a health behaviour. First are outcome expectancies, as outlined in SCT, which focus on the perceived consequences of performing a behaviour. These expectancies may also cover the notion of behavioural beliefs as considered in the TPB and include anticipated affective reactions.

Second are normative influences which are primarily tapped by the subjective norm and normative belief components of the TPB. This group of variables could also include moral norms and perceived social support. The third influence on individuals' intentions to perform a behaviour is self-efficacy. This variable would supersede the construct of perceived behavioural control from the TPB and may be based on a consideration of perceived barriers (HBM) and control beliefs (TPB). In the motivation stage, it is likely that other variables may have a more distal influence on behavioural intention via the variables outlined above. For example, health locus of control beliefs may help to shape self-efficacy expectancies, self-identity and health value may influence the interpretation of the potential consequences of a behaviour, and past behaviour or experience may provide information which is used to determine the ease or difficulty of performing a behaviour (i.e. self-efficacy).

Once a behavioural intention has been formed, it has to be translated into behaviour. In the third stage the individual is therefore concerned with planning; focusing on the specific actions, or instrumental acts, that need to be performed and the resources required to support them. Thus, a number of authors have highlighted the importance of action plans in this stage (Bagozzi and Warshaw 1990; Schwarzer 1992). Similarly, Gollwitzer (1993) focuses on implementation intentions which help to ensure performance of the target behaviour. Despite slight differences between definitions of these two concepts, both emphasize the need to construct fairly detailed plans of action in order to bridge the intention–behaviour gap. As Schwarzer (1992) argues, self-efficacy may have an important role to play in the development and implementation of such plans, as might self-identity (Sparks and Shepherd 1992) and a sense of commitment (Bagozzi 1993). The planning stage is brought to an end when the individual initiates behaviour.

In the fourth stage the individual has to ensure that the behaviour is successfully enacted. Various cognitive processes which are concerned with the monitoring of behaviour may be important in this stage. Schwarzer (1992), for example, highlights the need for action control in which the behaviour is re-evaluated against initial goals in order to regulate and maintain behaviour (see also Bagozzi and Warshaw 1990; Heckhausen 1991). As with the development of action plans, self-efficacy, self-identity and commitment may all be important variables in ensuring that behaviour is maintained. In addition, Kuhl (1981, 1985) has argued that there may be individual differences in people's propensity to engage in monitoring activities that may account for why behaviour is not always maintained. These monitoring activities help to ensure that the behaviour is successfully completed, and the same activities will be important in the maintenance stage for ongoing behaviours.

The above analysis of the social cognitive variables that may be important over the various stages of health behaviour adoption constitutes the basic components of a deliberative model of health behaviour. However, such a model may only be applicable when individuals are motivated and have the opportunity to engage in the systematic processing of information. In many cases, though, health behaviour may be more automatic or spontaneous in nature. It is therefore necessary also to focus on the spontaneous processes that may influence behaviour. One such model of spontaneous processing has been put forward by Fazio (1990), in which it is argued that certain cognitions (i.e. highly accessible attitudes) may guide behaviour through the selective perception and interpretation of a situation. This process is seen to be automatic and not to involve any conscious deliberations about the pros and cons of performing a behaviour. Highly accessible attitudes are likely to result from frequent and direct experience with the attitude object. As a result, certain environmental cues may trigger behaviour in a spontaneous manner through the activation of highly accessible attitudes. In this way, there may be a direct route from cues to action to behaviour. Clearly, further detailed work is needed on such spontaneous influences on behaviour if a full understanding of the social cognitive determinants of health behaviour is to be developed.

5 Conclusion

Over the past few decades there has been an ever increasing interest in social cognition models as predictors of health behaviour. This work has provided many insights into the determinants of people's motivations to adopt a whole range of health-related behaviours. We believe the challenge for future work in this area is two-fold: first, to develop, operationalize and test stage models of the contemplation, initiation and maintenance of behaviour; second, to outline the processes that may underlie a more spontaneous or automatic route to health behaviour. With these two goals in mind, and with the clear importance of health behaviour to morbidity and mortality, future research on social cognition models is likely to continue to attract considerable interest from researchers and health professionals alike.

References

Abraham, C. and Sheeran, P. (1993) Inferring cognitions, predicting behaviour: two challenges for social cognition models, *Health Psychology Update*, 14, 18–23.

Ajzen, I. (1985) From intention to actions: a theory of planned behavior. In J. Kuhl and J. Beckman (eds) *Action Control: from Cognitions to Behavior*. New York: Springer-Verlag, 11–39.

Ajzen, I. (1987) Attitudes, traits and actions: dispositional prediction of behavior in personality and social psychology. In L. Berkowitz (ed.) *Advances in Experimental Social Psychology, Volume 20*. New York: Academic Press, 1–64.

Ajzen, I. (1988) *Attitudes, Personality and Behavior*. Buckingham: Open University Press.

Ajzen, I. (1991) The theory of planned behavior, *Organizational Behavior and Human Decision Processes*, 50, 179–211.

Ajzen, I. and Driver, B.L. (1992) Prediction of leisure participation from behavioral, normative, and control beliefs: an application of the theory of planned behavior, *Leisure Sciences*, **13**, 185–204.

Ajzen, I. and Fishbein, M. (1974) Factors influencing intentions and the intention–behavior relation, *Human Relations*, **27**, 1–15.

Ajzen, I. and Fishbein, M. (1977) Attitude–behavior relations: a theoretical analysis and review of empirical research, *Psychological Bulletin*, **84**, 888–918.

Ajzen, I. and Fishbein, M. (1980) *Understanding Attitudes and Predicting Social Behavior*. Englewood Cliffs, NJ: Prentice-Hall.

Anderson, C.A. (1983) Imagination and expectation: the effect of imagining behavioral scripts on personal intentions, *Journal of Personality and Social Psychology*, **45**, 293–305.

Bagozzi, R.P. (1992) The self-regulation of attitudes, intentions and behaviour, *Social Psychology Quarterly*, **55**, 178–204.

Bagozzi, R.P. (1993) On the neglect of volition in consumer research: a critique and proposal, *Psychology and Marketing*, **10**, 215–37.

Bagozzi, R.P. and Warshaw, P.R. (1990) Trying to consume, *Journal of Consumer Research*, **17**, 127–40.

Bakker, A.B., Buunk, A.P. and Siero, F.W. (1994) Condom use of heterosexuals: a comparison of the theory of planned behavior, the health belief model and protection motivation theory, manuscript submitted for publication.

Bandura, A. (1986) *Social Foundations of Thought and Action: a Cognitive Social Theory*. Englewood Cliffs, NJ: Prentice-Hall.

Bandura, A. (1989) Human agency in social cognitive theory, *American Psychologist*, **44**, 1175–84.

Beck, L. and Ajzen, I. (1991) Predicting dishonest actions using the theory of planned behavior, *Journal of Research in Personality*, **25**, 285–301.

Becker, M.H., Haefner, D.P., Kasl, S.V., Kirscht, J.P., Maiman, L.A. and Rosenstock, I.M. (1977) Selected psychosocial models and correlates of individual health-related behaviors, *Medical Care*, **15**, 27–46.

Bentler, P.M. and Speckhart, G. (1979) Models of attitude–behavior relations, *Psychological Review*, **86**, 452–64.

Biddle, B., Bank, B. and Slavings, R. (1987) Norms, preferences, identities and retention decisions, *Social Psychology Quarterly*, **50**, 322–37.

Budd, R.J. (1986) Predicting cigarette use: the need to incorporate measures of salience in the theory of reasoned action, *Journal of Applied Social Psychology*, **16**, 663–85.

Calnan, M. (1984) The health belief model and participation in programmes for the early detection of breast cancer, *Social Science and Medicine*, **19**, 823–30.

Champion, V.L. (1984) Instrument development of the health belief model constructs, *Advances in Nursing Science*, **6**, 73–85.

Chaiken, S., Lieberman, A. and Eagly, A.H. (1989) Heuristic and systematic information processing within and beyond the persuasion context. In J.S. Uleman and J.A. Bargh (eds) *Unintended Thought*. New York: Guilford Press, 212–52.

Charng, H.W., Piliavin, J. and Callero, P. (1988) Role identity and reasoned action in the prediction of repeated behavior, *Social Psychology Quarterly*, **51**, 303–17.

Conner, M. (1993) Pros and cons of social cognition models in health behaviour, *Health Psychology Update*, **14**, 24–31.

Conner, M. and Norman, P. (1994) Comparing the health belief model and the theory of planned behaviour in health screening. In D.R. Rutter and L. Quine (eds) *Social Psychology and Health: European Perspectives.* Aldershot: Avebury, 1–24.

Cummings, K.M., Becker, M.H. and Maile, M.C. (1980) Bringing the models together: an empirical approach to combining variables used to explain health actions, *Journal of Behavioral Medicine*, 3, 123–45.

Davidson, A.R. and Jaccard, J.J. (1979) Variables that moderate the attitude–behavior relation: results of a longitudinal survey, *Journal of Personality and Social Psychology*, 37, 1364–76.

Davidson, A.R. and Morrison, D.M. (1983) Predicting contraceptive behavior from attitudes: a comparison of within- versus across-subjects procedures, *Journal of Personality and Social Psychology*, 45, 997–1009.

DeVries, H., Dijkstra, M. and Kuhlman, P. (1988) Self-efficacy: the third factor besides attitude and subjective norm as a predictor of behavioural intentions, *Health Education Research*, 3, 273–82.

DeVries, H. and Kok, G.J. (1986) From determinants of smoking behavior to the implications for a prevention programme, *Health Education Research*, 1, 85–94.

DiClemente, C.C. and Hughes, S.O. (1990) Stages of change profiles in outpatient alcoholism treatment, *Journal of Substance Abuse*, 2, 217–35.

DiClemente, C.C., Prochaska, J.O., Fairhurst, S.K., Velicer, W.F., Velasquez, M.M. and Rossi, J.S. (1991) The process of smoking cessation: an analysis of pre-contemplation, contemplation, and preparation stages of change, *Journal of Consulting and Clinical Psychology*, 59, 295–304.

Dishman, R.K. (1982) Compliance/adherence in health-related exercise, *Health Psychology*, 1, 237–67.

Dzewaltowski, D.A. (1989) Toward a model of exercise motivation, *Journal of Sport and Exercise Psychology*, 32, 11–28.

Eagly, A.H. and Chaiken, S. (1993) *The Psychology of Attitudes.* Fort Worth, TX: Harcourt Brace Jovanovich.

Epstein, S. (1979) The stability of behavior. On predicting most of the people much of the time, *Journal of Personality and Social Psychology*, 37, 1097–126.

Fazio, R.H. (1990) Multiple processes by which attitudes guide behavior: the MODE model as an integrative framework. In M.P. Zanna (ed.) *Advances in Experimental Social Psychology*, Vol. 23. San Diego: Academic Press, 75–109.

Fazio, R.H., Powell, M.C. and Williams, C.J. (1989) The role of attitude accessibility in the attitude-to-behavior process, *Journal of Consumer Research*, 16, 280–8.

Fazio, R.H. and Williams, C.J. (1986) Attitude accessibility as a moderator of the attitude–perception and attitude–behavior relations: an investigation of the 1984 presidential election, *Journal of Personality and Social Psychology*, 51, 505–14.

Fishbein, M. and Ajzen, I. (1974) Attitudes towards objects as predictors of single and multiple behavioral criteria, *Psychological Review*, 81, 59–74.

Fishbein, M., Middlestadt, S.E. and Chung, J. (1986) Predicting participation and choice among first time voters in US partisan elections. In S. Kraus and R. Perloff (eds) *Mass Media and Political Thoughts: an Information Processing Approach.* Beverly Hills, CA: Sage, 65–82.

Fredricks, A.J. and Dossett, D.L. (1983) Attitude–behavior relations: a comparison of the Fishbein–Ajzen and Bentler–Speckart models, *Journal of Personality and Social Psychology*, 45, 501–12.

Godin, G., Valois, P. and Lepage, L. (1993) The pattern of influence of perceived behavioral control upon exercise behavior: an application of Ajzen's theory of planned behavior, *Journal of Behavioral Medicine*, **16**, 81–102.

Gollwitzer, P.M. (1993) Goal achievement: the role of intentions. In W. Stroebe and M. Hewstone (eds) *European Review of Social Psychology*, Vol. 4. Chichester: Wiley, 141–85.

Gorsuch, R.L. and Ortberg, J. (1983) Moral obligation and attitudes: their relation to behavioral intentions, *Journal of Personality and Social Psychology*, **44**, 1025–8.

Harrison, J.A., Mullen, P.D. and Green, L.W. (1992) A meta-analysis of studies of the health belief model with adults, *Health Education Research*, **7**, 107–16.

Heckhausen, H. (1991) *Motivation and Action*. Berlin: Springer.

Hill, D., Gardner, G. and Rassaby, J. (1985) Factors predisposing women to take precautions against breast and cervix cancer, *Journal of Applied Social Psychology*, **15**, 59–79.

Hochbaum, G.M. (1983) *The Health Belief Model Revisited*. Dallas, TX: American Public Health Association.

Houston, D.A. and Fazio, R.H. (1989) Biased processing as a function of attitude accessibility: Making objective judgements subjectively, *Social Cognition*, **7**, 51–66.

Kendzierski, D. (1990) Decision making versus decision implementation: an action control approach to exercise adoption and adherence, *Journal of Applied Social Psychology*, **20**, 27–45.

Kok, G., DeVries, H., Muddle, A.N. and Strecher, V.J. (1991) Planned health education and the role of self-efficacy: Dutch research, *Health Education Research*, **6**, 231–8.

King, J. (1982) The impact of patients' perceptions of high blood pressure on attendance at screening, *Social Science and Medicine*, **16**, 1079–91.

Kruglanski, A.W. (1989) *Lay Epistemics and Human Knowledge: Cognitive and Motivational Bases*. New York: Plenum Press.

Kuhl, J. (1981) Motivational and functional helplessness: the moderating effect of state versus action orientation, *Journal of Personality and Social Psychology*, **40**, 155–70.

Kuhl, J. (1985) Volitional mediators of cognition–behavior consistency: self-regulatory processes and action versus state orientation. In J. Kuhl and J. Beckman (eds) *Action Control: from Cognition to Behavior*. New York: Springer, 101–28.

Kuhl, J. and Beckman, J. (1985) *Action Control: from Cognition to Behavior*. New York: Springer.

Lam, C.S., McMahon, B.T., Priddy, D.A. and Gehred-Schultz, A. (1988) Deficit awareness and treatment performance among traumatic head injury adults, *Brain Injury*, **2**, 235–42.

McConnaughly, E.A., DiClemente, C.C., Prochaska, J.O. and Velicer, W.F. (1989) Stages of change in psychotherapy: a follow-up report, *Psychotherapy*, **26**, 494–503.

Marteau, T.M. (1989) Health beliefs and attributions. In A.K. Broome (ed.) *Health Psychology: Processes and Applications*. London: Chapman and Hall, 1–23.

Mullen, P.D., Hersey, J.C. and Iverson, D.C. (1987) Health behavior models compared, *Social Science and Medicine*, **24**, 973–83.

Norman, P. (1993) Predicting the uptake of health checks in general practice: invitation methods and patients' health beliefs, *Social Science and Medicine*, **37**, 53–9.

Norman, P. and Conner, M. (1993) The role of social cognition models in predicting attendance at health checks, *Psychology and Health*, **8**, 447–62.

Norman, P. and Conner, M. (1994) Attendance at health checks and the role of past behaviour in attitude–behaviour models, paper presented at the 8th European Health Psychology Society Conference, Alicante, July.

Norman, P. and Fitter, M. (1989) Intentions to attend a health screening appointment: some implications for general practice, *Counselling Psychology Quarterly*, **2**, 261–72.

Norman, P. and Smith, L. (1995) The theory of planned behaviour and exercise: an investigation into the role of prior behaviour, behavioural intentions and attitude variability, *European Journal of Social Psychology*, **25**, 403–15.

Oliver, R.L. and Berger, P.K. (1979) A path analysis of preventive health care decision models, *Journal of Consumer Research*, **6**, 113–22.

Orbell, S. and Hodgkins, S. (1994) It's easy to change behaviour if you know when to: implementation intentions and behavioural enactment, paper presented at the BPS Special Group in Health Psychology Conference, Sheffield, September.

Parker, D., Manstead, A.S. and Stradling, S.G. (1995) Extending the theory of planned behaviour: the role of personal norm, *British Journal of Social Psychology*, **34**, 127–37.

Petty, R. and Cacioppo, J.T. (1986) *Communication and Persuasion: Central and Peripheral Routes to Attitude Change*. New York: Springer.

Pomazal, R.P. and Jaccard, J.J. (1976) An informational approach to altruistic behavior, *Journal of Personality and Social Psychology*, **33**, 317–26.

Prentice-Dunn, S. and Rogers, R.W. (1986) Protection motivation theory and preventive health: Beyond the health belief model, *Health Education Research*, **1**, 153–61.

Prochaska, J.O. and DiClemente, C.C. (1984) *The Transtheoretical Approach: Crossing Traditional Boundaries of Change*. Homewood, IL: J. Irwin.

Raats, M.M. (1992) The role of beliefs and sensory to milk in determining the selection of milks of different fat content, unpublished doctoral thesis, University of Reading.

Randall, D.M. and Wolff, J.A. (1994) The time interval in the intention–behaviour relationship: meta-analysis, *British Journal of Social Psychology*, **33**, 405–18.

Richard, R. and van der Pligt, J. (1991) Factors affecting condom use among adolescents, *Journal of Community and Applied Social Psychology*, **1**, 105–16.

Richard, R., van der Pligt, J. and deVries, N. (1993) Anticipated affective reactions and behaviour, paper presented at the 10th General Meeting of the European Association of Experimental Social Psychology, Lisbon, September.

Ronis, D.L., Yates, J.F. and Kirscht, J.P. (1989) Attitudes, decisions and habits as determinants of repeated behavior. In A.R. Pratkanis, S.J. Breckler and A.G. Greenwald (eds) *Attitude Structure and Function*. Hillsdale, NJ: Erlbaum, 213–40.

Rosenstock, I.M., Strecher, V.J. and Becker, M.H. (1988) Social learning theory and the health belief model, *Health Education Quarterly*, **15**, 175–83.

Rosin, S., Tuorila, H. and Uutela, A. (1992) Garlic: a sensory pleasure or a social nuisance?, *Appetite*, **19**, 133–43.

Rotter, J.B. (1966) Generalised expectancies for internal versus external control of reinforcement, *Psychological Monographs*, **80**, 1–28.

Rutter, D.R. (1989) Models of belief–behaviour relationships in health, *Health Psychology Update*, November, 8–10.

Rutter, D.R. and Bunce, D.J. (1989) The theory of reasoned action of Fishbein and

Ajzen: a test of Towriss's amended procedure for measuring beliefs, *British Journal of Social Psychology*, **28**, 39–46.

Sanbonmatsu, D.M. and Fazio, R.H. (1990) The role of attitudes in memory-based decision making, *Journal of Personality and Social Psychology*, **59**, 614–22.

Sandman, P.M. and Weinstein, N.D. (1993) Predictors of home radon testing and implications for testing promotion programs, *Health Education Quarterly*, **20**, 471–87.

Schuman, H. (1972) Attitudes vs. actions versus attitudes vs. attitudes, *Public Opinion Quarterly*, **36**, 347–54.

Schwartz, S.H. and Tessler, R.C. (1972) A test of a model for reducing measured attitude–behavior discrepancies, *Journal of Personality and Social Psychology*, **24**, 225–36.

Schwarzer, R. (1992) Self-efficacy in the adoption and maintenance of health behaviors: theoretical approaches and a new model. In R. Schwarzer (ed.) *Self-efficacy: Thought Control of Action*. Washington, DC: Hemisphere, 217–43.

Seydel, E., Taal, E. and Wiegman, O. (1990) Risk-appraisal, outcome and self-efficacy expectancies: cognitive factors in preventive behavior related to cancer, *Psychology and Health*, **4**, 99–109.

Shepherd, R., Sparks, P., Bellier, S. and Raats, M. (1993) Attitudes and choice of flavoured milks: extensions of Fishbein and Ajzen's theory of reasoned action, *Food Quality and Preference*, **3**, 157–64.

Sheppard, B.H., Hartwick, J. and Warshaw, P.R. (1988) The theory of reasoned action: a meta-analysis of past research with recommendations for modifications and future research, *Journal of Consumer Research*, **15**, 325–43.

Sparks, P. (1994) Food choice and health: applying, assessing, and extending the theory of planned behaviour. In D.R. Rutter and L. Quine (eds) *Social Psychology and Health: European Perspectives*. Aldershot: Avebury, 25–46.

Sparks, P. and Shepherd, R. (1992) Self-identity and the theory of planned behaviour: assessing the role of identification with 'green consumerism', *Social Psychology Quarterly*, **55**, 388–99.

Sparks, P., Shepherd, R. and Frewer, L.J. (1995a) Assessing and structuring public attitudes towards the uses of gene technology in food production: the role of perceived ethical obligation, *Basic and Applied Social Psychology*, **16**, 267–85.

Sparks, P., Shepherd, R., Wieringa, N. and Zimmermanns, N. (1992) Barriers to healthy eating: an examination of perceived behavioural control and unrealistic optimism, paper presented at the BPS Social Psychology Section Annual Conference, University of Hertfordshire, September.

Sparks, P., Shepherd, R., Wieringa, N. and Zimmermanns, N. (1995b) Perceived behavioural control, unrealistic optimism and dietary change: an exploratory study, *Appetite*, **24**, 243–55.

Stroebe, W. and Stroebe, M.S. (1995) *Social Psychology and Health*. Buckingham: Open University Press.

Sutton, S. (1994) The past predicts the future: interpreting behaviour–behaviour relationships in social psychological models of health behaviours. In D.R. Rutter and L. Quine (eds) *Social Psychology and Health: European Perspectives*. Aldershot: Avebury, 71–88.

Sutton, S. and Hallett, R. (1989) Understanding seat-belt intentions and behavior: a decision-making approach, *Journal of Applied Social Psychology*, **19**, 1310–25.

Towriss, J.G. (1984) A new approach to the use of expectancy value models, *Journal of the Market Research Society*, **26**, 63–75.

Triandis, H.C. (1977) *Interpersonal Behavior*. Monterey, CA: Brooks-Cole.

Valois, P., Desharnais, R. and Godin, G. (1988) A comparison of the Fishbein and the Triandis attitudinal models for the prediction of exercise intention and behavior, *Journal of Behavioral Medicine*, 11, 459–72.

Van den Putte, H. (1993) On the theory of reasoned action, unpublished doctoral dissertation, University of Amsterdam.

Van der Pligt, J. (1994) Risk appraisal and health behaviour. In D.R. Rutter and L. Quine (eds) *Social Psychology and Health: European Perspectives*. Aldershot: Avebury, 131–52.

Van der Pligt, J. and Eiser, J.R. (1984) Dimensional salience, judgement and attitudes. In J.R. Eiser (ed.) *Attitudinal Judgement*. New York: Springer-Verlag, 161–77.

Wallston, K.A., Wallston, B.S. and DeVellis, R. (1978) Development of multidimensional health locus of control (MHLC) scales, *Health Education Monographs*, 6, 160–70.

Warshaw, P.R. and Davis, F.D. (1985) Disentangling behavioral intention and behavioral expectation, *Journal of Experimental Social Psychology*, 21, 213–28.

Weinstein, N.D. (1988) The precaution adoption process, *Health Psychology*, 7, 355–86.

Weinstein, N.D. (1993) Testing four competing theories of health-protective behavior, *Health Psychology*, 12, 324–33.

Weinstein, N.D. and Sandman, P.M. (1992) A model of the precaution adoption process: evidence from home radon testing, *Health Psychology*, 11, 170–80.

Zuckerman, M. and Reiss, H.T. (1978) Comparison of three models for predicting altruistic behavior, *Journal of Personality and Social Psychology*, 36, 498–510.

INDEX